A WOMAN'S

MIDLIFE

COMPANION

A Woman's
Midlife
Companion

The Essential Resource for
Every Woman's Journey

NAOMI LUCKS AND MELENE SMITH, M.F.C.C.

PRIMA PUBLISHING

Library of Congress Cataloging-in-Publication Data

Lucks, Naomi.
    A woman's midlife companion : the essential resource for every woman's journey / Naomi Lucks, Melene Smith.
        p. cm.
    Includes index.
    ISBN 0-7615-1025-7
    1. Menopause—Popular works.   2. Middle aged women—Health and hygiene.
    I. Smith, Melene.   II. Title.
RG186.L835   1997
612.6'65—dc21   97-8883
                                                                       CIP

97 98 99 00 01 DD 10 9 8 7 6 5 4 3 2 1
Printed in the United States of America

HOW TO ORDER

Single copies may be ordered from Prima Publishing, P.O. Box 1260BK, Rocklin, CA 95677; telephone (916) 632-4400. Quantity discounts are available. On your letterhead, include information concerning the intended use of the books and the number of books you wish to purchase.

Visit us online at http://www.primapublishing.com

To our families, with love and appreciation:

Geoff, Marian, and Ken
M.S.

Helen and Larry Lucks, and Chuck and Ariel Sigal
N.L.

CONTENTS

part 1
THE GUIDEBOOK

part 2

YOUR PERSONAL COMPANION

Dear Reader,

Prepare to have as much fun reading *A Woman's Midlife Companion* as I had serving as the book's medical adviser. Naomi Lucks and Melene Smith have done a superb job providing you with an informative, well-written, user-friendly, compassionate, and, above all, *honest* book that addresses issues confronting women in their forties and fifties. The authors have successfully combined traditional Western medicine approaches with more holistic practices and beliefs, taking great care to separate fact from myth.

The authors also stress that no two midlife journeys will be alike. Whereas one woman may believe "midlife" signals a loss of womanhood, an end to romantic love, or a step closer to mortality, another woman will see midlife as a life without the drudgery of menstrual cramps, birth control concerns, and PMS. This *individualization* of patient care is, in my mind, the book's greatest strength.

Perhaps Naomi Lucks and Melene Smith will write a companion for younger women embarking on womanhood. Or maybe the authors will be the voice of women in their sixties and beyond. Until then, enjoy *A Woman's Midlife Companion.* You are in for a treat.

Margaret Owens Cuthbert, M.D.
Berkeley, California
1997

PREFACE

I always seem to get very involved in whatever interests me. When I was skiing all the time, I immersed myself in the ski business. When I wanted to buy a house, I ended up with a real estate license. Then I realized menopause was just around the corner, and here we are with a book.

MELENE, 53

Until Melene and I began talking about it, I never really thought "menopause" was a word that would apply to me.

NAOMI, 48

THIS BOOK began in a casual manner about five years ago. We thought that putting together a resource book for midlife women would be a good way to understand and participate in a life transition about which we knew little and around which there had been, until recently, much silence. We also wanted to write a book that would help women our own age find out what they needed to know to make the many decisions that seem to be the hallmark of midlife. We hope that we have done that. Writing *A Woman's Midlife Companion* has transformed and deepened our understanding of the midlife journey in ways that surprised us both.

Menopause is our wake-up call to the inevitability of transformation, but midlife is much more than menopause. Midlife is a crossroads, and crossroads are legendary places of power: a sacred ground to worshipers of the Greco-Roman crone goddess Hecate, a place to invoke deities in pre-Christian Europe, a clearing where the spirit of the Goddess as Earth Mother was said to dwell, a place of choice. As you approach this juncture in your own life, take a moment to honor the spirit of this important time of transition.

The crises and opportunities of this time of change can be difficult, but they can also open us to interior regions that are waiting to be explored. As author Ursula Le Guin said in "The Space Crone," "It seems a pity to have a built-in rite of passage and to dodge it, evade it, and pretend one is like a man. Men, once initiated, never get the second chance. They never change again. That's their loss, not ours. Why borrow poverty?"

We can't avoid making this journey, but we can plan our own itinerary. We can use the "pause" in menopause to stop for a moment and survey the terrain, check out the many paths, and pick up the reins of our own lives. We can honor the many changes of midlife for what they are: the biological event that marks a profound life transition, the chance to live life as fully and deeply as possible.

Bon voyage!

ACKNOWLEDGMENTS

A Woman's Midlife Companion turned out to be a much larger project than we first envisioned. Our names are on the cover, but it is also the product of many people's time, thoughts, work, and generosity. We owe a special debt to the many women, friends, and acquaintances who so generously shared their thoughts and experiences with us for the postcards and who made it abundantly clear that every woman's midlife journey is, indeed, her own.

This book might easily have remained just a good idea without the energy, good humor, and extraordinary editing skills of our agent, Sheryl Fullerton. Thanks especially to the staff at Prima for their accessibility and help in making this publishing process fun: acquisitions editor Georgia Hughes, project editor Betsy Towner, copy editor Joan Pendleton, associate publicist Jonna Pedrioli, and rights department manager Diane Durrett.

Our medical adviser, Margaret Cuthbert, M.D., has been unstinting in her enthusiasm for this project, and we have benefited from her support, interest, and delight during each phase of writing and production. Her focus on separating fact from myth when it comes to midlife was our guiding light in shaping this book, and her astute input and advice in the medical chapters were invaluable.

We want to thank all of our professional readers and reviewers for correcting errors, suggesting additions, and sharing their time to help make this a better book: Mona Reeva, Ph.D., who supported our project from the very beginning; China Galland, for her thoughtful input and life-changing ideas about the sacred fierce feminine; Terrie Heinrich Rizzo, manager of Health and Education Programs for the Stanford Health and Fitness Center, for her incredible energy and speed in responding to our questions; Camilla McCalmont, M.D., for helping us get the facts on skin care in midlife; Lee Ringlaro, for her support and for sharing her professional knowledge of skin, makeup, and hair in midlife; Ginny Howe, D.C., and Nancy Rakela, L.Ac., herbalist, and Doctor of Oriental Medicine, for their generous help regarding complementary therapies; Lani Simpson, D.C., director of the East Bay PMS and Menopause Clinic, for her insights into natural progesterone; Michael Castleman and Anki Gelb, R.D., for their astute input on diet and nutrition. Thanks also to Gaia Books in Berkeley, California, for allowing us to read and browse, and to Alkebulanian Books in Berkeley, California, for their help.

We are thoroughly indebted to our friends who volunteered their time to read drafts, make suggestions, and cheer us on throughout the process: Bonnie Jones, for always asking just the right question; Jessie Wood, for her discerning editorial skills; Marion Cowee, who encouraged us from the beginning; Jan Schreiber, for her sage advice; and Nancy Roberts, for sharing. Karen Lanphear and Chuck Sigal put in many grueling and unpaid hours on the phone to help us make sure our resources were up to date—we couldn't have done it without you. We are also indebted to Chuck for his quick and skilled response to our cries for technical computer support. Thanks to Linea, Carlene, Adele, Sandy, and Yana, our networking group, who pushed us to continue when we wanted to give up; and to fellow authors and exercisers Roberta Gould and Mani Feniger, for sharing the excitement.

Finally, we want to thank our families for being so wonderful over the course of this project, and for eating so much take-out food. Chuck, thanks for your support and understanding during this project, and for being so proud and happy at every new step. Ari, thanks for your patience and understanding. You really helped us get this work done. To my parents, Helen and Larry Lucks, thanks for your love and for always cheering me on. Thanks to Geoff for your enthusiasm and loving comfort; to Marian, my mother, for being there; to Dinnie for your support from afar; and to Karen for your focus.

YOUR ROAD MAP

*We've all, in the end, got to take care of
ourselves. Nobody else is going to do it.
We're each inside our own body alone,
and the final responsibility is our own.*

FAITH POPCORN, *The Popcorn Report*

If you could sign up for a package tour to the midlife journey, the brochure might read something like this:

> Women have been traveling through the sultry terrain of midlife for thousands of years. Of the countless travelers who have made this journey, none has returned unchanged. Yet, despite the well-trodden paths of this country, the precise nature of the journey has long been shrouded in a cloak of mystery, danger, and fear. Fortunately for today's traveler, groups of women are now journeying together into previously uncharted territory—and they are breaking with the old tradition of silence to leave oral, written, and even visual documents of their trip, invaluable guides for the new traveler. Dirt trails are being paved, shelters are being built, and the information highway is on the map. Why not plan your trip today?

The midlife journey isn't part of the Club Med package yet, but—thanks to the baby boomers, who are now turning fifty at the rate of one every eight minutes—it is being openly discussed. After so many years of youth and so much time spent doing all the things we need to do to get through each day, the arrival of midlife, with all its implications, can come as a surprise. As a consequence, many women wake one day to find themselves on the trail—with no itinerary, no reservations, no map, and no idea of what lies ahead.

Relax. True, the midlife journey is not on any map. But with a little preparation and thoughtful packing, you can find your own path and turn what may seem like a bad trip into a life-changing adventure. How? By getting to know yourself a little better, by taking charge of your choices, and by honoring your own unique wants and needs.

You've put in enough years to know what you like, what you don't like, who you are. That hasn't changed. On the midlife journey, as in everything else you do, you're unique. In a very real sense, you are your own clinical trial. What works for me may not work for you; what works for you may not work for your friend. And this is good. It means that the road is wide open: You have the opportunity to create your own unique vision of the rest of your life.

It's an exciting prospect, and one for which there is now an abundance of advice—from books, magazine articles, health practitioners, talk shows, friends, and relatives. Sometimes this can be too much of a good thing. If you're trying to decide what to do for hot flashes, for example, you may be bombarded with conflicting suggestions: One friend swears by her doctor's advice; another does everything her acupuncturist says; your mother tells you to tough it out. One book advises hormone replacement therapy to protect your heart; a TV doctor recommends against hormone therapy because of cancer risks; a third expert advises taking natural hormones made from yams. How can you possibly sort all this out? How can you figure out what *you're* supposed to do?

Take a few deep, relaxing breaths and consider your options with an open and inquiring mind. *A Woman's Midlife Companion* is intended to be your good friend on this journey. Part 1, The Guidebook, offers you a wealth of information and resources on the wide range of topics you may want to explore. Read it from cover to cover, or go straight to the chapter that most interests you—the chapters are written to stand alone. Enjoy the detours and alternative routes—explore to your heart's content. If you need help sorting through your options and making workable decisions about where you want to go, check out the workbook in Part 2, Your Personal Companion. Use this resource to help you get some perspective and reality on your needs and how you can meet them.

To get your bearings, take a quick look at the road signs that you'll come across in each chapter. Then pack your bags, take your *Companion* along for reference, and have a good trip!

PACKING FOR THE JOURNEY

Never underestimate the importance of packing correctly! Lugging around a suitcase full of useless items, or neglecting to take anything at all, can ruin any travel experience. That's why each chapter is packed with the information you need to make successful choices. Just look for your question and read the answer.

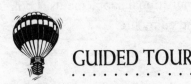

GUIDED TOUR

Is this a chapter you want to visit, or should you move on? Find out by taking the Guided Tour. This concise review covers the following topics:

Western Medicine

Midlife brings with it a few new health concerns that you may need help with. Western medicine has workable and tested solutions for a variety of health problems. This is a well-traveled road.

Complementary Therapies

Complementary therapies have been around for a long time—systems like traditional Chinese medicine and Ayurveda are thousands of years old. As Western doctors increasingly integrate alternative ideas into treatment plans, these concepts are coming into the mainstream.

Exercise

Giving your body the exercise it needs is one of the best things you can do to ensure your continued health and well-being. Moderate, regular exercise that incorporates aerobics, weight training, and stretching can help you feel better, look better, and live longer.

Mind–Body

Some kinds of exercise are designed as a workout for body *and* soul. Yoga, t'ai chi, qi gong, the Rosen method, massage, biofeedback, meditation, and many other systems can benefit you on all levels.

Nutrition

What you put into your body can make an enormous difference in your life: The medical community is becoming increasingly aware of the protective qualities of many foods and nutritional supplements. Look here for delicious ways to stay healthy and enjoy life.

Support

Finding emotional support on the rocky road of midlife can be a lifesaver. Getting counseling, joining a support group, or finding ways to be your own best friend can give you just the strength you need to continue.

SIDE TRIPS: OTHER PATHWAYS THROUGH THIS BOOK

Life is messy. It doesn't divide itself into perfectly contained compartments, and neither does the information in this book. That's why each chapter ends with a list of other chapters that can help you get a comprehensive perspective on the terrain. For example, you'll find information about healthy eating in Chapter 4, "Are You What You Eat?" But you'll also find specific information about food in the chapters on osteoporosis, hormone replacement therapy, appearance, stress, and breast cancer.

RESOURCES

You *can* find out what you need to know: Sometimes all you have to do is ask. The resources at the end of each chapter will help you with your search. We have made every effort to ensure that the information in each resource section is up to date. Please remember, however, that the nature of information is change!

ORGANIZATIONS AND SERVICES National resources, both government and private, can be extremely helpful, and many will send you invaluable information free of charge. Such materials helped us immeasurably in putting together this book. Some organizations have clearinghouses for information, and most have newsletters detailing their activities. For information, write, call, send e-mail, or visit the web sites.

HOTLINES When you need an answer in a hurry, call a hotline. It's free and fast, and the information is generally up-to-the-minute. You may be able to get the referral you need right away. Many organizations have toll-free numbers—just pick up the phone and call. Even if the organization you are interested in doesn't have a hotline, you can almost always call and talk to a live human being.

PRODUCTS AND CATALOGS Here's where you'll find things to buy and catalogs to send for. What could be more fun?

PERIODICALS Keep up to date on topics that interest you by subscribing to newsletters or magazines devoted to a particular topic. The next best thing to talking to a friend is reading some of these publications. Newsletters are perhaps the best way to keep up with changing information and new research, and they share the wealth of information that pours in from readers and news sources. Many newsletters will send you a complimentary copy. This is a good way to see if you like the publication before you sign up for a year's subscription!

BOOKS You can find a book on virtually any subject you're interested in knowing more about. It seems that at least one book has been written on every subject; and when it comes to women's midlife issues, it's safe to say another book is always on the way. Many bookstores carry books on women's issues, but women's bookstores carry more of them. You'll find the latest books and magazines on women's issues, as well as the old standbys. You'll also find something more: Most of these stores have become centers for women's issues, points of dissemination for information and activities. Many host readings that give you a chance to meet and ask questions of women writers. Some women's bookstores are politically oriented; some are more spiritually oriented. Wherever you fall on the spectrum, however, you will be welcome. To find one, ask your friends or look in the yellow pages under "Bookstores." If you still can't find one, contact Feminist Bookstore News (see the Resources in Chapter 18, "Bringing It Together").

AUDIO/VIDEO   You can find a surprising number of audiocassettes and videos on virtually every subject covered in this book. Tapes are a good way to get a lot of information quickly. Videotapes are also a great way to launch a support group discussion.

ONLINE   The Internet is a direct route to information on the midlife journey. It's a constantly changing, up-to-the minute route to answering virtually any question—and a good way to tap into ongoing support groups, real-time chat, advice, and ideas from other women from around the nation and the world. We've listed some of the sources that were available as of this writing, but new sources are added and removed every day.

If you've ever posted to a news group, you know that if you have a question, *someone* out there has an answer. You can find virtually anything from scholarly papers to a real-time discussion about hot flashes with a woman 3,000 miles away. Most organizations, government and private, now have web sites and e-mail addresses. One note: There are many gateways to the Internet, and it's not possible for us to cover them all. We've included web sites, mailing lists, and news groups that are available to most users. If you're a member of America Online, CompuServe, Prodigy, or another online service, check out local clubs and message boards.

If you're new to the Internet, remember that the commas and periods in the listings are for punctuation only—there are no commas or periods at the end of e-mail addresses or URLs (web site addresses). Also, for the sake of space, we have not included the beginning of each URL (in this book, it's always http://). Finally, if you want to subscribe to a mailing list, the general procedure is to send an e-mail note saying "subscribe [name of mailing list] [your name]" to the list server address provided. However, this varies slightly from list to list, so contact the list server for information on how to subscribe.

A WOMAN'S

MIDLIFE

COMPANION

part 1

THE GUIDEBOOK

Every transition begins with an ending. We have to let go of the

old thing before we can pick up the new—not just outwardly,

but inwardly. . . .

WILLIAM BRIDGES, *Transitions*

1

ENDINGS/BEGINNINGS
Midlife Transition

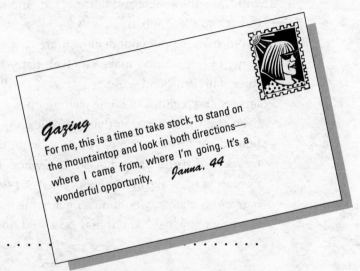

Gazing
For me, this is a time to take stock, to stand on the mountaintop and look in both directions— where I came from, where I'm going. It's a wonderful opportunity. *Janna, 44*

In midlife, just when everything seems to be running smoothly, the changes start coming thick and fast. Some changes are out of your control: You break into a drenching sweat in the middle of a business meeting; your children are bursting with adolescent angst while you're trying to understand your own hormonal ups and downs; your parents suddenly need full-time nursing care just when you thought you could get some time to yourself. If midlife has you feeling confused, you're not alone.

Just when we finally thought we had everything under control, it's all up in the air again. We're faced with choices about everything: whether to regulate our hormones, whether we need to put our parents into care homes, whether we should go back to school to get a degree (since a better-paying job would help put the kids through college), whether we should completely change our diet and exercise habits, whether a different wardrobe color scheme would go better with grayer hair, or . . . well, you get the idea.

In life, nothing is more certain than change. Why, then, do the changes of midlife sometimes come as such a shock? Like greatness, the midlife transition seems to be thrust upon us. One minute we're young women; the next we're women in the middle, looking back to where we've been, forward to the rest of our lives, and asking what it's all about.

The midlife journey has many surprises and detours. A path we thought we knew suddenly loops around and brings us face to face with something new and unexpected, and loops around again to bring us back to the familiar.

No matter how confident you are, the unpredictability and uncertainty of midlife may make you feel that you no longer understand the rules. This profound sense of *not knowing* may allow some long-forgotten images and feelings to come welling up: a sudden vision of who you've been and the realization that you're leaving at least part of that person behind. At the same time, you may begin to sense those unlived parts of yourself rising up and seeking a voice. It's tempting to close your eyes and say, Wake me when it's over! But sleepwalking through all this marvelous change would mean many missed opportunities: This is life wanting to be lived, and it may be a wild ride. Hang on!

 ## PACKING FOR THE JOURNEY

What's the Relationship Between Menopause and the Midlife Transition?

The first stirrings of hormonal change are unmistakable signs of the arrival of midlife, so it's not surprising that we tend to hang all of our thoughts and feelings about midlife on the experience of menopause. But there's much more to the midlife transition than this. The biological changes of this time of life give us a concrete metaphor for the

GUIDED TOUR: *Midlife Transition*

Midlife is a time of transition between youth and age. With the approach of menopause, change suddenly becomes more apparent, and we are forced to deal with what those changes mean. This is a time of uncertainty and unknowing, a time when we must deal with losses, perhaps for the first time; but it can also be a time of great promise, a time when we can put our accumulated knowledge to work to create our own vision of the rest of our lives.

EXERCISE

At midlife exercise is even more important to your health than it was earlier in life. Any kind of change is stressful, and the stresses of midlife are abundant. This is no time to leave your body in the lurch. Be sure to support your body with the exercise it needs to stay strong and healthy through this time and beyond.

MIND–BODY

Practices such as yoga, qi gong, t'ai chi, Alexander technique, Rosen work, and meditation are designed to help you come into balance. During this time of unknowing, grounding yourself in this way is a good idea.

NUTRITION

Hormonal imbalance may leave you bouncing between moods, and the stress of transition can rob your body of nutrients and weaken your immune system. Be sure you are eating the food your body needs to stay healthy, and eat often to keep your blood sugar steady.

SUPPORT

If midlife transition is raising more issues than you can deal with, remember you're not alone. Create a circle of friends, explore support groups, and, if needed, seek professional help. Professional counseling and structured support groups exist to address many needs.

Be an observer as well as an experimenter. Pay attention to other women your age: What do they look like? What are they doing? How are they are dealing with this transition? Observe yourself. What makes you comfortable or uncomfortable? What gets your juices going? What awakens your passion? How do you see yourself living and being in the coming years? A project notebook can help you give some form to this time of change. Keep a small notebook that you can carry with you and write down thoughts, quotes, things you might like to try, areas you might want to explore.

many other changes we begin to experience at this time: changes in how we regard ourselves, how we relate to others, and how we look at the world. In the midst of this kaleidoscope of change, the physical instabilities and changes of menopause can't help but create a shifting, disorienting sensation.

In some ways, midlife has a lot in common with puberty. We're concerned with changing bodies, changing roles, with how the world sees us and how we want to present ourselves to the world. We're preoccupied with hormonal ups and downs, and we're wondering, again, what we're going to do with our lives. This time around, however, we can draw from rich stores of experience and view life from a far different perspective. Midlife, like puberty, is a time to try on different ideas—not to become someone completely different, but to give some growing room to parts of ourselves we've had to put aside. Explore, take risks, have fun. Recreate yourself, and let what is there unfold.

I was thirty-five years old before I understood that there is no ending without a beginning. That beginnings and endings are always right up against each other. Nothing ever ends without something else beginning or begins without something else ending. Perhaps this would be easier to remember if we had a word for it. Something like "endbegin," or "beginend."

RACHEL NAOMI REMEN, *Kitchen Table Wisdom*

What Are the Stages of the Midlife Transition?

For all its unpredictability, the midlife transition can be seen to have three stages: a time of ending, a time of unknowing and re-forming, and a time of renewal. If this seems familiar, it's not surprising, for it is the pattern of life itself. The plant dies back in fall; the seed germinates underground in winter; the flower buds forth in spring. William Bridges, one of the seminal thinkers on the complex nature of transition, explains in *Transitions*, "Adulthood unfolds its promise in a rhythm of expansion and contraction, change and stability. In human life as in the rest of nature, change accumulates slowly and almost invisibly until it is made manifest in the sudden form of fledging out or thawing or leaf-fall. It is the transition process rather than a thing called a mid-life transition that we must understand."

Stage 1, Endings: What Are the Changes of This Time?

During Stage 1 you may become acutely aware that some familiar aspects of your life will be ending. Even when you know that something new will be born out of the process, the loss of the familiar can feel like the loss or ending of your own being rather than preparation for a next step. It's important to remember that most of the experiences of this time are common to all women. Being familiar with the possibilities may allow you to think about them more easily. Trying to hang on is tempting, but only when you let yourself acknowledge endings and loss can you begin to let go and see the road ahead.

MENSTRUATION ENDS   Whether you think menstruation is a blessing or a curse, the monthly cycle lends a rhythm to life. When it suddenly becomes unpredictable, you may feel surprisingly disoriented. The potential to reproduce life is a source of power. The loss of this ability may leave you feeling temporarily empty and aimless.

ROLE AS MOTHER CHANGES   Historically, women have been valued for their role as mothers. If you have spent the last decade or two raising children, you probably think of yourself as a "mom." You'll always be a mom, of course, but as you launch your children into their own adult lives, the degree of control you've had in this position will change.

SELF-IMAGE CHANGES   As a child you probably couldn't wait to grow up. And for at least twenty years, you lived as a "young woman." But when it's time to put that image behind you, you may have the disconcerting feeling that you are no longer the same person.

YOUTH IS SEEN AS FLEETING   The approach of menopause tells you in no uncertain terms that aging is inevitable. In our society, which values youth and beauty and devalues age, the loss of youth can mean loss of a

Some Good Movies About Midlife Transition and Aging

Believe it or not, a number of movies deal—for better or for worse—with women in transition. Here are a few to get you started; you should be able to find them at video rental stores:

All About Eve (1950) Bette Davis as the aging star beset by the aspiring young actress, Anne Baxter.

Another Woman (1988) Woody Allen directs Gena Rowlands in a drama about a woman who must suddenly reconsider her life.

Enchanted April (1991) Joan Plowright and Miranda Richardson join two other women in a funny, romantic, and life-changing visit to an Italian villa.

Fried Green Tomatoes (1991) Kathy Bates, Jessica Tandy, Mary Stuart Masterson, and Mary-Louise Parker in a sweet, sad, and funny movie about the relationships between women.

Marvin's Room (1996) Diane Keaton and Meryl Streep as two very different sisters who come together over issues of life and death.

Ordinary People (1980) Mary Tyler Moore as a repressed wife and mother whose life unravels around the death of her son.

Shirley Valentine (1989) Pauline Collins as a midlife woman who finds renewal on a solo trip to Greece.

Steel Magnolias (1989) Sally Field, Dolly Parton, Shirley MacLaine, and a number of others in this story of relationships between women in a beauty parlor.

(continued)

sense of power and worth with little to replace it. This realization can be unsettling, especially if you've depended on youthful charm as a bargaining tool.

RELATIONSHIPS MAY CHANGE The inevitable changes of this time often sweep in other changes. Some, such as divorce, a breakup, or a change in friendships, may have fermented for many years. Some are part of life: Your partner and friends are also aging, and illness and death may become a new factor.

PARENTS AGE Your parents are getting older too, and this is another reminder of your own life journey. You may find yourself taking care of your parents or an aging relative or having to deal with more than one serious illness or death at the same time. All of this can add to your stress and make you feel that life is unfair.

CAREER CHANGES If you've been a full-time mother, you may recognize that your children are older and more independent, and so you may decide to reenter the job market or go back to school. If you've worked all your life, you may decide to think about retiring, changing jobs, or even beginning over with a new career. Corporate downsizing may displace you from a long-held job and force you to reconsider your work life.

AWARENESS OF MISSED OPPORTUNITIES Regrets are common in this stage of midlife. You become aware of the sacrifices you've made for the life you have; you realize that your opportunity to bear children has passed, that some of your dreams will be unfulfilled.

Stage 2, Unknowing:
What Are the Feelings of This Time?

During Stage 2 you may feel confused, uncertain, adrift. Don't despair. You are doing very deep work, whether you know it or not: You are re-forming yourself in preparation for the time of renewal that is to come. During this time, when everything you were and will be is up in the air, you may experience feelings of emptiness, chaos, and isolation, along with startlingly powerful glimpses of the future. Be patient. In the words of psychologist Stanley Kelemen, "The unknown offers many mysteries from which newness springs."

TRAVEL TIP (continued)

Strangers in Good Company (1991) A Canadian film about women who must get to know each other when their bus breaks down.

Terms of Endearment (1983) Shirley MacLaine and Debra Winger in a movie about the relationship between a mother and daughter.

An Unremarkable Life (1989) Patricia Neal and Shelley Winters in a movie about the relationship between two sisters.

BETRAYAL BY THE BODY   Your menstrual cycle, which was once as predictable as the seasons of the year, is now unpredictable. You may be overcome by hot flashes. Although you used to sleep through the night, your sleep is now disturbed. Although you used to count on your body to support your sexual arousal with moisture, you encounter a sudden dryness. These changes may make you feel out of control and may make you want to turn on your body and beat it back into submission with any remedy that comes to hand. While there are remedies for the changes of this time, it's also a good idea to relax around these changes and not betray your body in misguided retaliation.

A NEED FOR INFORMATION ABOUT MENOPAUSE   Confusion about your changing body may lead to a desire for more understanding of the biological process. You can't stop the process, but understanding more about what's going on can give you back some sense of control.

FEAR OF SERIOUS DISEASE   At midlife the years of living may begin to accumulate and take their toll. You may suddenly realize that you are at risk for heart disease and osteoporosis. You may take menstrual irregularities and lumpy breasts as signs that something is dreadfully wrong. Fears like these can be allayed by facts. If you are worried, see your doctor.

DRAWING INWARD During this confusing time we often draw inward; it's almost a time of hibernation. We pull back to sort things out, think things through, reconcile old feelings. If you feel like this, revel in it and enjoy the cocoon of thoughtfulness. But also recognize that wanting to be alone can sometimes lead to a sense of isolation, the feeling that no one but you is experiencing this turmoil and upheaval. At these times it can be lifesaving to reach out and connect with other women who are experiencing the same sorts of changes.

SEEKING COUNSELING At midlife you may decide to seek counseling. Some women find that their usual ways of doing things don't work anymore and they need help changing them. Other women may have unfinished emotional business that they're now ready to deal with. The confusing emotions of this time leave many women feeling out of control and panicked or depressed. It's good to remember that the same transition that leaves you feeling vulnerable also opens the door to great leaps in insight and understanding. Therapy can be the place to explore what it is you want from life.

SPIRITUAL CONNECTIONS This time of unknowing and re-forming often leads to a deeper appreciation of life's mysteries and a surrendering to the movement of life itself. You deepen and begin to feel more connected with the cycles of change that underlie everything.

Stage 3, Renewal: What Are the New Directions of This Time?

From the pain of loss and endings and the upheaval of the unknown comes the birth of a new self who may surprise the old self with her sense of wholeness and confidence, with her impetus to move in directions the old self never thought possible, and with an energy that is entirely new. The work of Stage 2, where we touch and explore and nurture our deeply held ideas, needs, and desires, begins to bloom and come to fruition in Stage 3.

COMING TO TERMS WITH THE BODY   After menopause, you may feel a sense of relief, freedom, and newness. You no longer have to be concerned with pregnancy or discomfort. You have spent a number of years in transition coming to terms with your body. Now, finally, you can go forth into the world as a new person with your own lived experience of change.

POSTMENOPAUSAL ZEST   Anthropologist Margaret Mead once said, "The most creative force in the world is the postmenopausal woman with zest." Many women are surprised to discover that after the fatigue and exhaustion of the midlife transition they have a renewed sense of vigor and vitality, emotionally as well as physically.

RENEWED INTEREST IN SELF-CARE   Many women find that attention to their changing body forced on them by approaching menopause leaves them with the desire to pay more attention to its care. We are indeed living on, and we might as well live in the healthiest body possible.

BIRTH OF SELF   During Stage 2, you have the chance to really get to know yourself, perhaps for the first time. Your true self comes home after years spent wandering in the wilderness of growing up and living daily life. During Stage 3, you may have a powerful feeling of wholeness and three-dimensionality that you have not felt since you were a small child.

SENSE OF CONNECTION   As the sense of isolation of the time of unknowing recedes, you

POINT OF INTEREST
Creating a New Vision of Aging

Coming to terms with the fact that once we have reached menopause, we will continue to get older can be a formidable task, especially in the United States. In a society where older women have been devalued for so long, it's no wonder few women truly look forward to getting older.

Older women seem to fare better in traditional cultures. According to *The Menopause, Hormone Therapy, and Women's Health,* "The position and power of the shaman are available to women only after the menopause in both the Plains Cree and Winnebago Indian cultures," and "The Bemba of East Africa reserve many leadership roles, both political and social, for older women." Asian cultures traditionally venerate elders.

One challenge for women in our society is to create a new vision of aging. As the baby-boomer generation, we've moved through life like Moses parting the Red Sea, making a cult of youth and an industry of motherhood, changing the way society looks at whatever issue we happen to be dealing with. Our mothers either moved quietly through the change, not wanting to upset anyone, or angrily asserted their right to be emotional wrecks—remember Edith Bunker? But this is our change and, by the looks of it, we're going to do it *our* way.

The social role of older women is changing, and we are the ones transforming it. Our society has few good definitions of age for women, few guidelines for those who find themselves following the natural and inevitable pattern. We're on our own here, with a once-in-a-lifetime chance to redefine our vision of aging, of what it means to be an older woman. It will take hard work on our part to fight the cultural stereotypes and return the older woman to her rightful role as the wise and powerful elder, but it will be satisfying work.

are welcomed back into the community. Once you have come home to yourself, you may find a new empathy that allows you to connect more deeply with others.

How Can I Begin to Think About the Future?

Many of us grew up believing that we'd never live past thirty. When we did, we figured surely forty would be the limit. At some point, however, it becomes clear that we are actually going to live out a life. Then we wonder: How in the world can I do that? Worries about health, finances, and housing suddenly take on a pressing reality. We worry whether we will be healthy enough to enjoy the rest of our lives, whether we will have enough money to live with dignity, and whether we will be able to live in a place of our own choosing.

These are serious, practical questions that deserve attention. Part 2 of this book, Your Personal Companion, is a workbook designed to help you figure out where you are now and where you'd like to be in five years, ten years, or more. As you read this book, you may want to use this workbook to help you personalize your own journey and start thinking and even acting on some of these issues.

HEALTH Sooner or later, midlife changes will bring your attention to your health. Take advantage of this intensified interest to assess how your health is now and how you can keep yourself healthy as you get older. You can use the Personal Health History form in Part 2, Your Personal Companion, as a beginning. We address issues of health and support throughout this book, and you'll find many sources of information on women's health in the Resources section of each chapter.

HOUSING As you watch your parents growing older and less able to take care of themselves, you may begin to think about your own future. Planning ahead about where and how you will live can be disconcerting, but it's a good issue to begin working on now. As

Back to School

I am nearing fifty, my daughter is going off to college soon, and I was feeling less and less fulfilled in my job. I needed to explore what might be, and felt that if I didn't do it now, it would be too late. I was really scared when I quit my job to return to grad school, but it's been an expansive decision. At times I am overwhelmed. I think, What have I done? Maybe I should just quit. But those feelings pass, and I'm sure I'm on the right track. *May, 48* more and more of us are growing older, the question of housing and care is getting more attention. Many people are exploring alternatives such as cohousing and group living. Some friends buy property together now and make plans to live together in supportive, cooperative homes. You'll find a number of options you haven't thought about if you begin looking and thinking now. See the Resources in this chapter and in Chapter 15, "Everybody Needs Me Now," for ideas.

MONEY   Jobs come and go; you may be forced to retire on a small pension or you may be self-employed and have no pension; your partner may fall ill and need care; you may divorce or be widowed . . . you've probably already given thought to the many ways your nest egg can dwindle. The prospect of being older and without financial resources is not a pleasant one. Will you have enough money to live on when you get older? You can take steps now to ensure that surprises down the road don't drain your bank account. See Resources for ideas on how to start planning.

TAKING ACTION   Worrying about the future is useful only up to the point that it gets you to take action. You may have already given these issues a lot of thought and perhaps have begun taking steps. If not, there's no time like the present to begin looking into how you can structure your future. Many women's advocacy groups and groups on aging have already given attention to other issues, and they are set up to answer your questions. See the Resources at the end of this chapter for organizations, periodicals, books, and even videos that can help you begin to think about these practical and vital life issues.

What Are the Personal Growth Issues of the Midlife Transition?

Making decisions about how we are going to live out this middle life and preparing for what lies ahead are natural preoccupations of

When you turn fifty, you will automatically get mail from the American Association of Retired Persons (AARP). Your first response may be, I'm not that old yet, I'm sending this back, they've obviously made a mistake! When you calm down, take another look. This membership organization publishes a lot of very helpful information on many subjects—including divorce, widowhood, status of older women, health care, financial management, housing options, employment planning, exercise, returning to the job market, and consumer rights—that can help you start thinking about the future. They also offer many services to their members and are a powerful force in lobbying for change in age-related areas. You don't have to be fifty *or* a member to order their very good books and videos. For more information, see Resources.

the woman in the middle. Beyond the basic questions of survival are questions of personal growth and change: What work will I do? How will my relationships change? Should I go in a new direction, or grow more in my present role? How will I keep my mind stimulated? Who am I now? Who do I want to be in ten years, in twenty years? These are important questions, and it is in the process of answering them that you begin to take yourself seriously as an older woman and reaffirm your worth.

HOW OTHERS SEE US   The transformation of roles in midlife seems to fall into two categories: how others see us and how we see ourselves. Most women are shocked into the awareness that they have grown older the first time a store clerk calls them "ma'am." Yet in this time of re-forming, when we are most self-conscious, it sometimes seems as if we have suddenly become invisible. We no longer get as many looks from strangers or whistles (welcome or not) from construction workers. Some women find this sudden withdrawal of attention disconcerting, if not disturbing; others breathe a sigh of relief, feeling that their social invisibility allows them to become more authentic.

RETHINKING ROLES   We can't do too much about how others see us, but we do have control over how we see ourselves. During this time many women rethink their roles. Some role transformations, such as mother to grandmother, young lover to older lover, seem to take care of themselves. Others leave us with many choices. Some women who have worked all their lives are able to retire, but many are not; some women choose to keep working at jobs they love; some change careers. Still other women decide to reenter the workforce or return to school and find new roles as workers or students.

RETHINKING RELATIONSHIPS   For most women, relationships are the focal point of their lives, but the relationships they have may change profoundly in midlife. At this time of life, women may have fewer family-related demands, giving them time to struggle with how to remain in or establish a relationship and also be genuinely themselves. Divorce, death, or choice may compel a woman to form new partnerships. Many women at this time feel the need to connect more meaningfully with other women who are on the same journey. They begin to look beyond traditional family and intentionally build a new family of friendships.

DEVELOPING NEW INTERESTS Midlife is a time to try out a new self—or selves. Who are you beyond the many roles you, as a woman, have and will have in your life? Do you have a fantasy to pursue? It's not too late. Don't just say, When I retire, or, When I have the time. Go more deeply into yourself *now*. Have something budding for the future. Water it, nurture it, watch it grow. If you don't have a clue as to what this new direction might be, think about what gives you delight and awakens your passion. See Chapter 17, "The Inner Journey," for ideas about exploring your creativity.

INTELLECTUAL STIMULATION Many women put off their educational plans to care for children or to bring in enough money to support the family. When you go back to school with the experience of adulthood behind you, it's an adventure very different from your earlier years in school. Now you're really ready to learn, and you have a life context in which to fit your learning. To start, look at various school catalogs to see what's being taught these days (your library should have a collection of these). Many community colleges and state universities have reentry programs for

POINT OF INTEREST
Getting Together: Forming a Networking Group

When we first contemplated writing this book, the project seemed overwhelming. Left to our own devices, we would soon have talked ourselves out of it. Fortunately, a friend pulled us (somewhat reluctantly) into an informal networking/support group. It was just the right thing at the right time. We were a group of women with a mission: Each of us had a project in mind that we wanted to see to fruition. Some, like ours, were work projects. Other women were dealing with the practical issues of changing direction in life. We have to credit this group with encouraging us and keeping us going when we could barely talk out loud about what we were doing. Here are some of the guidelines from the group we formed. Feel free to improvise—it works!

- Form a group of six to eight women. You do not have to be good friends or see each other outside the group.

- Meet once a month at someone's home or, better yet, at a cafe—that's what we did. That way you're not creating more work for yourself; you're freeing up time to work on your own projects and goals. Schedule about an hour and a half for the meeting.

- Allow time at the beginning for a check-in around the table. This is a quick update on how you are doing with your project and goals.

- Choose two people to take time at the next meeting to give a thorough update about their project, ask for feedback, discuss what is going well and where the stumbling blocks are.

- If your group is open to deeper exploration, have someone in the group lead an exercise in visualizing what it is you want to happen. Write, draw, or talk about what you visualized.

Work to Improve Life for Older Women

Many women in midlife want to work for political or social change. Some are drawn to issues that will affect children's lives, such as the environment or children's advocacy. Others enjoy working within the political system to bring about change on issues that interest them. Another choice is to work for the women we will become, as advocates experimenting with new and visionary ways to grow old together: developing housing alternatives and medical services for women or working on issues like the status of older women in the workplace and more visibility for the aging woman. Action and assistance groups offer advocacy, political action, resources, networking, and assistance with a wide range of issues. Some have clearinghouses for information, and most have newsletters detailing their activities. See Resources for some places to begin.

older students. Call to find out. Here are some other points to consider: Does the school offer any grants or scholarships for returning students or specifically for female students? Does it have an already established support or networking group for returning older students? Does it have a work–study program?

How Can I Survive This Transition?

The transition process—through changing a career, going back to school, surviving the loss of a relationship, or coming to terms with growing older—sometimes seems as if it will never end. You wonder if you can keep it together long enough to find out. Part 2, Your Personal Companion, includes questions that can help you gain some perspective on yourself and your needs so that you can decide what you really want to do. Meanwhile, here are some suggestions for getting yourself grounded in rough weather.

INFORM YOURSELF   Find out all you can about whatever transition you are making, be it a change in relationship, career, health, or role. Knowledge is empowering. When you have at least some idea of what to expect, you can begin to gain back some control.

SET SOME GOALS BUT LIVE THE PROCESS   A single-minded attack on the future may get you where you intend to go, but when you arrive you may discover that it's the wrong place. Paradoxically, to attain your goal you must almost let go of it and become immersed in the process of getting where you are going. When you arrive, you will not only know where you are, but also how you got there.

WORK WITH OTHERS   Other people can help ease and even speed a transition. Consider forming a networking group if, for example, you are making a career change or working on a project. Support groups that address the emotional change you are confronting are very helpful. Talking about what is happening is important. Knowing you are not alone and that you are learning with and from others is rewarding and can deepen your experience. For ideas, see this chapter and Chapter 16, "Getting Help."

Seeking Inspiration

Aging is definitely new and scary territory for me. I do not have a mother whom I consider to be a good role model. I want to be vital and interested and interesting as I grow. I am visualizing aging as a chance to continue to grow, so I try to seek out older women whom I admire and who seem to be leading fulfilling lives. I hope they will want to share with me what they know, and I want to let their enthusiasm and spirit be my inspiration. *Joanne, 43*

TAKE CARE OF YOURSELF You may become so engrossed in the process of transition that you neglect yourself. To ensure that you do not fly apart during this stressful time, pay attention to your body's needs. Make sure you have the proper nutrition to support you through the transition. You may be less interested in preparing food and have less time to cook, but eating right is even more important during times of stress. Exercise also contributes to good health and is a great stress reducer. Don't stop now! Finally, do all you can to reduce the effects of stress on your system. Take the time you need for yourself—listen to music you enjoy, take warm baths, get a change of scene, take up meditation.

WRITE IN A JOURNAL Writing about what is going on and how you are proceeding can help you recognize the cycle of change. Record your feelings, reactions, and dreams. Read them for internal clues to what is happening. You may see that you already know what your next step will be.

TAKE SOME DOWN TIME Make room in your schedule for some quiet time to reflect and evaluate. Let yourself acknowledge any losses, and integrate what is happening. Play.

FIND A MENTOR Making friends with someone who has gone down the road you are about to travel can bring great comfort, learning, and inspiration. You don't have to reinvent every wheel.

GET SUPPORT Some changes may be best addressed with the help of a professional. If you decide to use professional services, try to choose someone who has experience in the area you are dealing with and who comes recommended by friends or other professionals you trust. See Chapter 16, "Getting Help," for more ideas on choosing a therapist.

> Most folks think getting older means giving up, not trying anything new. Well, we don't agree with that. As long as you can see each day as a chance for something new to happen, something you never experienced before, you will stay young.
>
> SARAH DELANEY, age 105, *The Delaney Sisters' Everyday Book of Wisdom*

 ## SIDE TRIPS: OTHER PATHWAYS THROUGH THIS BOOK

CHAPTER 2: WHY IS THIS HAPPENING TO ME? Menopause is the biological marker of midlife transition. Look here to learn more about this powerful and unsettling time.

CHAPTER 3: KEEP ON MOVING Exercise is a great way to relieve some of the stress of the midlife transition. Look here to learn more about what constitutes a good exercise program.

CHAPTER 4: ARE YOU WHAT YOU EAT? What are the nutritional needs of midlife? Look here to find out.

CHAPTER 5: BREATHE EASY The stresses of midlife don't have to get the best of you. Look here to learn some easy ways to give yourself a break.

CHAPTER 16: GETTING HELP If the midlife transition is more than you can bear alone, find support. Look here to learn more about the kinds of support available.

CHAPTER 17: THE INNER JOURNEY The midlife transition inevitably brings us face to face with issues of mortality, and the urge to go more deeply into your spiritual nature may be strong. Look here to learn more about the inner midlife journey.

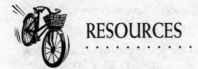

RESURCES

Organizations and Services

WOMEN'S ADVOCACY/AGING/POLITICAL ACTION

American Association of Retired Persons (AARP), 601 E St. N.W., Washington, DC 20049. Voice: (202) 434-2277. Hotline: (800) 424-3410. E-mail: member@ aarp.org. Internet: www.aarp.org. AARP is an organization for people fifty or older. Membership brings you the monthly bulletin, *Modern Maturity* magazine, and many benefits, including legislative advocacy on important issues, home delivery pharmacy, discounts for travel and lodging, insurance, and investment programs. Members and nonmembers can order from AARP's extensive collection of publications, fact sheets, and videos on topics ranging from aging to working options. AARP's Women's Initiative Network (WIN) works to improve the status of midlife and older women. The Widowed Persons Service is part of AARP's Social Outreach and Support Service.

Gray Panthers, 2025 Pennsylvania Ave. N.W., Suite 821, Washington, DC 20006. Voice: (202) 466-3132. This membership organization advocates for older people's rights, international peace, and a universal health care system. Request a brochure on ageism, get in touch with a local chapter, or find out how to start one if there isn't one in your area.

National Action Forum for Midlife and Older Women (NAFOW), P.O. Box 816, Stony Brook, NY 11790. This membership organization is a clearing-house of information for women at midlife and beyond who want to take charge of their physical, economic, and social well-being. Contributions of any amount are welcome and will bring you the always informative *Hot Flash* newsletter (see Periodicals).

National Caucus and Center on the Black Aged, 1424 K St. N.W., Suite 500, Washington, DC 20005. Voice: (202) 637-8400. Fax: (202) 347-0895. Call or write regarding advocacy services and other resources concerning health, housing, and employment.

National Coalition Against Domestic Violence, P.O. Box 18749, Denver, CO 80218-0749. Voice: (303) 839-1852. Fax: (303) 831-9251. This national information and referral service publishes a national directory of domestic violence programs and will put you in touch with a program in your area. It also has a public policy branch.

National Domestic Violence Hotline, 3616 Far West Blvd., Suite 101–297, Austin, TX 78731. Voice: (512) 453-8117. Fax: (512) 453-8541. Hotline: (800) 799-SAFE. E-mail: ndvh@admin.inetport.com. Internet: www.inetport.com/~ndbh. This group provides information, referrals, and resources for victims of domestic violence. It also operates a hotline for emergency information and help.

National Institute on Aging, National Institutes of Health, Information Center, P.O. Box 8057, Gaithersburg, MD 20898-8057. Voice: (800) 222-2225. TDD: (800) 222-4225. Fax: (310) 589-3014. E-mail: niainfo@access.digex.net. Internet: www.nih.gov/nia. The NIA, part of the National Institutes of Health, conducts research in all aspects of aging—medical, biological, and social. Call the 800 number to discover the wide range of published information available.

National Pacific/Asian Resource Center on Aging, Melbourne Tower, Suite 914, 1511 3rd Ave., Seattle, WA 98101. Voice: (206) 624-1221. Fax: (206) 624-1023. This organization provides employment counseling for people over fifty-five years of age.

Older Women's League (OWL), 666 11th Street N.W., Suite 700, Washington, DC 20001. Voice: (202) 783-6686 or (800) TAKE-OWL. Fax: (202) 638-2356. This national membership organization develops educational materials on health issues for women and promotes legislative advocacy, providing information to state, local, and national legislators on issues affecting women at midlife and beyond. Low-cost publications cover such topics as caregiving and elder abuse; reports are available on economic status, Social Security, and pension information. The organization also has audiotapes on different topics, including widowhood and financial planning. If you become a member, you will have access to a telephone number that keeps you updated daily about legislative issues, and you will receive the newsletter, *OWL Observer.* Call to find out about local chapters.

Parents and Friends of Lesbians and Gays (PFLAG), 1101 14th St. N.W., Suite 1030, Washington, DC 20005. Voice: (202) 638-4200. This organization provides referrals and information about local support groups. Pamphlets are available in several languages.

Senior Activism in a Gay Environment (SAGE), 305 7th Ave., 16th Floor, New York, NY 10001. Voice: (212) 741-2247. Fax: (212) 366-1947. Lesbian and gay senior services, workshops, educational materials, socials, and other resources for the aging.

White House Women's Office, 708 Jackson Place N.W., Washington, DC 20503. Voice: (202) 456-7300. Fax: (202) 456-7311. Internet: www.eop.gov. Contact this office for information on a range of women's issues, including health.

EDUCATION

AAUW Career Development Grants, American Association of University Women, Educational Foundation, P.O. Box 4030, Iowa City, IA 52243-4030, or 2201 North Dodge St., Iowa City, IA 52245. Voice: (319) 337-1716. Fax: (319) 337-1204. E-mail: recogprog@Act-Act4-PO.act.org. Internet: www.aauw.org. The AAUW awards grants to women preparing for reentry into the workforce, career changes, and career advancements. Call to get additional information on grants and an application form.

National Women's Studies Association, University of Maryland, 7100 Baltimore Ave., #301, College Park, MD 20740. Voice: (301) 403-0524. Fax: (301) 403-4137. E-mail: nwsa@umail.umd.edu. Internet: www.feminist.com/nwsa.htm. This organization fosters dialogue and collective action among women committed to feminist education at every level. It sponsors caucuses on such topics as aging, Jewish women, women of color, and women's centers, as well as task forces on peace, eco-feminism, scholarship, and other issues. The organization's publications include *Guide to Graduate Work in Women's Studies.*

HEALTH

For health advocacy organizations, see Resources in Chapter 8, "What's Up, Doc?"

HOUSING

CoHousing Company, 1250 Addison St., #113, Berkeley, CA 94702. Voice: (510) 549-9980. E-mail: coho@cohousingco.com. Internet: www.cohousingco.com. This architectural design and consulting firm specializes in cohousing communities. It also offers resources, such as books, printed material, slides, videos, and sample documents. Call or write for the resource and price list.

Women's Housing Task Force, c/o McAuley Institute, 8300 Colesville Road, Suite 310, Silver Spring, MD 20910. Voice: (301) 588-8110. Fax: (703) 716-7349. Internet: www. housinglink.com/unlock.htm. This is a coalition of groups interested in creating opportunities in housing for women. Its publication "Unlocking the Door" discusses many women's housing issues, including housing for the displaced homemaker, community housing, welfare housing, and more. It's free if you order it through the fax number (punch in "500") or over the Internet.

Women's Institute for Housing and Economic Development, Inc., 14 Beacon St., 6th Floor, Boston, MA 02108. Voice: (617) 367-0520. This group works with nonprofit organizations to develop housing and economic opportunities for low-income women and their families. It has helped develop battered women's shelters, transitional housing, and cooperative housing for a variety of organizations. The group does not offer housing placement.

RELATIONSHIP CHANGE

NOW Legal Defense and Education Fund, 99 Hudson St., New York, NY 10013. Voice: (212) 925-6635. Send a written request and $5 to receive a Divorce and Separation Legal Resource Kit; the small donation covers reproduction and mailing costs. The kit contains a divorce-planning guide for women, divorce-planning resources, and a bibliography covering such topics as mediation and alimony, all aimed at helping you understand and protect your rights.

Parents Without Partners. Voice: (800) 637-7974. This organization has many chapters throughout the country to provide support and activities for single parents and their children. It also publishes a newsletter and offers education and information about single parenting. Leave a message and the group will send you information and a referral to a chapter in your area.

THEOS Foundation, 322 Boulevard of the Allies, Suite 105, Pittsburgh, PA 15522. Voice: (412) 471-7779. This organization provides support and outreach to widowed men and women. It can put you in touch with a local organization to help with bereavement and building a new life. It also publishes the periodical *Survivors*, dealing with the stages of grief.

Widowed Persons Service, AARP Social Outreach and Support, 601 E St. N.W., Washington, DC 20049. Voice: (202) 434-2260. Fax: (202) 434-6474. The Widowed Persons Service is a national outreach program that puts newly widowed men and women of any age in touch with local volunteers. You can also request the publication "Directory of Services for the Widowed in the United States and Canada," which contains about 500 assocation and agency names that offer support and counseling for widows. The organization will help you establish a Widowed Persons Service in your area if there isn't one already. Ask about the publication "Divorce After Fifty," which emphasizes finding local resources.

RETIREMENT

National Center for Women and Retirement Research, Long Island University, Southampton Campus, Southampton, NY 11968. Voice: (800) 426-7386. Fax: (516) 283-4678. E-mail: NCWRR@southampton.liunet.edu. Internet: www. southampton.liunet.edu/ncwrr/brochure.htm. The National Center for Women is a life-planning organization that researches and prepares educational handbooks, videos, cassettes, and seminars to help women address various issues related to aging. Topics include financial planning, retirement, social/emotional changes, divorce, employment, and retirement. It also offers videos on divorce and finance (see Audio/Video). The Center's PREP program offers seminars around the country to help women develop secure retirement plans. Call for a directory of information.

Pension Rights Center, 918 16th St. N.W., Suite 701, Washington, DC 20006. Voice: (202) 296-3776. Fax: (202) 833-2472. E-mail: pnsnrights@aol.com. This group will refer your calls about pension rights to the appropriate office and will provide literature on pension, retirement, and the ways divorce may affect pensions. It also offers a state-by-state list of lawyers who deal with pension issues. There is a charge for printed material.

Setting Priorities for Retirement Years (SPRY), 200 K St. N.W., Suite 800, Washington, DC 20006. Voice: (202) 223-7779. Fax: (202) 223-7246. E-mail: RLFSYSOP @compuserve.com. Internet: www.spry.org. This nonprofit foundation was established in 1991 to help older adults plan for a healthy and financially secure future. It conducts research and develops education programs that respond to consumer needs. The web site has many great links.

WORK

Association of Part-Time Professionals, 7700 Leesburg Pike, Suite 216, Falls Church, VA 22043, or 7655 Old Springfield Road, McLean, VA 22102. Voice: (703) 734-7975. If you are currently working part-time or thinking about it, this nonprofit organization can help you with planning, resources, and information about flexible work options. Membership will bring you the newsletter *Working Options* and a discount on the group's publications.

Business and Professional Women USA, 2012 Massachusetts Ave. N.W., Washington, DC 20036. Voice: (202) 293-1100. Fax: (202) 861-0298. This professional activist membership organization brings together working women to promote equal opportunity, self-sufficiency, networking, conferences, and training.

Catalyst, 250 Park Avenue South, Fifth Floor, New York, NY 10003. Voice: (212) 777-8900. Fax: (212) 477-4252. This organization helps businesses encourage women in leadership roles. It also has an extensive library on women and work.

Coalition of Labor Union Women, 1126 16th St. N.W., Washington, DC 20036. Voice: (202) 466-4610. Fax: (202) 776-0537. This organization offers programs and resources, referrals, and printed material on issues affecting women in the workplace. It also has a committee for older and retired women workers.

National Board for Certified Counselors, 3 Terrace Way, Suite D, Greensboro, SC 27409. Voice: (910) 547-0607. Fax: (910) 547-0017. This organization can provide you with a list of certified career counselors in your area.

National Clearinghouse on State and Local Older Worker Programs, NASUA, 1225 I Street N.W., Suite 725, Washington, DC 20005. Voice: (202) 898-2578. Fax: (202) 898-2583. E-mail: staff@NASUA.org. This group provides consultation to agencies on aging and offers training for businesses on recruiting, training, and hiring older workers. It offers publications and sponsors an annual older worker conference.

National Commission on Working Women, 1325 G St. N.W., Washington, DC 20005. Voice: (202) 737-5764. This organization is committed to promoting the rights of working women. It is especially concerned with ageism and provides information about employment rights and older working women.

National Committee on Pay Equity, 1126 16th St. N.W., Room 411, Washington, DC 20036. Voice: (202) 331-7343. Fax: (202) 331-7406. E-mail: NCPE@essential.org. NCPE offers information about women and people of color and discrepancy in pay; some of its publications are free.

National Foundation for Women Business Owners, 1100 Wayne Ave., Suite 830, Silver Spring, MD 20910. Voice: (301) 495-4975. Fax: (301) 495-4979. E-mail: NFWBO@worldnet.att.net. Internet: www.nfwbo.org. This organization does research on women business owners, including the latest statistics on women and business, how women buy and use technology, and women and capital credit and financing. These research reports are published and available for a fee.

Score, 409 3rd St. S.W., Washington, DC 20024. Voice: (800) 634-0245. Fax: (202) 205-7636. This is the national office of Score, which is sponsored by the Small Business Administration. Call for help with your small business or for a referral to a Score office in your area, which will provide free business consultations from retired executives.

Wider Opportunities for Women, 815 15th St. N.W., Suite 916, Washington, DC 20005. Voice: (202) 638-3143. Fax: (202) 638-4885. WOW advocates for the needs and rights of women workers and sponsors several national and local projects. The Nontraditional Employment Project offers education and skills training for nontraditional and technical jobs; the Workplace Solutions Project provides assistance to employers and unions to integrate and retain women in nontraditional occupations and prevent sexual harassment in the workplace. The Women's College Assistance Project helps women receiving welfare enter college.

Women Work National Network for Women's Employment, 1625 K St. N.W., Suite 300, Washington, DC 20006. Voice: (202) 467-6346. Fax: (202) 467-5366. E-mail: womanwork@worldnet.att.net. This nonprofit membership organization provides financial aid, counseling, job training, and child care for women who are divorced, separated, or widowed and reentering the workforce. Call for a referral to an affiliated program in your area.

Hotlines

National Domestic Violence Hotline: (800) 799-SAFE. This twenty-four-hour hotline will refer you to counseling services or battered women's shelters in your area and will do some crisis intervention.

Small Business Administration: (800) 767-0385. Call for recorded information about business administration plans and programs for starting a small business. This organization offers programs especially for women starting a small business.

Score: (800) 634-0245. Call for counseling assistance for small businesses from retired business executives, free of charge. If possible, the organization will make an appointment for you to talk with a person who has experience in the business in which you are interested. You can also get information on local seminars on starting a business.

Social Security Administration: (800) 772-1213. Get the answers to your questions about Social Security benefits.

Periodicals

Hot Flash. NAFOW, Box 816, Stony Brook, NY 11790-0600. This publication for members of the National Action Forum for Midlife and Older Women includes information on public policy affecting older women as well as articles covering issues of midlife. It's always lively and very informative.

MidLife Woman. MidLife Woman's Network, 5129 Logan Ave. South, Minneapolis, MN 55419-1019. Voice: (800) 886-4354. E-mail: MDLFWOMAN@aol.com. Internet: users.aol.com/mdlfwoman/info.htm#MidLife. This bimonthly newsletter covers many midlife issues in depth and informatively. Areas of interest include emotional changes, spirituality, successful transitions, menopause, and health.

National Center for Women and Retirement Research. Long Island University, Southampton Campus, Southampton, NY 11968. National Center for Women, Long Island University, Southampton Campus, Southampton, NY 11968. Voice: (800) 426-7386. Fax: (516) 283-4678. E-mail: NCWRR@southampton.liunet.edu. Internet: www.southamption.liunet.edu/ncwrr. This newsletter, which comes with membership in the National Center for Women, features a national workshop calendar and many interesting tidbits about women, work, and retirement.

Books

Greg Anderson. *Living Life on Purpose: A Guide to Creating a Life of Success and Significance.* San Francisco: HarperSanFrancisco, 1997. This is a small, concise book that includes a self-scoring life mission skills test. Vision, Service, Passion, and Mission are the clearly named sections of this easy-to-use book.

William Bridges. *Transitions: Making Sense of Life's Changes.* Reading, MA: Addison-Wesley, 1980. This book explores the pattern of transitions, suggesting ways to understand and cope with them while coming to a better knowledge of who we are. It's a thorough and enlightening look at the role of change in our lives.

Janis Fisher Chan. *Inventing Ourselves Again: Women Face Middle Age.* Portland, OR: Sibyl Publications, 1996. Women-to-women stories of making transitions and aging. The personal stories are engaging and honest. It's like being with a circle of friends.

Paula B. Doress-Worters and Diana Laskin Siegal, with Boston Women's Health Collective. *The New Ourselves, Growing Older.* New York: Simon and Schuster, 1994. A wonderful and useful book to have as we age. This is an invaluable resource that gives much attention to the many aspects of women and aging—physical, social, psychological, and spiritual. It has great resources and stories of women's experiences.

Betty Friedan. *The Fountain of Age.* New York: Simon and Schuster, 1993. In this best-seller, Friedan paints the new possibilities of intimacy and purpose as we age: career, recreation, retirement, and learning. A new look at what's possible.

Marion E. Hayes. *Primelife: Planning Guide for the 40+ Generation.* Springdale, AK: Primelife Publications, 1996. This workbook provides information on such topics as relationships, career, learning, recreation, and retirement. It has a good section on education and some ways to pursue educational interests outside the classroom.

The Hen Co-op. *Growing Old Disgracefully: New Ideas for Getting the Most Out of Life.* Freedom, CA: The Crossing Press, 1994. Irreverent and innovative ideas for growing older with a vengeance. Great fun and inspiring.

Gerda Lerner. *The Creation of Feminist Consciousness.* New York: Oxford, 1993. Documents the historical struggle of women to free their minds, to create Women's History and feminist consciousness.

Joan Steinau Lester. *Taking Charge: Every Woman's Action Guide to Personal, Political, and Professional Success.* Berkeley, CA: Conari Press, 1996. This book encourages women to set goals, to network with other women, and to support each other in becoming who we want to be. It's packed with good ideas.

Letty Cottin Pogrebin. *Getting Over Getting Older: An Intimate Journey.* Boston: Little Brown, 1996. The author writes in a straightforward and humorous style to debunk aging myths and the culture of youth. She encourages women to move toward the path of acceptance and comfort "as time speeds up and the body slows down."

Gail Sheehy. *New Passages: Mapping Your Life Across Time.* New York: Random House, 1995. In this bestseller, Sheehy looks at how men and women can take the opportunity of midlife to "map out" the direction of the life yet to be lived.

Barbara Sher, with Anne Gottlieb. *Wishcraft: How to Get What You Really Want.* New York: Ballantine, 1997. How to find out about what you want and how to get it. This book has lots of ideas about networking, support, creative thinking, and brainstorming.

HOUSING

Kathryn McCaman and Charles Durrett. *Cohousing: A Contemporary Approach to Housing Ourselves.* Berkeley, CA: Ten Speed Press, 1994. Cohousing is a cooperative approach that brings to reality the dreams and intentions of those who want to live together in their later years. This book looks at how it can be done.

LITERATURE/PERSONAL STORIES

Lydia Lewis Alexander, Marilyn Hill Harper, Otis Halloway Owens, and Mildred Lucas Pattersen. *Wearing Purple: Four Long-Term Friends Celebrate the Joys and Challenges of Growing Older.* New York: Crown, 1996. These women met at one of the country's historically African American colleges and formed a lasting friendship that is documented by their letters over the years. They share thoughts and feelings about life experiences—joy, sadness, loss, fulfillment, laughter—as they age. This book illustrates the value and joy in female relationships.

Doris Lessing. *The Summer Before the Dark.* New York: Knopf, 1973. Lessing's classic book about a woman's observations of her midlife transformation. Meticulous, piercing, and relentlessly honest.

Lee Lynch and Akia Woods, eds. *Off the Rag: Writings on Menopause.* Norwich, VT: New Victoria Publications, 1996. A collection of stories about menopause and aging in the words of lesbians.

Sandra Martz, ed. *When I Am an Old Woman I Shall Wear Purple*. 2d ed., Watsonville, CA: Papier-Mache Press, 1991. A collection of poems, short stories, and photos about women aging, mostly by women. Humorous, courageous, and, of course, outrageous.

Cathleen Rountree. *On Women Turning Fifty: Celebrating Midlife Discoveries*. San Francisco: HarperSanFrancisco, 1993. Eighteen women examine what it means to grow older in many aspects of their lives, including work, family, creativity, love, and spirituality. The women exemplify many positive ways to see aging; this book is a good way to enter the topic of aging and women.

Barbara Sang, Joyce Warshaw, and Adrienne J. Smith, eds. *Lesbians at Midlife: Creative Transition Anthology*. Minneapolis, MN: Spinsters Inc., 1991. A collection of inspiring stories of women and midlife from the lesbian perspective.

Dena Taylor and Amber Sumrall, eds. *Women of the 14th Moon: Writings on Menopause*. Freedom, CA: The Crossing Press, 1991. Women share their stories through essays, poems, and stories about the many experiences and dimensions of the menopausal journey.

Velma Wallis. *Two Old Women: An Alaska Legend of Betrayal, Courage, and Survival*. New York: HarperCollins, 1993. A woman recounts the story her mother told her: an Alaskan legend about two elderly women expelled by their tribe and how they survive and learn in the process. A sweet and inspiring story.

MONEY

Francis Leonard. *Money and the Mature Woman*. Reading, MA: Addison-Wesley, 1993. This book is written by a former legal counsel for the Older Women's League. She sees women's financial needs and concerns as being different from men's and urges women at midlife and beyond to look at their financial situation and understand what their retirement might look like. She also includes ideas on how to plan.

Ralph Wainer. *Get a Life: You Don't Need a Million to Retire Well*. Berkeley, CA: Nolo Press, 1996. This book addresses planning for retirement without sacrificing the best years of your life by overworking for something in the future. It looks at what it takes to live well on what you have.

RELATIONSHIP CHANGE

Charlotte Foehner and Carol Cozart. *The Widow's Handbook*. Colorado: Fulcrum, 1988. Two women who were widowed combine their experiences and what they have learned in a helpful and compassionate way. Very practical and inspirational.

Philomene Gates. *Suddenly Alone*. New York: Harper & Row, 1990. This is another practical guide to the problems of widowhood. It addresses such issues as choosing a lawyer, friendships, work, travel, and self-care.

Penny Kaganoff and Susan Spano. *Women on Divorce: A Bedside Companion.* New York: Harcourt Brace, 1995. Fourteen women tell their stories of divorce. This book is sometimes humorous and always interesting.

Sheila Kitzinger. *Becoming a Grandmother: A Life Transition.* New York: Scribner, 1996. Welcome to a new vision of grandmothers that acknowledges this important life transition. This valuable book addresses stereotypes, grandmothering skills, new relationships with one's own children, and learning all about this new role.

Rita Robinson. *When Women Choose to Be Single.* Van Nuys, CA: Newcastle Publishing, 1992. Robinson explores the issue of being single at any age—it is always an option. The book encourages the reader to develop a strong and satisfying relationship with herself and gives suggestions on having a successful life as a single woman.

Violet Woodhouse, J.D., C.F.P., and Victoria F. Colby, Ph.D., C.F.P., with M. C. Blakeman. *Divorce and Money: How to Make the Best Financial Decisions During Divorce.* 3d ed., Berkeley, CA: Nolo Press, 1996. If you're getting divorced, take a look at this book. It explores more aspects of divorce and money than you may have thought of, including planning for the future, what to do about your house and property, establishing retirement benefits, and other long-term financial consequences of divorce.

WORK

Rebecca Maddox. *Inc. Your Dreams.* New York: Penguin, 1995. This book is full of ideas for women in career transition—from starting your own business to improving what you already have. It includes exercises aimed at helping you become more specific.

Deloss L. Marsh. *Retirement Careers: Combining the Best of Work and Leisure.* Charlotte, VT: Williamson Publishing, 1991. Many women are not able to retire—for financial reasons or just because they enjoy working. This book offers ideas and how-to's on developing one or even several enjoyable retirement careers.

Audio/Video

Some of the agencies listed in Organizations and Services, in particular **AARP** and the **National Center for Women and Retirement Research**, have excellent audiocassettes and videotapes available for sale or rental. You'll find other good tapes for issues of transition in the following catalogs:

Films and Video About, For, and By Women, Pennsylvania State University Audio-Visual Services, 127 Fox Hill Road, University Park, PA 16803-1824. Voice: (800) 826-0132. Internet: www.libraries.psu.edu/avs/. This is a good source for a variety of tapes about women.

Pacifica Radio Archive, P.O. Box 8092, Dept. F, Universal City, CA 91609-0092. Voice: (800) 735-0230. The archive has audiotapes from over forty years of Pacifica radio shows, many on women's issues.

Terra Nova Films, 9848 S. Winchester Ave., Chicago IL 60643. Voice: (800) 779-8491. E-mail: tnf@terranova.org. Internet: www.terranova.org. This company distributes more than 200 videos on aging, many specifically about women. The videos range from industrial films for training and education to documentaries.

VIDEOS

Whisper the Women. Available from Terra Nova Films. A close look at seven women, ages fifty-eight to ninety-one, who are active and enjoying their lives. Focuses on positive aspects of aging.

Widows. Available from Terra Nova Films. A film about women who are widowed and the many feelings that arise from this situation. Has been used as a lead-in to discussion for support groups.

Women and Divorce. 60 minutes. Available from the National Center for Women and Retirement Research. This video, based on research done by the National Center for Women, explores divorce and women's rights, legal issues, finances, and other issues.

Women and Money. 60 minutes. Available from the National Center for Women and Retirement Research. This video, based on research done by the National Center for Women, looks at issues of women and money, including budgeting, investing, and retirement.

Online

Many of the organizations listed in Organizations and Services, above, have home pages on the Internet. For specific issues of transition, such as finances, education reentry, or career transition and retirement, use a search engine to find interesting web sites.

MAILING LISTS

Gender-Related Electronic Forums, at www-unix.umbc.edu/~korenman/wmst/forums.html, is a good place to find mailing lists on women and gender-related issues. Search categories include activist lists, education lists, health lists, Internet information lists, religion/spirituality lists, women of color lists, and women's studies lists.

NEWS GROUPS

For women's news and issues, try **clari.news.women** (a moderated discussion about women's issues, such as sexism); **soc.women** (women's problems and relationships); or **tnn.interv.women** (information exchange on women's issues). To discuss retirement and other aging issues, try **soc.retirement.** For support to see you through a breakup, try **alt.support.divorce.**

WEB SITES

Jumping-off points for women's sites include **WWWomen** at www.wwwomen.com, a search directory for women, with categories that include publications, diversity, education, arts and entertainment, health and safety, and many more. **Women Online,** at www.women-online.com/, has links to web resources for women's online columns and publications, web site reviews, and more. **ElectraPages,** at www.electrapages.com, is a huge, searchable database of names and addresses of more than 7,500 women's organizations and businesses. In fact, it's the web site of the National Women's Mailing List (see Resources in Chapter 18, "Bringing It Together: Gathering Information").

Women's Wire, at www.women.com, is a pioneer online women's magazine. It covers just about everything of interest to women, including breaking news, sports and fitness, sex, health issues, quizzes, entertainment, shopping, appearance, and even comic strips. Updates are ongoing, so each day's issue is slightly different. Check it out.

For feminist resources, go to **Feminist Activist Resources on the Net** at www.igc.apc.org/women/feminist.html. This is a good starting place to find links to women's organizations, general resources for political activism, feminism, global issues, women's health advocacy, and more. If you want to explore activism, go to **WomensNet** at www.igc.apc.org/igc/wnl and do as the site suggests: "Select an issue/Press button." Issues include everything from activism, atmosphere, and climate to the Green movement, labor, indigenous peoples, toxins, and women.

AARP's web site offers a number of online brochures, including "Life Transitions," www.aarp.org/programs/transitions/home.html, a guide to midlife transitions and thinking ahead, with information on dealing with death, divorce, and estate planning. For information about an unusual housing alternative, explore **CoHousing** at www.cohousing.org.

Here's a good collection of government sites that offer an abundance of information: **Administration on Aging,** www.aoa.dhhs.gov/aoa/pages/aoa; **Health Care Financing Administration,** www.hcfa.gov/; and, of course, the **Social Security Administration,** www.ssa.gov/. If you want to go straight to the top, try the **White House** at www.whitehous.gov/; **Cap Web,** a guide to the U.S. Congress, is at congress.org/; the **U.S. House of Representatives** is at www.house.gov/; and the **U.S. Senate** is at www.senate.gov/.

For issues of aging, head for these general sites: **Interactive Aging Network,** at www.ianet.org, or **Senior.com,** at www.senior.com. Both have lots of links to other web resources. Finally, try SPRY—Setting Priorities for Retirement Years—at www.spry.org. This is a wonderfully helpful site with links to pages dealing with health, retirement, finances, and many other sources of ideas and information.

2

WHY IS THIS HAPPENING TO ME?
Menopause

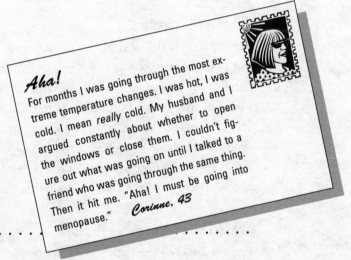

Aha!
For months I was going through the most extreme temperature changes. I was hot, I was cold. I mean *really* cold. My husband and I argued constantly about whether to open the windows or close them. I couldn't figure out what was going on until I talked to a friend who was going through the same thing. Then it hit me. "Aha! I must be going into menopause."
Corinne, 43

One thing is certain: As long as we are alive, we will get older. As attorney Gloria Allred once said, "As far as aging goes, the hope is that I *will* age, given what the alternative is." Nonetheless, the undeniable signs that we are growing older can come as a great shock. Steeped in the culture of youth, we are somehow able to believe that the changes we have witnessed in our mothers, aunts, grandmothers, and friends have no relation to us. So when change begins to be undeniable, we may find ourselves unprepared to deal with it.

Change of life, menopause, means something different to each of us: the end of youth and the beginning of age. The end of childbearing and the beginning of sexual freedom. The end of taking care of children and the beginning of taking care of our parents. The end of doing so much for others and the beginning of doing more for ourselves. The end of wondering what life's all about and the beginning of wisdom.

Whatever it means to you, the hot flashes, the menstrual irregularities, and all the changes that accompany it tell you unmistakably that you are continuing on life's path. Menopause, for all that it puts us through, is the biological event that marks a profound transition. Why not take hold of it and make it your own?

 ## PACKING FOR THE JOURNEY

What Is Menopause?

Menopause is the end of menstruation and hence the end of fertility, but it is more of a journey than an event. When we speak of "going through menopause," we're talking about dealing with the many changes that occur before menstruation ends, as our bodies produce less and less of the sex hormones, estrogen and progesterone. We generally mark these changes in two phases: menopause, when a woman has stopped having her period for at least a year, and perimenopause, the years of transition that precede this time.

When Does Menopause Begin?

Each woman's experience with menopause is uniquely her own. The time it takes and the age at which it begins vary from woman to woman. According to the North American Menopause Society (NAMS), the average age for menopause in the West seems to be unchanged since ancient times—about fifty-one. But menopause can occur at any age. "Premature ovarian failure" can occur any time after menstruation, even as early as seventeen. By sixty, however, virtually all women will have experienced menopause. A number of factors may influence the timing.

perimenopause A catch-all term for the time before menopause when a woman experiences physical symptoms due to the effects of declining hormones.

menopause The stage of life reached when a woman's menstrual periods have stopped for one year.

Your Age When You Had Your First Period It doesn't matter if you were the first

GUIDED TOUR: *Menopause*

Menopause is the end of menstruation and hence the end of childbearing. A woman is considered to have experienced menopause if she has not had her period for at least one year. Perimenopause, the years leading up to menopause, may be marked by a number of physical and emotional changes related to declining levels of reproductive hormones, increased PMS, natural aging, and general stress.

WESTERN MEDICINE

Consult your physician about your risks for osteoporosis and heart disease, which are health concerns to women after menopause. Always see your doctor if you have unusual bleeding or pain. Your doctor can answer your questions about hormone replacement therapy.

COMPLEMENTARY THERAPIES

Complementary therapies may be able to help you work toward balance during this time of bodily unpredictability. Practitioners of homeopathy, acupuncture, Ayurveda, traditional Chinese medicine, and other healing systems work with people to find personalized treatments to help balance the hormonal system and relieve hot flashes, insomnia, and other problems.

EXERCISE

A regular program of daily aerobic exercise can even out mood swings, lift depression, help you sleep better, and help prevent cardiovascular disease. Strength training can help prevent or retard osteoporosis, and stretching your muscles can help keep them from injury.

MIND–BODY

Practices such as yoga, t'ai chi, qi gong, Alexander technique, and Rosen work may help balance hormones, relieve stress, and improve flexibility and balance. Meditation, biofeedback, massage, and other stress-reduction techniques can reduce the severity of hot flashes and other problems.

NUTRITION

Soy products and other vegetables containing phytoestrogens may help curtail problems related to hormonal imbalance, such as hot flashes. Aim for a diet low in saturated fat and rich in vegetables, fruits, whole grains, and adequate protein.

SUPPORT

Self-help, peer support, or professional counseling can help you get over the rough spots of your midlife transition. You're not in this alone.

All at Once

I turned forty-five, and blam. It hit me all at once: lumpy breasts, heavy bleeding, hot flashes, reading glasses. I always thought I'd have time to have children, and now they tell me I can't have children anymore.

Kathy, 45

girl on your block to get your period or the last. Recent research shows that there is no connection between age at first menstruation and age at menopause.

YOUR MOTHER'S AGE WHEN SHE EXPERIENCED MENOPAUSE There may be some connection here. Chances are, you'll experience menopause around the same time your mother did. But beware of anecdotal evidence: Until recently, women didn't discuss menopause as much as they do now, and your mother may not remember precisely how old she was at the time.

CIGARETTE SMOKING   Cigarette smokers tend to experience menopause somewhat earlier than average. According to NAMS, "Smokers, and even former smokers, can experience menopause up to three years earlier than nonsmokers."

How Long Does Perimenopause Last?

On average, perimenopause begins three to five years before your periods stop. During this time your body begins to gear down, producing less and estrogen and progesterone. Reproductive hormone levels keep getting lower and lower during the change of life, but they don't just drop off suddenly or slow down evenly. The rate and style of decline is different for each woman, and it's also different from day to day. Menopause is not official until you have not had a period for at least one year—thirteen months is the magic number. After that, you're considered postmenopausal. Your body is still producing estrogen, but at a much lower level and with fewer fluctuations.

woman of the fourteenth moon A postmenopausal woman; the fourteenth month, or moon, is considered the first official month marking one's new beginning as a woman who has passed through the journey of menopause.

What Are the Signs of Perimenopause?

Some women ask, "How will I know I'm approaching menopause?" The quick answer is, "Don't worry, you'll know!" The real trick is separating out the signs of declining hormones from the signs of increased PMS and the signs of stress and normal aging. For the most part, indications of approaching menopause that the medical community recognizes are: hot flashes and profuse sweating, feeling very hot and then very cold, vaginal dryness, and an increased risk of heart disease and osteoporosis. These signs are tied to declining reproductive hormone levels and are treatable with hormone replacement therapy.

If That's All There Is, What Are All These Other Signs I'm Experiencing?

Good question. What about the lengthy collection of problems we call "this menopause stuff"? (For a complete list, see the Point of Interest "Hot Flash: Signs of Midlife Found!") Why do so many women have similar complaints?

SIGNS CONNECTED TO HORMONAL DECLINE Declining hormones may affect much more than current thinking shows—for example, researchers have recently linked memory problems to low levels of estrogen. Some problems are clearly connected—if you are bothered by hot flashes and sweating at night, you will very likely have trouble sleeping and thinking clearly; and if you are experiencing vaginal dryness, a loss of interest in sex should not be surprising.

SIGNS CONNECTED TO EXAGGERATED PMS Many of the discomforts we attribute to menopause are really increased PMS, which is common to women in midlife. Even if you have never had PMS before, you may have it now. And if you have always suffered from PMS, it may worsen. Bloating,

I Still Love Paul
I'm a baby boomer. I saw the Beatles live in 1964. I still love Paul. I still wear blue jeans! How can I be going through menopause?

Tracy, 48

POINT OF INTEREST
Historical Menopause

1845: Columbat de l'Iesere, in his *Treatise on the Diseases of Females,* included a chapter on the menopause that contained the following: "Compelled to yield to the power of time, women cease to exist for the species and henceforward live only for themselves."

1882: Tilt determined that the menopause is "always a time of trial, often of suffering and danger."

1887: Farnham summarized the relationship between the menopause and psychiatric disorder in this way: "The ovaries, after long years of service, have not the ability of retiring in graceful old age, but become irritated, transmit the irritation to the abdominal ganglia, which in turn transmit the irritation to the brain, producing disturbances in the cerebral tissue exhibiting themselves in extreme nervousness or in an outburst of actual insanity."

Source: Office of Technology Assessment, Congressional Board of the 102nd Congress, *Menopause, Hormone Therapy, and Women's Health* (Washington, DC: U.S. Government Printing Office, May 1992).

headaches, irritability, mood swings, cramping, and other premenstrual problems may get worse during this time.

SIGNS CONNECTED TO STRESS Some problems are signs of stress, which is certainly a factor in this time of powerful physical and emotional transition. In fact, if you put a list of the so-called "common signs of menopause" next to a list of the "common signs of stress," you'll see that they're virtually identical. For example, trouble concentrating, trouble sleeping, exhaustion or fatigue, loss of interest in sex, and irritability are listed in both.

SIGNS OF NORMAL AGING   Still other problems are signs of (gasp!) normal aging. This includes skin sensitivities, dry skin, and digestive upsets. Sometimes we forget that menopause isn't an isolated phenomenon; it's part of natural aging. Men have similar changes and stresses in midlife (minus the hot flashes)— they just don't have the cue of menopause to hang them on. When we don't lump all these issues together as "this menopause stuff," we can more quickly find the true cause of discomfort and do something about it.

What Is Surgical Menopause?

Premenopausal women who have both ovaries removed surgically will not have the luxury of a leisurely journey through menopause. For more on surgical menopause, see Chapter 14, "Is This Really Necessary?"

What Are the Special Health Concerns of Menopause?

First of all, it's important to remember that menopause is not a disease: It is part of the natural aging process. You do not have to run to your doctor when you begin to experience perimenopausal changes, but you may want to discuss what's going on with your body and explore your options. If you're experiencing pain or heavy bleeding, it's a good idea to have a medical evaluation. Even though menopause itself is not a medical condition, lowered hormonal levels affect almost every area of the body. This is especially true for the heart and bones: An increased risk of cardiovascular disease (heart problems) and osteoporosis (thinning bones) are the two major health concerns for women at midlife and beyond.

What?

Difficulty concentrating and problems with memory worry a lot of women during the menopausal years. If this is a problem for you, you're in good company. The hormonal declines that create havoc in other parts of our bodies also seem to affect thinking and can affect short-term memory. This may make it difficult to remember that word you need or just why you walked into the kitchen. You may feel as if you're losing your mind, but you're not. Here are some things you can do to help yourself.

ESTROGEN   Recent research indicates that estrogen therapy has a good effect on some types of memory and concentration in menopausal and postmenopausal women. As a bonus, research indicates that it may protect against the onset of Alzheimer's disease and seems to slow its progression.

EAT YOUR BRAIN CHEMICALS Choline and inositol (both components of lecithin) are brain chemicals that aid in learning and understanding. When these are low, our brains just don't work as well. Food sources for both include egg

The Menstrual Migraine

A couple of years ago, I began to have these horrendous headaches whenever my hormones were going through a major change—in the middle of my cycle, or right before I got my period. It's always over my left eye, there's nothing I can do about it, and it lasts for thirty-six hours. When it's over, I feel like I've been kicked in the head. My mother said she had the same headache around my age, but it disappeared after her menopause.   *Maria, 39*

Okay, so they're not all signs of approaching menopause. But they're also not signs that you're losing your mind or seriously ill. Rest easy: *No one* experiences every symptom on this long, long list. And, as you'll see, you can find ways to cope. Here are the more common and less common signs that may mark your midlife passage.

- Body (more common): Hot flashes, profuse sweating, night sweats, feeling very hot then very cold, headaches, sleep disturbance, exhaustion or fatigue, weight changes, breast tenderness, fibrocystic breasts, bone loss, weight gain

- Body (less common): Muscle or joint pain, leg cramps, increased cholesterol levels, heart palpitations associated with hot flashes, easy bruising, dizziness, change in body odor

- Menstrual irregularities: Heavy bleeding or spotting during periods, bleeding that lasts longer than usual, irregular menstrual cycles

- Sex (more common): Change in sexual interest (more often dampened but sometimes heightened)

- Sex (less common): Pain or bleeding during or after intercourse

- Skin and hair (more common): Acne, dry skin, "shrinking" lips, dry hair

- Skin and hair (less common): Unusual skin sensitivity; itchy, crawly, or burning skin; thinning hair; hair loss; facial hair growth

- Emotions: Mild depression, mood swings, nervousness, irritability, anger, panic

- Memory and thinking: Forgetfulness, fuzzy thinking, memory loss, difficulty concentrating

(continued)

yolks, soybeans, wheat germ, oatmeal, brewer's yeast, peanuts, green peas, green leafy vegetables, and lean meat. Inositol is also found in cantaloupe, grapefruit, raisins, unrefined molasses, and cabbage. Manganese, which helps the body use choline, is found in whole-grain cereals, nuts, green leafy vegetables, peas, and beets.

GET SOME EXERCISE   As we all know, exercise improves blood circulation, and the blood can't help but flow through your brain. According to studies, aerobic exercise helps memory and reasoning. It also helps improve your mood, which may make you more inclined to remember things.

LAY OFF PASTA/EAT WHOLE GRAINS   Large meals of complex carbohydrates can make you feel less than alert. In fact, they can make you feel like taking a nap. Save these meals for the end of the day. If you're going to a business lunch, eat light protein and less pasta. Whole grains like brown rice and bulgur wheat have the B vitamins, folic acid, and magnesium you need for energy, memory, and stable moods.

FIGHT DEPRESSION   Depression, a feeling of deep sadness that lingers on, can also interfere with memory and thinking. If you think depression is a problem for you, seek help to turn it around. Exercise also helps fight depression.

GET SOME SLEEP   Lack of sleep makes fuzzy thinking a certainty, even in the absence of other problems. Sleep deprivation over a period of days is even worse. See "How Can I

Get a Good Night's Sleep?" for ideas on getting some rest.

TRY AN HERBAL REMEDY Preparations made from the leaves of *Ginkgo biloba* increase blood flow to the brain and are thought to have a positive effect on memory. Research is ongoing and promising. Ginkgo is popular in Europe, where use of herbal remedies is more popular. The strength of various preparations varies from brand to brand, so you will have to experiment. Ginkgo doesn't work overnight; allow a couple of months for results.

EXERCISE YOUR MIND Your mind needs exercise to stay in shape. Keep it active—read, take a class, solve problems, do crossword puzzles, have lively discussions. If you practice remembering the interesting and fun things, you'll probably have better luck recalling the boring stuff.

USE MEMORY TRICKS Make a real effort to remember things. This means trying not to let your mind wander down two or three thought roads at once. Let a pencil be your friend: Make a list of the things you intend to do during the day, and refer to it. Leave notes for yourself around the house as reminders. And always put your keys and glasses away in the same place.

RELAX If all else fails, forget about it. With a little relaxation, that elusive memory will probably pop right back into your mind. Sleep on it!

How Can I Get a Good Night's Sleep?

Most women say they could deal with the itching, they could deal with the irritability, they could even deal with the

POINT OF INTEREST (continued)

- Vaginal/urinary changes: Loss of lubrication, thinning tissues, vaginal dryness, pain with intercourse, vulvar itching or burning, urinary tract infections, urinary incontinence, frequent urination

- Digestion: Digestive upsets, flatulence, bloating

- Eye and vision changes: Dry eyes (burning, itching, redness), tearing, swollen or red eyelids, focusing problems, sensation of having something in your eye

- Mouth and teeth: Dry mouth, pain inside of mouth, inflamed and bleeding gums, changes in taste

Dress for Success

The temperature changes were driving me crazy until I figured out how to dress. I found that my temperature fluctuations calmed down when I wore sandals that let my feet breathe—it's like wearing a hat to keep your body heat in, only backwards! And I also started wearing vests and light T-shirts, keeping my core warm just like you do when you're skiing. *Pat. 41*

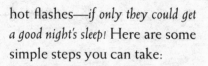

hot flashes—*if only they could get a good night's sleep!* Here are some simple steps you can take:

Cut Down on Caffeine

You may need to avoid caffeine altogether. If this doesn't seem like an option to you, determine your limit and stick to it. Drink your latté earlier in the day rather than with dinner. One woman may be able to drink coffee up to six o'clock in the evening with no sleep disturbance, while another can drink coffee only in the morning.

Cut Down on Alcohol

Alcohol would seem to be the perfect substance to relax you and help you sleep, and it may be—for a while. But it can also interfere with sleep, making it fitful. If you're having sleep problems, alcohol may be a cause.

Avoid Heavy Meals Late at Night

When you go to sleep, your body goes to work. If it has to work really hard at digesting, you'll be awake. Eat protein, but eat larger amounts earlier in the day, when it will help you be alert and awake. Eat a smaller, lighter meal at night.

Eat Complex Carbohydrates Later in the Day

Complex carbohydrates, like potatoes and whole-grain bread, increase levels of serotonin in the brain. This makes you feel good *and* sleepy.

Take a Warm Bath with Epsom Salts

Two for the price of one: The warm bath promotes relaxation. The magnesium in the Epsom salts (use about 1 cup to a full bath) relaxes your muscles and is a pleasant way to absorb some of the magnesium you need for calcium absorption.

EXERCISE EARLIER IN THE DAY   Exercise can dissipate anxiety and tension, which can help you get a good night's sleep. But vigorous exercise a few hours before bedtime can make you feel raring to go just when it's time to get some rest. Be sure to exercise earlier to avoid interfering with sleep.

DEVELOP A SLEEP RITUAL   Have cues that remind your body that it's time to go to sleep. Try to go to sleep at the same time every night. Relax with a book, a hot bath, or restful music.

TRY AN HERBAL REMEDY   The plant world has a number of helpful sleep inducers. Try tea made from hops (*Humulus lupulus*), spearmint, or chamomile (remember Peter Rabbit?) or a few drops of tincture of valerian or passionflower (*Passiflora incarnata*).

TRY ACUPUNCTURE   This can be an effective treatment for insomnia. Be sure to tell your practitioner all of your symptoms.

TRY RELAXATION TECHNIQUES   Visualization, guided imagery, and similar practices can help you relax into sleep. Establish a relaxation routine you can call on whenever you need a cue to fall asleep.

TRY CALCIUM AT BEDTIME   Calcium is another sleep inducer. Take your calcium supplement before you go to bed rather than in the morning. Or try this warm milk drink: Warm up a cup of nonfat milk and mix it with honey to taste (or blackstrap molasses, for added calcium and a rich flavor), a dash of vanilla, and a sprinkle of nutmeg, cinnamon, or cardamom. This is also a great drink for putting you *back* to sleep in the middle of the night.

When you're taking a long journey, it's always good to be prepared!

Tours: Package tours are not available. Each woman's journey is uniquely hers.

Transportation: Plan to provide your own transportation. Walking, cycling, dancing, and jogging are all ways to make this trip a healthy one.

Climate: Changeable, unpredictable; often hot and humid, sometimes very cold.

Clothing: The best way to cope with the unpredictable climate is to dress in layers. If you need to take off your sweater to cool off from a hot flash, you'll want to be wearing a light cotton shirt underneath! Natural fibers whisk moisture away from the body more effectively than most synthetics. (Polypropylene is the exception: Try it in cold weather.)

Food: Drink plenty of water. Eat a wide variety of fresh fruits and vegetables, including soy foods.

Time out: This journey is always interesting, but it can be exhausting. Take a refreshing detour from time to time: Meditate, take a nap, visit a spa, go on vacation.

Traveling companions: Solitary travel can be enriching, but sometimes it gets lonely out there. Fortunately, there are plenty of other women on this journey. Meet them through support groups or talk to them on the Internet.

When you're feeling out of balance, you may find relief in the wisdom of complementary therapies and mind–body practice, which generally aim to balance mind, body, and spirit. Some non-Western systems, like traditional Chinese medicine and Ayurveda, have been used by millions of people for thousands of years. Alternative therapies, including homeopathy, naturopathy, aromatherapy, and acupuncture, offer women many ways to smooth the uncomfortable physical effects of hormonal fluctuation. Here's a sampler:

Aromatherapy: Calm your anxiety with lavender oil. Put a few drops on a handkerchief and tuck it into your bra to surround yourself with scent all day long.

Acupressure: Gentle pressure on the correct points can help ease headache, insomnia, anxiety, cramps, fatigue, and more.

Acupuncture: Many women swear by acupuncture's ability to help balance the hormonal system, minimizing insomnia, hot flashes, and many other complaints.

Traditional Chinese medicine: Try dong quai tonic for general hormonal balancing, ho shour wu (*Polygonum multiflorum*) for insomnia, wu wei zi for hot flashes.

Homeopathy: Remedies for hot flashes and flushing include *Lachesis, Pulsatilla,* and *Kreosotum*. See a practitioner to determine which remedy is best for you.

Herbs: Licorice root, chasteberry, black cohosh, red sage, and false unicorn root all have estrogenic properties.

Reflexology: According to reflexologist Roberta Kirschenbaum, quoted in Dee Ito's *Without Estrogen:* "The area between the ankle bone and the heel on both the inside and outside of the foot, can be rubbed every day. Some women find that it helps lessen mild hot flashes and relieves tension if done regularly."

TRY HORMONE REPLACEMENT THERAPY If your sleep disturbance is the result of being rudely awakened by hot flashes at 2 A.M., you may want to assess the risks and benefits of hormone replacement therapy. HRT can eliminate hot flashes and night sweats and help you get some rest. Talk to your health practitioner.

BREATHE If you're too tense to sleep, chances are your chest is tight and your breathing is shallow, or you may even be holding your breath. Slow, conscious breathing can relax you and put your body in the mood for sleep. See Chapter 5, "Breathe Easy," for more.

So, What Are My Options?

There are as many alternate routes on the midlife journey as there are women walking the path. Here's an overview of the territory.

EXERCISE AND DIET It's this simple: The foundation of good health is a healthy diet—low in saturated fat, with plenty of whole grains, a variety of fresh fruits and vegetables, and light protein—and a good program of exercise. Many of the problems that women feel are an inevitable part of perimenopause can be moderated or even avoided completely with change in these two areas. For more on why, see Chapter 3, "Keep on Moving," and Chapter 4, "Are You What You Eat?"

MIND–BODY PRACTICES AND COMPLEMENTARY THERAPIES For thousands and thousands of years, women all over the world have been finding ways to cope with the changes of menopause. This wealth of information is alive today in mind–body techniques like yoga and t'ai chi, in medical systems like traditional Chinese medicine and Ayurveda, and in plant-based folk remedies. See the Point of Interest "Seeking a Natural Balance" for some ideas; and see Chapter 3, "Keep on Moving," and Chapter 7, "The Holistic Kit and Caboodle," for more information.

HORMONE REPLACEMENT THERAPY   HRT helps balance your system by replacing the estrogen and progesterone in your body. Not all women can tolerate it, and you may have to experiment with dosage and types of medication; but when it works, it works well and relatively quickly. To learn more about the risks and benefits of HRT, see Chapter 9, "Yes or No?"

TAKE CARE OF YOURSELF   Balancing your system really means seeking balance in your life. Midlife offers a wonderful opportunity to learn how to relax, to nourish yourself and see to your emotional and psychological needs, to open yourself to new opportunities for growth, to deepen your spiritual understanding of the journey, and to create your own positive image of aging.

ALL OF THE ABOVE   You can take more than one route through menopause. Allow yourself to explore as many new and old ideas as you like: Try acupuncture *and* get some good exercise. Take HRT, eat well, lift weights, *and* do yoga. This is a huge opportunity for change and growth: Don't let it get away!

What Is a Hot Flash?

A hot flash is the sudden feeling of heat spreading over your body, often accompanied by profuse sweating and sometimes by palpitations or feelings of panic. According to the National Institute on Aging, more than 60 percent of perimenopausal American women will experience hot flashes. (Hot flashes are uncommon among perimenopausal women in Japan, possibly because of their high

POINT OF INTEREST
Out of Control?

Midlife changes can be disorienting and disturbing. We don't feel like ourselves, we don't feel right. We want to be who we used to be—the person it has taken us this long to get comfortable with. We want to do something to make it all go away *right now.* We've survived adolescence and spent decades learning how to make a life: Do we really have to struggle some more?

Being compelled to keep growing by a process that is out of our control, and being made to feel out of control by the uncertainties of hormonal fluctuation, can be difficult emotionally as well as physically. The pressure to "fix" ourselves can be strong. But before you plunge headfirst into a sea of decisions, take a step back and survey the territory. Your biology is out of your hands, but how you choose to respond to these changes is well within your control. Educate yourself, ask questions, share your experiences, get support. You *do* have options.

Get the Most Out of Your Hot Flash

Whether you like it or not, hot flashes are part of many women's experience. Here are a couple of thoughts that might improve your attitude:

It's a power surge: Whether it's kundalini energy or some other kind of energy, some women report a feeling of renewal following a hot flash.

It's a purifying mechanism: As noted by Vicki Noble in *Shakti Woman,* our body uses high fevers during illness to burn up viruses. It's possible that hot flashes may be performing a similar cleansing function.

It's a spiritual cleansing tool: In *Anatomy of the Spirit,* medical intuitive Carolyn Myss says that hot flashes may be releases of untapped sexual energy.

consumption of soy foods.) A hot flash can last a few seconds, a few minutes, or even a half hour. Hot flashes are connected with declining estrogen levels, but no one really knows why we experience them.

When Will the Hot Flashes Stop?

There's really no way to know. You may experience hot flashes for a couple of months to a number of years. A small but beleaguered percentage of women report hot flashes continuing ten years after their periods have stopped.

How Can I Cool Down That Hot Flash?

Hot flashes are not pleasant. Fortunately, you may find relief in a number of ways. If one remedy doesn't work for you, try another. Here are some tried and true suggestions for coping:

FOODS   Foods high in vitamin E (nuts and seeds), boron (broccoli), bioflavonoids (in the pith of citrus fruits), and magnesium (spinach, sunflower seeds) are helpful. Recent research suggests that soy and other foods containing phytoestrogens can help alleviate symptoms of lowered estrogen levels. Sage tea may help prevent hot flashes for some women. Make it a daily beverage and see what happens. Caffeine (in coffee, tea, sodas) alcohol, hot drinks, spicy foods, and salt can all trigger hot flashes. Finally, eat several small meals throughout the day: A drop in blood sugar can bring on a hot flash.

Help!
My body's not my body any more. I'm tired all the time. I'm dry where I used to be wet. I'm wet where I used to be dry. I never know when I'm going to start bleeding, or sweating, or screaming. I don't think I like this.

Julie, 45

HORMONE REPLACEMENT THER-APY Ask your doctor about

the risks and benefits of hormone replacement therapy. Since hot flashes are the result of decreasing estrogen levels, replacing that estrogen can relieve hot flashes.

TRADITIONAL CHINESE MEDICINE Acupuncture, acupressure, and associated dietary treatments can be effective in preventing hot flashes.

VITAMIN E SUPPLEMENTS Supplements of between 400 and 800 International Units daily have been shown to prevent hot flashes in some women.

BREATHING EXERCISES Stress may bring on a hot flash. Recent studies show that women who practice deep breathing exercises (such as in yoga), biofeedback, meditation, and muscle relaxation significantly reduce hot flashes, day and night.

HOMEOPATHY *Salvia*, sulfur, metallic gold, and calcium carbonate are all used to treat hot flashes. For best results, let a homeopath prescribe the specific remedy for your symptoms.

DRINKING WATER Staying hydrated is great for your system overall—try to drink six to eight glasses of water a day. Drinking a glass of cool (not cold) water when you first feel a hot flash coming on may actually prevent it. Keep water by your bed for middle-of-the-night relief.

BAKING SODA BATH One cup of baking soda in a warm bath once or twice a week may help circulation and prevent hot flashes. Stay in the water until it cools down.

EXERCISE According to recent studies, active women report fewer hot flashes than inactive women.

EVENING PRIMROSE OIL CAPSULES Some women find these very effective in reducing hot flashes, although little research has been done.

> I lay awake a long time that night, watching the gray, starless sky through the gaps in the canopy. The outside world felt very far away, and I felt very sealed off from it. The gorge had turned opaque, damp, and airless, as if it were inside a giant Tupperware box. And everything was hot. Either hot or wildly hot. About once an hour I would start to sweat so profusely I'd have to flap the sheets to dry off.
>
> These heat episodes were beginning to come with such uncomfortable regularity that I could no longer ignore them. I couldn't talk about them; in fact, I could barely think about them. But I knew what was happening. The rain forest wasn't changing temperature in an hourly cycle, I was. I was entering menopause.
>
> TRACEY JOHNSTON, *Shooting the Boh*

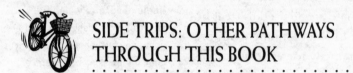

SIDE TRIPS: OTHER PATHWAYS THROUGH THIS BOOK

CHAPTER 3: KEEP ON MOVING Regular exercise can strengthen your bones, improve you mood, slow down the aging process, and preserve your good health. Look here to learn more about what constitutes a good program of exercise.

CHAPTER 4: ARE YOU WHAT YOU EAT? What you eat can't help but affect your health and the way you feel. Look here to learn more about soy and phytoestrogens and what constitutes a good diet for midlife.

CHAPTER 5: BREATHE EASY The unpredictability of perimenopausal changes makes stress virtually inevitable. Look here to learn how you can relieve the pressure.

CHAPTER 6: LOOKING GOOD How you look (and how you look at yourself) begins to change in midlife. Look here to learn how to be kind to your hair and skin and how to maintain a healthy weight.

CHAPTER 7: THE HOLISTIC KIT AND CABOODLE An integral approach to midlife health and balance incorporates a world of alternatives. Look here to learn about the many treatment options.

CHAPTER 8: WHAT'S UP, DOC? Menopause is not a disease, but it brings certain health concerns. Look here for some suggestions about how to find a health practitioner you can work with.

CHAPTER 9: YES OR NO? Wondering whether or not to take hormone replacement therapy? Look here to learn more about the risks and benefits.

CHAPTER 10: THE WORLD DOWN UNDER Hormonal decline has a big impact on vaginal health. Look here to discover what you can do about vaginal dryness and incontinence and to learn about menopause and sex.

CHAPTER 11: BONING UP Menopause is one risk factor for osteoporosis that applies to all women. Look here to find out about your risks and what you can do to prevent and retard osteoporosis.

CHAPTER 12: AND THE BEAT GOES ON Look here to see what you can do to prevent heart disease, the number-one killer of women in the United States.

CHAPTER 13: WHAT ARE MY CHANCES? More and more women are becoming concerned about breast cancer. Look here to learn more about this disease and what you can do if you or a loved one are diagnosed with it.

CHAPTER 16: GETTING HELP Sometimes you just need a little help to get over the rough spots. Look here for some ideas on finding emotional support.

CHAPTER 17: THE INNER JOURNEY Menopause is an initiation into a new world. Look here to learn more about spirituality and the introspective aspect of your life.

RESERVES

. . . .

Organizations and Services

For general medical organizations, see the listings in Chapter 7, "The Holistic Kit and Caboodle," and Chapter 8, "What's Up, Doc?"

American College of Obstetricians and Gynecologists, Office of Public Information, 409 12th St. S.W., Washington, DC 20024-2188. Voice: (202) 638-5577. Fax: (202) 484-5107. Internet: www.acog.com. Contact this professional organization for pamphlets on menopause, midlife, and other aspects of women's health.

American Menopause Foundation, Inc., P.O. Box 2013, New York, NY 10010. Voice: (212) 475-3107. This organization has information about issues of menopause. It can put you in touch with support groups in your area that deal with menopause and alternative treatments.

National Headache Foundation, 428 W. St. James Place, 2nd Floor, Chicago, IL 60614. Voice: (800) 843-2256. Fax: (773) 525-7357. Internet: www.headaches.org. A good place to go for information about headaches. This foundation educates the public about the seriousness of headaches, promotes research, and provides information to sufferers and family members. It also has information about migraines and menopause.

National Institute on Aging, National Institutes of Health, Information Center, P.O. Box 8057, Gaithersburg, MD 20898-8057. Voice: (800) 222-2225. TDD: (800) 222-4225. Fax: (310) 589-3014. E-mail: niainfo@access.digex.net. Internet: www.nih.gov/nia. Send for the free booklet "Menopause." It's informative, comprehensive, and very clear.

National Sleep Foundation, 1367 Connecticut Ave., Suite 200, Washington, DC 20036. Voice: (202) 785-2300. Fax: (202) 785-2880. Call for information about everything from how to get a good night's sleep to understanding sleep disorders.

National Women's Health Network, 514 10th St. N.W., Suite 400, Washington, DC 20004. Voice: (202) 347-1140, Fax: (202) 344-1168. With membership in this woman's advocacy organization, you'll get a newsletter that updates you on all activities. Call or write for more information on the group's wealth of resources, including the Women's Health Clearinghouse and the Women's Health Information Service Library. You do not need to be a member to purchase, for a low fee, the informative packets.

North American Menopause Society (NAMS), c/o Department of OB/GYN, University Hospitals of Cleveland, 11100 Euclid Ave., Cleveland, OH 44106. Voice: (216) 844-8748. Fax: (216) 844-8708. E-mail: nams@atk.et. Internet:www. menopause.org/all.html. The North American Menopause Society is a nonprofit professional organization of physicians, clinicians, scientists, and researchers.

NAMS promotes the study and exchange of information about the climacteric in women. It also offers educational programs and maintains a list of menopause care providers. Send for a list of doctors in your area who specialize in menopause.

Research Reports

Keep up to date on breast cancer research by sending for the latest research reports. See the listings in Chapter 8, "What's Up, Doc?," for resources.

Periodicals

Harvard Women's Health Watch, P.O. Box 420234, Palm Coast, FL 32141-0234. Voice: (800) 829-5921. E-mail: HWHW@warren.med.harvard.edu. This eight-page newsletter covers virtually every health topic of interest to women, including many articles on subjects related to menopause and hormones.

Menopause, The Journal of the North American Menopause Society, 12107 Insurance Way, Hagerstown, MD 21740. Voice: (800) 638-3030. Internet: www.menopause. org/journal.htm. This quarterly journal has an impressive assortment of research articles on various aspects of menopause. If you want to read the unadulterated versions, start here. The web site has review abstracts of articles for you to peruse.

Menopause News, 2074 Union St., San Francisco, CA 94123. Voice: (800) 241-MENO. This is a terrific newsletter about menopause, midlife, and other women's health issues, from one woman to another.

MenoTimes: Alternative Choices to Menopause and Osteoporosis, c/o The Menopause Center, P.O. Box 6558, San Rafael, CA 94903. Voice: (415) 459-5430. E-mail: mtimes@nbn.com. Internet: www.aimnet.com/~hyperion/meno/menotimes.index. html. This newsletter covers the latest information on complementary approaches to menopause. The web site has samples and information about ordering tapes.

MidLife Woman, 5129 Logan Ave. South, Minneapolis, MN 55419-1019. Voice: (800) 886-4354. Fax: (612) 925-5430. Internet: users.aol.com/mdlfwoman/ info.htm. This information-packed newsletter thoroughly explores issues of importance to midlife women. It covers one topic in depth each issue, along with news updates and book reviews. You can also order training/seminar materials on menopause and osteoporosis. The web site lets you take a look at back issues.

Books

Lonnie Barbach. *The Pause*. New York: Penguin, 1995. A personal look at the experience of menopause. Barbach, a therapist, speaks from her own experience and suggests many ways to treat the signs of perimenopause that can plague women and often catch them by surprise.

Deepak Chopra, M.D. *Restful Sleep: The Complete Mind/Body Program for Overcoming Insomnia.* New York: Random House, 1994. Chopra combines Ayurvedic and mind–body techniques with medical research to create this program for getting a good night's sleep.

Sandra Coney. *The Menopause Industry: How the Medical Establishment Exploits Women.* Alameda: Hunter House, 1994. Read this book if you are trying to make sense of research studies. Coney explains the different types of studies and what they mean, and explores the vested interest groups that constitute the menopause industry—hormone manufacturers, ad agencies, researchers, universities, national societies, and the medical establishment.

Robert Dosh, M.D., Susan W. Fukushima, M.D., Jane E. Lewis, Ph.D., Robert L. Ross, M.D., Lynne A Steinman, Ph.D. *The Taking Charge of Menopause Workbook.* Oakland: New Harbinger Press, 1997. This in-depth workbook includes many self-tests and has a good section on medical tests for women.

Paula B. Doress-Worters and Diana Laskin Siegal, with the Boston Women's Health Collective. *The New Ourselves, Growing Older.* New York: Simon and Schuster, 1994. A wonderful and useful book to have as we age. This large book addresses many topics concerning women and aging. The chapter on menopause talks about the signs of menopause and ways to cope.

Gillian Ford. *Listening to Your Hormones.* Rockin, CA: Prima Publishing, 1997. This book is especially for women with severe hormonal problems that affect their physical and emotional well-being. Ford experienced severely incapacitating hormonal problems and tells her story along with those of other women. Also includes treatments.

Sadja Greenwood, M.D. *Menopause Naturally.* San Francisco: Volcano Press, 1996. The latest edition of this classic, informative, and highly readable book on menopause and self-care offers even more complementary approaches. Also available in a Spanish-language edition.

Charles B. Inlander and Cynthia K. Moran. *67 Ways to Good Sleep.* New York: Ballantine Books, 1995. Strategies for getting a good night's sleep. The book includes a glossary of terms; what to eat, do, think; and the side effects of drugs.

Dee Ito. *Without Estrogen: Natural Remedies for Menopause and Beyond.* New York: Crown, 1994. This book looks at a number of alternative approaches for controlling menopausal symptoms, including Chinese herbal medicine, acupuncture, chiropractic, aromatherapy, diet and nutrition, and exercise. It also includes a section of women's stories about how they approached this passage in their own lives.

Susan Love, M.D., with Karen Lindsey. *Dr. Susan Love's Hormone Book.* New York: Random House, 1997. Menopause often leads to directly to thoughts about hormone replacement. If you're contemplating HRT, you couldn't do better than this intelligent, thoughtful, and clearly written book. Love explains all the issues, including how to understand the research. She covers menopause and all related medical topics, and her discussion of the alternatives to HRT is especially strong. A very good book.

John R. Lee, M.D. *What Your Doctor May Not Tell You About Menopause.* Warner Books, 1996. If you're interested in natural progesterone, this is a more user-friendly version of Lee's first book, *Natural Progesterone, The Multiple Roles of a Remarkable Hormone.* Lee talks about menopause and the role of progesterone, and he explains natural progesterones. He also discusses lifestyle and menopause.

Judy Mahle Lutter and Lynn Jaffee. *Bodywise Woman.* 2d ed. Champaign IL: Human Kinetics Press, 1996. This big book is filled with solid information about physical activity and women's health, including chapters on menopause and its associated health concerns.

Christiane Northrup, M.D. *Women's Bodies, Women's Wisdom: Creating Physical and Emotional Health and Healing.* New York: Bantam Books, 1994. Dr. Northrup is a holistic physician who combines Western medicine and mind–body approaches to health. This book is not specific to midlife women, but does include a good chapter on menopause and its associated health concerns, natural and synthetic hormone replacement therapy, and how to do a "trial run" of replacement therapy.

Linda Ojeda. *Menopause Without Medicine.* Alameda, CA: Hunter House, 1992. This book emphasizes nutritional supplementation and has a major nutrient guide. Ojeda also offers some herbal treatments for the signs of menopause

Susan Perry and Katherine A. O'Hanlan, M.D. *Natural Menopause: The Complete Guide to a Woman's Most Misunderstood Passage.* Rev. ed. Reading, MA: Addison-Wesley, 1997. The newly revised edition of this comprehensive book on menopause includes the latest information on all the issues.

Judith Reichman, M.D., *I'm Too Young to Get Old: Health Care for Women After Forty.* New York: Times Books, 1996. Dr. Reichman is straightforward, humorous, and informative and doesn't hedge on her views. She has a lot to say about menopause and is heartily in favor of hormone replacement therapy.

Russell J. Reiter, Ph.D., and Jo Robinson. *Melatonin.* New York: Bantam, 1995. This book, written by one of the leading researchers on melatonin, explores all aspects of this brain chemical: its effect on immune function, PMS, sleep, and mood as well as ways to stimulate your body to produce more on its own.

Carol R. Schulz with Mary Jenkins, M.D. *Sixty Second Menopause Management.* Far Hills, NJ: New Horizon Press, 1996. An easy-to-use reference guide that offers simple techniques for handling the signs of hormonal change.

Gail Sheehy. *Silent Passages.* New York: Pocket Books, 1993. This look at the passage of menopause through the eyes of the author and other women drew a lot of attention to the topic. If you read the stories you'll also find ideas on how to cope with the signs of hormonal fluctuation.

Honora Lee Wolfe. *Second Spring: A Guide to Healthy Menopause Through Traditional Chinese Medicine*. Boulder, CO: Blue Poppy Press, 1990. A good book if you're interested in traditional Chinese medicine. Wolfe explains the theories of Chinese medicine and how it applies to menopause; she includes therapies for menopause as well as information on diet, exercise, and supplements.

Audio/Video

Some of the agencies listed in Organizations and Services, above, have excellent audiocassettes and videotapes available for sale or rental. **Meno Tapes** is a good source for audiocassettes on many issues of menopause, most from the perspective of complementary therapies. You'll find catalogs for this company and other good sources of health tapes listed in Chapter 7, "The Holistic Kit and Caboodle," and Chapter 8, "What's Up, Doc?"

AUDIO

Creating Health, Christiane Northrup, M.D. 5-tape set. Available from Women to Women (see Audio/Video, Chapter 8). This set includes tapes on Menopause, Whole Nutrition, and Creating Breast Health. Dr. Northrup, author of *Women's Bodies, Women's Wisdom*, integrates Western medicine with a mind–body approach to creating health.

VIDEOTAPES

Approaching the 14th Moon, Women and Health Professionals Discuss Menopause. Available from Elizabeth Sher, P.O. Box 8123, Berkeley, CA 94707-8123. Voice: (510) 528-8004. This upbeat, informative documentary video puts together interviews with forty very different women, including doctors Sadja Greenwood and Margaret Cuthbert, to shed light on menopause and the process of becoming an older woman in contemporary America.

Menopause: Dispelling the Myths, Telling the Truths, Exploring Possibilities. Available from Moondancer Productions, 1767 Goodyear Ave., Suite 101, Ventura, CA 93003. Voice: (800) 760-7775. A video that brings the subject of menopause out into the open.

Menopause: Taking Charge. Available from The Learning Lane (see Audio/Video, Chapter 8). Author, psychoanalyst, and fitness researcher Veryl Rosenbaum presents ways to approach menopause with creativity and vigor.

PMS: An Answer, the Harris PMS Program. 60 minutes. Available from The Learning Lane (see Audio/Video, Chapter 8). Self-help for women with PMS, developed by the National PMS Association. Touches on lifestyle changes and the Endorphin Release Technique.

Straight Talk on Menopause. 120 minutes (two-tape set). Available from the VideoFinders Collection (see Audio/Video, Chapter 8). Gynecologist Judith Reichman, author of *I'm Too Young to Get Old*, discusses many aspects of menopause in a straightforward, humorous, and informative style. An understandable presentation of how hormones work, as well as a discussion of HRT and its relationship to other health issues.

When Women Go Through Menopause, Where Do Men Go? The Other Side of the Moon. Available from Elizabeth Sher, P.O. Box 8123, Berkeley, CA 94707-8123. Voice: (510) 528-8004. This documentary video explores men's reactions to getting older as well as how menopause affects them. It explores hormone use for women and men and looks at couples aging together.

What's New About Menopause. Available from the VideoFinders Collection (see Audio/Video, Chapter 8). This video profiles research on menopause and looks at ethical issues related to what happens when science enables women to bear children after menopause.

Online

You can find an enormous amount of basic information about menopause online. Check web sites for newsletters, interviews with stars in the world of menopause, and links to organizations. Chat in real time or subscribe to news groups and mailing lists to share your experience with other women. Many of the organizations and newsletters listed above have web sites, and you can also search for menopause information on the web sites listed in Chapter 7, "The Holistic Kit and Caboodle," and Chapter 8, "What's Up, Doc?"

NEWS GROUPS

For wide-ranging discussions about all aspects of perimenopause and menopause, check out **alt.support.menopause.**

MAILING LISTS

The **MENOPAUS** mailing list is the place to discuss all things menopause and more, including travel ideas. Exchange ideas and information with women all over the United States and the world. Send subscription messages to LISTSERV@PSUHMC.HMC.PSU.EDU—and note that MENOPAUS is spelled without the final "E."

WEB SITES

All of the web sites cited here have more links than you can shake a stick at. **Power Surge,** located at members.aol.com/dearest, is an online newsletter with attitude and an all-around great resource for menopause. Browse through back issues of the entertaining and informative *Power Surge Newsletter,* read about or be there for interviews with stars of the menopause world such as Sadja Greenwood and Lonnie Barbach, search through the amazing list of links, and more.

All About Menopause, www.menopause.org/index.html, is sponsored by NAMS. It includes breaking news, a menopause FAQ, and abstracts of articles that have appeared in the NAMS journal, *Menopause*. **Menopause—Doctor's Guide to the Internet**, at www.pslgroup.com/MENOPAUSE.HTM, will keep you up to date on the latest medical approaches, including information on hormone replacement therapy.

3

KEEP ON MOVING
Exercise, Movement, and Mind–Body Practice

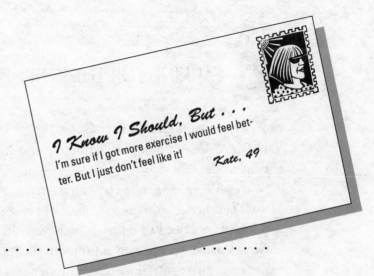

I Know I Should, But . . .
I'm sure if I got more exercise I would feel better. But I just don't feel like it!   *Kate, 49*

Like Kate, many of us run around like mad to avoid exercising. We feel too tired or too rushed to make time to work out, and then we feel guilty on top of everything else. Ironically, the more exercise you get, the better you feel and the more you want. So why do we spend so much time not exercising?

We put this chapter up front for a reason. When we first outlined the chapters for this book, this was Chapter 11—after one chapter on menopause and nine on various diseases and health conditions of midlife. What's wrong with this picture? In midlife, it seems, we spend an inordinate amount of time worrying about what illness is going to get us and then trying to ward it off by doing "good" things. As authors, we were sucked right in. But after some months of feeling bogged down by reading and writing about disease, it occurred to us that doing good things for our bodies—exercising, eating right, and feeding our spirit—was much more fun, and more productive, than fixating on illness.

Along with this realization came a change in our attitude toward exercise. It changed from a chore that we had to cram into our work day to a gift we were giving to our bodies. Exercise is one of the most important components of continued good health and well-being. Our bodies are made to move, and movement improves everything: from how we look to how we feel to how long we'll live. Hitting midlife is no excuse to stop dead in your tracks. In fact, in midlife you have every reason to *make* tracks by making exercise a regular and enjoyable part of your life.

 ## PACKING FOR THE JOURNEY

What's So Good About Exercise?

In *Fresh Start*, physiologist and nutritionist Joyce Adams Hanna, president of the Fifty-Plus Fitness Association, says, "Most things that get worse with aging get better with exercise." And, we might add, aging itself gets better with exercise. Being fit means you're in better shape to do what you need to do every day—carry the groceries into the car, climb up and get the cans off the top shelf, clean out the garage, walk the dog, chase after kids. Exercise benefits every part of your body, from your bones to your cardiovascular system to your digestion to your complexion. It aids weight loss and helps put you in a good mood.

I Love Yoga

Even when I have to drag my tired body to a yoga class after work, within a few minutes I remember why I'm there. I leave the world of my mind and enter the world of my body: breath and blood, muscle and joint, bending and standing and stretching. You can change your life in an hour. *Raina, 41*

What's the Right Kind of Exercise for Me?

The best exercise for you is an activity that you enjoy and that you can—and will—do three

GUIDED TOUR: *Exercise, Movement and Mind–Body Practice*

Our bodies change in midlife, but change doesn't necessarily entail falling apart. Exercise is a vital part of staying well and strong in midlife and beyond. A moderate program of regular exercise that works on aerobics, strength training, and flexibility can improve just about everything, from signs of hormonal imbalance, to your mood, to your risk of having osteoporosis and cardiovascular disease.

WESTERN MEDICINE

Virtually every woman can benefit from regular exercise, even women with chronic health problems. Consult your doctor before you begin an exercise program if you have any reservations or any of the following symptoms: chest pains, history of heart disease, dizzy spells, bone or joint problems, or high blood pressure. If you have other medical problems or disabilities you think may prevent you from exercising, consult your physician or physical therapist for customized exercise guidelines.

EXERCISE

A good program of exercise includes aerobic activity for the cardiovascular system, stretching for flexibility and balance, and strength training for strong muscles, improved balance, and stronger bones. Choose from a long list of aerobic activities, including walking, running, dancing, swimming, cross-country skiing, and cycling; work out at home or in a gym.

MIND–BODY

Practices such as yoga, qi gong, t'ai chi, Alexander technique, Feldenkrais, Rosen method, and Pilates integrate mind and body, stimulating awareness of how you are using your body. Regular practice can improve balance, strength, flexibility, and mood and may help balance hormones

NUTRITION

Combine exercise with a healthy diet (a variety of fresh fruits and vegetables, whole grains, and light protein; minimal intake of saturated fat) that gives you the energy you need to work out. Drink plenty of water before, during, and after exercise.

Twelve Good Reasons to Exercise

1. To improve your overall health
2. To slow down the aging process
3. To reduce or eliminate hot flashes
4. To sleep better
5. To improve your mood
6. To reduce your risk of heart disease, breast cancer, and osteoporosis
7. To improve your balance and reduce your risk of falling
8. To maintain your weight more easily
9. To look better and feel better
10. To improve your ability to perform your daily activities
11. To improve your digestion
12. To give yourself more energy and stamina

TRAVEL TIP
When to Stop

If exercise is good, is too much exercise better? No! You will not achieve physical fitness by pushing yourself past your body's endurance, and you may injure yourself.

- Warm up first with a walk or slow version of your aerobic activity (stretching should be done *after* muscles are warmed up).

- Try the talk test: In the thick of your aerobic workout, try singing a verse of your favorite song or reciting a verse of your favorite poem. If it's no problem, you're not working hard enough. If you can't complete the first line easily, slow down.

- When you're exercising, pain is *not* good! If you're in pain, stop.

or four times a week for at least a half an hour. But why limit yourself to just one? A good way to make sure you keep up an exercise program is to vary it—don't give up the whole idea just because you've burned out on one activity.

DO WHAT YOU LIKE   The important thing is to discover what motivates *you* and then modify the exercise to match your ability or make it more aerobic. For example, if you play golf, consider walking the course briskly instead of sauntering or taking a cart. If you like to swim, consider swimming laps and trying to increase your speed and endurance over time. If you like setting records, try speed walking or counting the miles you walk or swim each week. If you like to dance, take a class or go to a club. If you like to exercise your spirit and your mind together, try all-around body awareness activities such as yoga or martial arts.

MAKE MODIFICATIONS   Modify your activities according to your abilities. If you've been sitting around for the last five or ten years, for example, don't try to do forty-five minutes on the treadmill right away. And, in the same vein, don't go easy on yourself if you're in good shape. If you walk, try varying your walk by going up and down hills or up and down stairs. If you climb stairs, jog up the stairs next time. If you swim laps, challenge yourself by trying to increase your speed and endurance.

Am I Too Old Too Start Exercising Now?

Too old to exercise? Not! According to Terrie Heinrich Rizzo, Manager of Health and Fitness Education Programs for the Stanford

Health Improvement Program, you can start a fitness program—and see gains—at virtually any age:

> Recent research shows that people of all ages can improve muscle strength and tone—and slow or even reverse some of the losses due to the natural aging process. Our muscle mass and strength tends to peak naturally in our twenties. The natural decline starts at about age thirty to thirty-five, as lean body mass gradually begins to shrink. The rate of decline usually speeds up after about forty, when people notice a steady decline in muscle mass, tone, strength, and stamina. Typically, by age sixty-five, strength declines by at least 20 percent. By eighty, about half of total muscle mass is lost. The great news is that, with exercise, you can greatly slow or even reverse this natural decline and gain back muscle strength and tone—even if you are ninety. A well-conditioned sixty-five-year-old may possess far better muscle tone than a thirty-year-old who doesn't exercise!

EXERCISE SLOWS DOWN THE AGING PROCESS Studies by Harvard University comparing people in their sixties and seventies who exercise with people of the same age who don't exercise found the exercisers to be physiologically ten to twenty years younger. In addition, a Tufts University study found that women who complete one year of strength training are fifteen or twenty years younger physiologically than they were when they began.

I HAVEN'T FALLEN/I CAN GET UP! Many of the falling injuries that seem to plague older women can be prevented by a regular program of exercise. Stronger muscles and more flexibility mean you're more likely to retain your balance, and stronger bones (the result of strength training) mean you're less likely to fracture a bone if you do fall. The Tufts study results

TRAVEL TIP

How to Exercise in Spite of Yourself

You don't have to go to a gym or run a marathon to get exercise. Here are some simple ways to get exercise without even knowing it:

1. Take the stairs instead of the elevator.

2. Take a walk at lunch instead of sitting and eating for an hour.

3. Walk to the corner store—leave your car at home.

4. Do your own gardening and save money on the gardener.

5. Park at the far end of the parking lot and walk to the store.

6. If your job is near home, walk or ride your bike instead of driving or taking public transportation.

7. Do what you normally do, but do it faster!

TRAVEL TIP

Exercise + Calcium = Strong Bones

If you want to build strong bones, combine your exercise with at least 1,000 milligrams of calcium a day. According to epidemiologist Bonny Specker of the University of Cincinnati Medical Center, as quoted in *Health* magazine, "You need both. You can walk two miles a day, but if you're not getting enough calcium, the exercise won't help your bones. And calcium doesn't have any effect if you're sedentary."

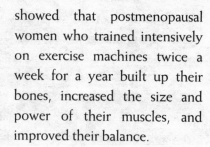

showed that postmenopausal women who trained intensively on exercise machines twice a week for a year built up their bones, increased the size and power of their muscles, and improved their balance.

GET MOVING, KEEP MOVING

The Tufts study also showed an interesting side benefit of exercise: You want *more* exercise. "The women who trained developed an appetite for exercise, increasing their spontaneous physical activity an average of 27 percent. The untrained [control] group slacked off by nearly that much."

Do I Have to Consult My Doctor Before I Start Exercising?

If you're in reasonably good health, you can probably begin a program of moderate exercise right now, even if you haven't exercised for years. In fact, if you've been sedentary, you'll see more progress sooner. Just remember to start slowly and don't push yourself too hard. If you have any of the following problems, however, consult your doctor for guidelines before you plunge in: a history of heart problems, chest pains, dizzy spells, bone or joint problems, high blood pressure.

What's a Good Exercise Program?

A good exercise program works the whole body. The Stanford Medical School Health and Fitness Program recommends including moderate-intensity exercises in three areas: aerobics, flexibility, and strength.

AEROBICS   Aim for between twenty and sixty minutes of aerobic activity, three or four times a week. Keep the intensity moderate and vary the activity to keep your interest up.

TRAVEL TIP
Water, Water Everywhere

It's easy to remember to drink water during a workout, but it's just as important to drink water before and after a workout. Tea, coffee, and soda don't count! Here are the latest guidelines from the American College of Sports Medicine:

Two hours before you begin your workout: Drink two glasses of water (about five ounces each).

During your workout: Drink five to twelve ounces every twenty minutes.

Replace lost water: Weigh yourself before and after exercise, and drink two glasses of water for every pound you've lost.

FLEXIBILITY Include ten to fifteen minutes of controlled stretching daily ("controlled" means no bouncing and holding the stretch gently for at least fifteen seconds). When your muscles are cold, you can hurt them with stretches, so stretch during or after your aerobics workout.

STRENGTH TRAINING Two to four strength-training sessions a week—of twenty to thirty minutes each—will help build bone as well as muscle. Don't do strength training two days in a row—you need to give muscles a chance to repair themselves between workouts.

Why Should I Do Aerobic Exercise?

Aerobic activities keep the heart rate above normal for a sustained period of time. Aerobic means "with oxygen," and aerobic activities help your cardiovascular system (heart and lungs) bring oxygen to all parts of your body more efficiently.

What Are Some Aerobic Activities?

Aerobic activities are everywhere. You don't have to buy an expensive leotard and pay for a class to do aerobics—you have plenty of other choices.

OUTDOORS If you can get outdoors, you're getting the added boost that comes from exercising in the fresh air. If possible, try to avoid working out in heavily polluted areas. (If you live in a city, for example, walk in a park rather than on a street clogged with traffic.) Aerobic activities you can do outside include brisk walking, hiking, jogging, running, cycling, rowing, cross-country skiing, aqua aerobics, swimming, and gardening continuously.

Owning a dog is a great excuse for exercise. If you live in the country, you probably have your choice of wonderful walks just outside your door. If you live in an urban area, however, finding a good walk may take a little more effort. There's nothing to prevent you from putting the leash on your pet, packing some plastic bags for cleanup and a water bottle for refreshment (for you *and* your dog), and setting out to explore the city streets. Some areas even have dedicated "dog parks," where you and your dog can run free and socialize with other dogs and dog owners.

INDOORS You can do the following activities at a gym or at home with your own equipment or a video. Try low-impact aerobics, step aerobics, aerobic dancing, or fast dancing; use the treadmill, stair-climbing machine, stationary bike, rowing machine, or cross-country skiing machine.

INDOORS/OUTDOORS Martial arts routines, yoga (especially power yoga), and other movement programs can also be aerobic when poses are performed briskly and continuously.

What About Walking?

Walking is terrific exercise, and the possibilities are endless: Walk fast, walk slow, walk on flat roads, walk up and down hills, walk your dog, walk with a friend, take a nature hike. Wear good-quality shoes and have fun! As exercise goes, walking can't be beat. It's free, it requires minimal preparation, you can do it at your own speed and in virtually any setting, and it's right outside your door. According to the Melpomene Institute, all you need to do to get aerobic benefits from walking is "walk long enough, walk often enough, walk without stopping, and walk fast enough."

Aerobics classes (step aerobics, dance aerobics, low-impact aerobics, and others) are so popular it's hard *not* to find one. If you need the motivation of a class and the encouragement of an instructor to get going, this is a fine way to start. Many types of classes are available. Low-impact aerobics gives you a great workout with less chance of injury than high-impact aerobics. Check with your local YMCA, parks and recreation department, community college, Jewish community center, or church organizations.

What About Running?

Like walking, running is an exercise you can do almost anywhere. It does not require expensive facilities—just some properly fitting and well-cushioned running shoes, lightweight and comfortable clothing, and an attitude! Many women who were runners in their twenties and early thirties are not sure if this is an activity they can continue. If you feel that running is for younger people, think again. If running brings you joy, continue. You might have to adapt your program—run on a track instead of on the sidewalk, or join a running club for motivation and companionship. If you have health issues, your physician can help you determine the appropriateness of your running program.

What About Swimming and Aqua Aerobics?

Moving around in water is perhaps the most egalitarian and benign way to exercise—swimming can be good for you no matter how old you are or what kind of physical condition you are in, and it's really difficult to hurt yourself doing it. Classes are available in everything from gentle water exercise for people with arthritic problems to water aerobics, which gives you a workout without putting stress on your joints. You can join a Masters swimming group if you like directed workouts or want to compete. Whether or not swimming acts as a resistance exercise is still an area of dispute, so if you're a swimmer don't forget to do some strength training too.

Masters Swimming

You don't have to be a great swimmer to be on a Masters team. You just have to be able to swim across the pool and back—fifty yards. When I started, I knew how to swim and that was about it. But Masters was great. They work with you at your own level. I'm good at getting in the pool but I'm not so good at making myself swim hard, so I really enjoyed having a structured workout. The exercise is great, my swimming has improved, I've made a lot of friends, and I'm always clean! *Justine, 52*

Why Should I Stretch?

Flexibility exercises keep your muscles stretched and toned. Working on stretching, reaching, and bending keeps the body supple, improves balance, and actually protects muscles against injury. To prevent injury, do your stretching in the middle of your workout or as a cooldown—*after* your muscles are warmed up, not before.

What Are Some Flexibility Exercises?

Exercisers fall into two groups: Those who work on flexibility and neglect strength and those who would rather do anything but stretch. If you fall into the second group, remember that stretching your muscles can

TRAVEL TIP
Crunch!

When you're planning your strength-training program, don't forget to tone your stomach. Properly done, abdominal exercises like crunches help support your spine, alleviate or prevent back problems, and improve your posture. Let your abdominals do all the work. If you're straining your back or neck, you're not getting the full benefit of the exercise and you will likely hurt yourself. If you have back problems, consult a physical therapist for exercises that will help you rather than hurt you.

actually help protect them from injury during the rest of your workout. And it feels so good.

INDOORS/OUTDOORS Any kind of controlled stretch: Stretch slowly, don't bounce, and hold the stretch for at least fifteen seconds. Join a class, consult an exercise book, or watch a video for a variety of stretches. Remember to stretch *all* muscle groups. Yoga, qi gong, t'ai chi, and other martial arts and movement programs such as Pilates, Rosen work, and Alexander technique all incorporate stretching.

Why Should I Work on My Strength?

Activities that work your muscles against increased resistance build, tone, and shape muscles, and they also increase bone mass and improve balance—important considerations for midlife women. More women are taking up weight training as a way to gain more endurance and to shape up and tone muscles that are heading south with time and the force of gravity.

What Are Some Strength-Training Exercises?

Strength-training exercises work your muscles against resistance. You can go to the gym of your choice or work out at home. Be sure you get instruction in the proper use of weights before you begin. Many gyms offer access to personal trainers who will meet you at the gym or come to your home.

TRAVEL TIP

Yes, Movement Work and Mind–Body Practices Count As Exercise

Yoga, qi gong, Rosen work, and many other practices can be aerobic, and even build strength. If your mind–body workouts tend to be for stretching only, make sure that you supplement with the necessary amount of aerobics and strength training.

INDOORS You may have to join a gym to use weight machines and strength-training machines such as Nautilus. At home you can take advantage of free weights, home rowing machines, and floor exercises such as modified push-ups, crunches, and side leg lifts. The Pilates reformer and some yoga poses (such as Downward-Facing Dog) can build strength as well as flexibility.

OUTDOORS   Aerobic activities like rowing and cross-country skiing will also strengthen bones and muscles.

What Are Movement and Mind–Body Practices?

Many movement and mind–body practices have their roots in ancient Eastern traditions that did not differentiate between medicine, exercise, and spirituality. The integral nature of these and other practices survives to this day, and they can be a terrific antidote to our tendency to compartmentalize. All of these activities improve flexibility and balance, relieve stress, and encourage you to be more aware of how you are using your body in your daily life. Here's a brief sampling of some of the more popular programs. For information on finding a class near you, see Resources.

ALEXANDER TECHNIQUE   Alexander was originated by an actor and orator who felt that correcting problems with posture and movement could help his voice and on-stage technique. Alexander teachers use a hands-on technique to identify individual movement and posture problems and help students learn to self-correct. No exercise at home is involved; problems can usually be resolved in eight to ten sessions.

FELDENKRAIS   Developed by Moshe Felden-krais, a nuclear physicist, Feldenkrais is based on the principle that correcting movement in the

You don't have to spend a lot of money to outfit yourself correctly. But even if you do opt for the high-end product, you'll more than make up for the expense in comfort and injury prevention.

Small investments/big returns: *Comfortable shoes* that are designed for the activity you're doing can be crucial in whether or not you stick with it. Make sure you go to a store whose employees understand how to make sure you've got the right shoe and the right fit for your needs. *Comfortable clothing* that is appropriate for your activity can also make a surprising difference. You don't have to buy expensive designer activewear, but do make sure you're wearing fabrics that breathe and styles that give you room to move.

Larger investments/big returns: *Feedback devices* can help you stick to your exercise plan, especially if lack of motivation is a problem for you. There are devices for general fitness, such as heart monitors, and devices for particular activities, such as pedometers for walking or running and mileage monitors for bikes. Many home exercise machines come with feedback devices that measure time, distance, calories burned, and a lot more.

body means becoming mentally aware of what your body is doing. This is done in two ways: "awareness through movement," which involves understanding how your body performs complex movements, and "functional integration," storing the memories in your muscles. If your neck is always tense and you don't know why, try Feldenkrais.

PILATES   Not quite a gentle exercise, Pilates is done in a studio on specialized equipment—notably, a machine called the reformer—that creates variable resistance for muscles. This exercise system is particularly good for women in midlife because it exercises abdominal organs and encourages both resistance work and flexibility. If you do Pilates and Pilates-based exercises properly, you will be engaging your lower abdominals and pelvic floor, much as Kegel exercises do (see Chapter 10, "The World Down Under"). The Pilates method has been around for years (it was used by dancer Martha Graham and choreographer George Balanchine) but is only now becoming popular. It develops a long, lean muscle rather than a bulky one and emphasizes breathing and abdominal support in every movement.

QI GONG   This ancient Chinese practice literally means "the practice of the life force." *Qi,* or *chi,* is the life force, similar to the Indian concept of *prana* or the Greek *pneuma.* This practice is a series of graceful, gentle, yet vigorous movements designed to create balance by enhancing the circulation of qi in the body. It is similar to t'ai chi, but with an added emphasis on breathing and movement of the body's vital energy. Both meditative and active, this practice is great for stress relief and calming, wonderful for strength and balance; it is said to bring health and strength to the internal organs and claims to enhance healing by mobilizing our own natural healing capacities.

ROSEN METHOD MOVEMENT Rosen method has been developed by physical therapist Marion Rosen over the past fifty years. Marion is a good example of her work: She's been teaching a class for thirty years. Classes are lively and enjoyable and encourage sociability. Students explore and improve their flexibility, muscular function, and breathing. Stretching and jumping exercises done to the rhythms of natural breathing are designed to improve body alignment and ease of movement. The gentle swinging exercises are often done to music.

T'AI CHI The Chinese martial art t'ai chi is very graceful and visually beautiful. You may have seen t'ai chi classes in the park practicing what looks like slow motion dancing. Like qi gong, this practice consists of a series of continuous movements, with attention given to breathing and the ebb and flow of internal energy. T'ai chi develops flexibility, balance, concentration, and inner awareness, and it is very relaxing.

YOGA Hatha yoga is an ancient system of breathing and movement that originated in India. Its concentration on breathing, awareness, and attention to movement makes it a true integration of mind and body. Because yoga is a great stress reducer, it's used in cardiac rehabilitation programs and sleep disorder clinics. It is terrific for developing flexibility and strength; poses that offer resistance may help build bones; and regular practice can help keep your spine limber. Some styles of yoga are languid

YMCA

I'm a great fan of the YMCA. Over the years, I've taken advantage of aerobics classes, weight machines, and cardiovascular equipment. I've played racquetball and gone swimming, and taken yoga and t'ai chi. Recently, I've noticed that they are offering health care classes—breast self-exam, menopause, getting your back in shape. I love it. It doesn't cost a lot, and there's always something going on.

Sandy, 50

and relaxing; others, such as Iyengar-style yoga, require concentration and some exertion; other systems, such as power yoga, are both aerobic and strength building.

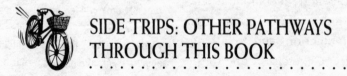

SIDE TRIPS: OTHER PATHWAYS THROUGH THIS BOOK

CHAPTER 6: LOOKING GOOD   Exercise not only helps you feel better but also helps maintain weight and keeps you looking good. Read this chapter for more suggestions on skin care and body image.

CHAPTER 11: BONING UP   Exercise that puts stress on the bones, such as strength training, can help retard osteoporosis. Look here to learn more about what you can do to retard bone loss.

CHAPTER 12: AND THE BEAT GOES ON   Lower levels of estrogen after menopause leave the heart vulnerable to cardiovascular problems. Exercise is one of the major recommendations for preventing heart disease. Look here to learn more about your heart and how to protect it.

CHAPTER 13: ARE YOU WHAT YOU EAT?   A healthy diet combined with a good exercise program can go a long way toward keeping you healthy. Look here to learn more about how what you eat affects you.

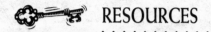

RESOURCES

Organizations and Services

American College of Sports Medicine, P.O. Box 1440, 401 W. Michigan St., Indianapolis, IN 46206-1440. Voice: (317) 637- 9200. E-mail: pipacsm@acsm.org. Internet: www.acsm.org/sportsmed. This group is dedicated to enhancing physical performance, fitness, health, and quality of life. Members apply scientific research about sports medicine and exercise science to real sports to achieve these enhancements. Contact this organization for membership information and a list of publications, including "Fit Over Forty."

American Council of Exercise, 5820 Overland Drive, Suite 102, San Diego, CA 92121. Voice: (800) 529-8227. Fax: (888) 348-3299. Internet: www.acefitness.org. Can't seem to get up that hill on your own? Call the ACE for names of certified fitness instructors in your area. Free health and fitness information is also available.

Melpomene Institute for Women's Health Research, 1010 University Ave., St. Paul, MN 55104. Voice: (612) 642-1951. Internet: www.melpomene.org. The Melpomene Institute (pronounced "mel-*pom*-uh-nee") is interested in the relationship between women's health and exercise. Currently, the institute is conducting research on exercise and menopause. Write or call to request resource packets, brochures, and videos. The organization has a very good thirty-two-page publication, "Let's Get Moving," for the fifty-plus woman who wants to exercise as well as information on sports and fitness specifically for women of color. Check out the web site.

President's Council on Physical Fitness and Sports, 701 Pennsylvania Ave. N.W., #205, Washington, DC 20004. Voice: (202) 272-3421. Fax: (202) 504-2064. The U.S. government wants *you* to be physically fit. Write or call for free copies of articles and booklets on the benefits of many different exercise programs.

Senior Fitness Association, P.O. Box 2575, New Smyrna Beach, FL 32170. Voice: (800) 243-1478. Fax: (904) 427-0613. This training, education, and certification organization can refer you to a fitness professional who works with low-fitness fifties or retirement-age adults. The organization also specializes in working with people who have some physical limitations. Instructors are trained not only in exercise techniques, but also in such things as physiology of aging and effects of medication.

YMCA–USA, 101 N. Wacker Drive, Chicago, IL 60606. Voice: (800) USA–YMCA. Fax: (312) 977-9063. Internet: www.ymca.net. The Y is a great facility for exercise in many forms—gyms, swimming, yoga, aerobics, and more. In addition, educational services and health programs are offered. Call the 800 number to find the Y nearest you.

AEROBICS

Aerobics and Fitness Association of America, 15250 Ventura Blvd., Sherman Oaks, CA 91403. Voice: (800) 446-2322. Fax: (818) 990-5468. Internet: www.afaa.com. Send a stamped, self-addressed business-size envelope to receive a list of certified fitness instructors in your area.

Cooper Wellness Program, Cooper Aerobics Research Institute, 12230 Preston Road, Dallas, TX 75230. Voice: (800) 444-5192. Fax: (977) 386-0039. A recent Cooper Institute study found that people who incorporate physical activity into their daily lives (taking the stairs instead of the elevator, walking their dog, and so on) were doing as well as people who got their exercise in a gym program. Write or call for information about wellness programs with a special emphasis on aerobics.

Jazzercise, 1050 Joshua Way, Vista, CA 92083. Voice: (800) 348-4748. If you like to dance, Jazzercise may be for you: This popular aerobics technique is based on jazz dancing. Call for location and more information about classes in your area. Videotapes geared to various fitness levels are available.

ALEXANDER TECHNIQUE

North American Society of Teachers of Alexander Technique, P.O. Box 517, Urbana, IL 61801. Voice: (800) 473-0620. Fax: (612) 822-7224. E-mail: nastat @ix.netcom.com. This organization has information on teacher training and books. Ask for a directory of Alexander teachers in your area.

DISABLED SPORTS ORGANIZATIONS

Arthritis Foundation, 1330 Peachtree St., Atlanta, GA 30309. Voice: (800) 283-7800. Internet: www.arthritis.org. The Arthritis Foundation has information about arthritis, local chapters, exercise videos, and publications. Call or write for videos and materials about exercises and water classes for people with joint problems. Programs include PACE: People with Arthritis Can Exercise; Joint Efforts: An Arthritis Movement Program; and Arthritis Foundation Aquatic Program.

Disabled Sports USA, 451 Hungerford Drive, Suite 100, Rockville, MD 20850. Voice: (301) 217-0960. Fax: (301) 217-0968. TDD: (301) 217-0963. E-mail: dsusa@dsusa.org. Internet: www.nas.com/~dsusa. This network of eighty-three community-based chapters in forty states provides year-round sports, recreational, and social activities for people with all sorts of disabilities.

National Sports Center for the Disabled, P.O. Box 36, Winter Park, CO 80482. Voice: (970) 726-5514. E-mail: infor@nscd.org. Internet: www.nscd.org/nscd. Call about summer and winter recreational sports programs customized for more than forty-five different disabilities. Winter programs include full-service ski programs; summer programs include visually impaired or blind rock climbing, hiking on wheelchair-accessible trails, and much more.

Wheelchair Sports USA, 3595 E. Fountain Blvd., Suite L-1, Colorado Springs, CO 80910. Voice: (719) 574-1150. E-mail: WSUSA@aol.com. This group provides athletic experiences for the disabled athlete. Call or write for information.

FELDENKRAIS

The Feldenkrais Guild, 524 Ellsworth St. S.W., P.O. Box 489, Albany, OR 97321. Voice: (800) 775-2118. Fax: (541) 926-0572. Write or call to request articles about the Feldenkrais method and a list of local practitioners. A free catalog of tapes and books is available.

PILATES

Current Concepts, Ken Endelman, 7500 14th Ave., #23, Sacramento, CA 95820. Voice: (800) 240-FLEX. Call or write for a list of instructors of Pilates-based exercise in your area and a brochure about the home reformer (a machine!). Also available are instructional tapes on Pilates and Pilates-based exercises.

Physical Mind (A Pilates-Based Exercise), 1807 2nd St., #28, Santa Fe, NM 87501. Voice: (505) 988-1990. Fax: (505) 988-2837. E-mail: piltd@mcimail.com. Call or write for a list of instructors in your area. You can also request information on a home reformer and a videotape for home practice.

The Pilates Studio, 2121 Broadway, #201, New York, NY 10023. Voice: (800) 474-5283. Call or write for a brochure and a list of trainers certified in the Pilates training program.

QI GONG

Health Action, 243 Pebble Beach, Santa Barbara, CA 93117. Voice: (805) 685-4670 or (800) 824-4325. This is a resource center for books, audiotapes, and videotapes on qi gong. Roger Jahnke, teacher and author, offers workshops throughout the country. Call to get a list of workshops and resources.

ROSEN METHOD MOVEMENT

Rosen Method Professional Association, 2550 Shattuck Ave., Box 49, Berkeley, CA 94704. Voice: (510) 644-4166. Call for information about Rosen Centers, body workers, and movement classes in your area.

SWIMMING/AQUA AEROBICS

Aquatic Exercise Association, Box 1609, Nokomis, FL 34274. Voice: (914) 486-8600. Fax: (941) 486-8820. E-mail: AEA@ix.netcom.com. Internet: www.youth.net/aeal/aea/aea. This nonprofit association has a consumer network. Call or write for its newsletter on the benefits of water exercise.

US Masters Swimming, 261 High Range, Londonderry, NH 03053. Voice: (603) 537-0203. E-mail: tracyswims@aol.com. This national organization will refer you to a local Masters swimming program, fitness swimming at any level or age over eighteen. If you're interested in competitive swimming, Masters has meets on all levels. Membership brings you *Swim* magazine and your local newsletter.

T'AI CHI

Patience T'ai Chi Association, P.O. Box 350532, Brooklyn, NY 11235. E-mail: taichiptc@aol.com. T'ai chi instructor William C. Phillips has put together a national referral service for t'ai chi instructors. He also offers a videotape for home instruction.

WALKING

Dynamic Health and Fitness Institute, 17 Blue Rock Court, Corte Madera, CA 94925. Voice: (415) 924-4013. Fax: (415) 924-5342. E-mail: dynamic@well.com. This institute offers individual instruction, group classes, seminars, and teacher training in walking, with emphasis on postural alignment. The institute will send you information about its approach to walking and can refer you to an Institute-trained instructor in your area.

Prevention Walking Club, 33 East Minor, Emmaus, PA 18098. This "paper club" offers encouragement through information. It also sponsors an annual walker's rally, where hundreds of people come together to walk, talk, and learn. For a fee, you will receive (among other things) a year-long walker's log, product discounts, and a bimonthly eight-page newsletter with articles on such diverse subjects as race walking and walking meditation. Inquire by mail only.

Sierra Club National Headquarters, 85 Second St., San Francisco, CA 94105. Voice: (415) 977-5500. E-mail: information@sierraclub.org. Internet: www.sierraclub.org. If you like walking outdoors, check out the Sierra Club, which organizes walks, hikes, bike tours, and skiing trips for people of all ages and levels. Call or write for the name, address, and telephone number of the chapter nearest you.

Walking the World, P.O. Box 1186, Fort Collins, CO 80522. Voice: (800) 340-9255. Call to get a brochure and to find out about walking and hiking programs.

YOGA

B. K. S. Iyengar Yoga National Association of the United States, 1676 Hilton Head Court, #2288, El Cajon, CA 92019. Voice: (800) 889-9642. Call this national headquarters to find a teacher in your area, for information about membership and programs, or to order hard-to-find books.

Products and Catalogs

Jazzertogs, 1050 Joshua Way, Vista, CA 92083. Voice: (800) 348-4748. Fax: (800) 2-FAX-TOG. Call for a catalog of fitness supplies—videos, clothing, and more.

Living Arts Catalog, P.O. Box 2939, Venice, CA 90291. Voice: (800) 254-8464. Fax: (800) 582-6872. A great place for yoga supplies (blankets and other props) and instructional tapes.

Title Nine Sports, 5743 Landregan, Emeryville, CA 94608. Voice: (510) 655-5999. Fax: (510) 655-9191. E-mail: t9sports@aol.com. This woman-owned mail-order company is devoted to selling reasonably priced workout gear for women only. The company will answer questions about its products as well as questions about women and sports.

Yoga International's Guide to Yoga Teachers and Classes. To order, call: (800) 821-YOGA. RR 1, Box 407, Honesdale, PA 18431. Looking for a yoga teacher? This guide lists yoga teachers across the United States and internationally, as well as certification programs and yoga associations.

Yoga Journal's Yoga Teachers Directory, 2054 University Ave., Suite 600, Berkeley, CA 94704. (800) 359-YOGA. Directory of yoga teachers in the United States.

Periodicals

Fitness Walking, 1010 University Ave., St. Paul, MN 55104. Voice: (612) 642-1951. This magazine for walkers has helpful articles, such as how to pick shoes and how to develop a walking program.

National Masters News, P.O. Box 50098, Eugene, OR 97405. Voice: (503) 343-7116. Fax: (503) 345-2436. This is the official publication for Masters track and field, long-distance running, and race walking. To compete, you must be over thirty—there are no other qualifications. You can work out on your own or join an organized club. There's very little pressure. Information on events and clubs is printed in the magazine.

Swim, P.O. Box 863, El Segundo, CA 90245-9961. A magazine for the adult fitness-oriented swimmer. You'll find all sorts of swimming tips in this glossy magazine.

T'ai Chi, P.O. Box 26156, Los Angeles, CA 90026. Voice: (213) 665-7773. Fax: (213) 665-1627. E-mail: taichi@tai-chi.com. This magazine has articles about (what else?) t'ai chi. You'll find articles by martial arts masters and good resources.

The Walking Magazine, P.O. Box 56561, Boulder, CO 80322-6561. Voice: (800) 678-0881. This magazine offers a variety of articles on walking and everything related to it. It also contains a calendar of walking events.

Women's Sports and Fitness, WSF Inc., 2025 Pearl St., Boulder, CO 80302. Voice: (800) 877-5281. This magazine is all about women's fitness. Its stories of women in sports are inspiring.

Women's Sports Traveler, 167 Madison Ave, Suite 405, NY, 10016. Voice: (212) 686-6480. Fax: (212) 685-6240. E-mail: sporttravl@aol.com. This quarterly publication celebrates the sporting and traveling life with a decidedly female slant. Emphasis on a variety of sports, including walking, hiking, water sports, cycling.

Yoga Journal, California Yoga Teacher's Association, 2054 University Ave., Berkeley, CA 94704. Voice: (510) 841-9200. The *Yoga Journal* is for readers at every level of familiarity with yoga. Articles range from interviews with New Age personalities to illustrated yoga *asanas* to self-care and nutrition.

Yoga International Guide to Yoga Teachers and Classes—Resource Directory, RR1, Box 407, Honesdale, PA 18431. Voice: (800) 253-6243.

Books

Covert Bailey, *Smart Exercise*. Boston: Houghton Mifflin, 1994. The author of *Fit or Fat* has produced a comprehensive guide to exercise and training in which his prejudice, "Fit muscles rule the body," is right up front. His sense of humor and great sense of self-respect give readers the confidence they need to get started and stick with a new fitness program.

Pat Lyons and Debby Burgard. *Great Shape*. Palo Alto, CA: Bull Publishing, 1990. Exercise for women of all shapes and sizes, especially those who are larger or over their ideal weight. The theme: Don't let your size stop you from exercising.

Judy Mahle Lutter and Lynn Jaffee. *Bodywise Woman.* 2d ed. Champaign, IL: Human Kinetics Press, 1996. This big book, available through the Melpomene Institute and elsewhere, is filled with solid information about physical activity, women's health, menopause, body awareness, and much more.

Stanford Medical School Health and Fitness Program. *Fresh Start: Real Health, Real Results for Real People.* San Francisco: KQED Books, 1996. An exercise book for everyone, with chapters on everything from back health to customizing exercise for special needs. Plenty of easy-to-follow exercises illustrated by midlife and older men and women.

ALEXANDER TECHNIQUE

John Gray. *The Alexander Technique: A Complete Course in How to Hold and Use Your Body for Maximum Energy.* New York: St. Martin's Press, 1990. This reader-friendly book covers many of the Alexander techniques. It also gives some theory behind the Alexander technique and has good illustrations on how to use your body to maximize your energy.

Judith Leibowitz and Bill Connington. *The Alexander Technique.* New York: Harper Perennial, 1990. Using her twenty years of experience at the Juilliard School of Music, Liebowitz's book takes the reader from the theory to the practical aspects of the Alexander program. Well illustrated; easy to use as a beginning resource.

BICYCLING

Susan Weaver. *A Woman's Guide to Cycling.* Berkeley, CA: Ten Speed Press, 1991. The editor of *Bicycling* magazine has written a comprehensive guide for women. It includes the joys of riding, repairs, and a list of where to find bicycle gear for women.

FELDENKRAIS METHOD

Moshe Feldenkrais. *Body Awareness as Healing Therapy: The Case of Nora.* Berkeley, CA: Frog Books, 1977. This classic study is the foundation of Feldenkrais's work. It provides the reader with the basics of the theory as well as inspiration to move beyond existing physical limitations through body awareness and action.

MARTIAL ARTS

Richard Strozz Heckler. *The Anatomy of Change: A Way to Move Through Life's Transitions.* Berkeley, CA: North Atlantic Books, 1984. Drawing on Aikido and Lomi body work, the author brings the reader to a new level of body awareness and a process to help center and focus energy for life's changes.

Carol A. Wiley, ed. *Women in the Martial Arts.* Berkeley, CA: North Atlantic Books, 1992. This how-it-feels book rather than how-to book is filled with personal stories from women in the martial arts who express the physical and spiritual aspects of these disciplines.

Qi Gong

Roger Jahnke. *The Healer Within: The Four Essential Self-Care Methods for Creating Optimal Health.* San Francisco: HarperCollins, 1997. This book, written by a practitioner of traditional Chinese medicine and teacher of qi gong, addresses the power of qi gong to prevent disease and promote healing. It discusses breathing, massage, meditation, and movement.

Michael Tse. *Qi Gong for Health and Vitality.* New York: St. Martin's, 1995. Michael Tse offers easy-to-follow instructions for beginners. He also includes a section on movements for specific ailments.

Running

Joan Benoit Samuelson. *Running for Women.* Emmaus, PA: Rodale Press, 1995. This book, written by an Olympic gold medal winner, offers information on all aspects of running. The author addresses running and its effect on women's health and also talks about PMS and menopause.

Swimming

American Lap Swimmer's Association. *Swimmers Guide.* To order, call (800) 431-9111. If you're a swimmer on vacation, you'll want this guide that lists 1,200 pools across the country—maps and information about hours, prices, pool size, and temperatures.

Walking

Don and Debbie Lawrence. *Walklog: Diary and Guide for the Exercise Walker.* Indianapolis: Masterpress, 1995. This log lets you keep track of your walks and also offers tips. The authors address footwear, technique, and stretching.

Weight Training

Karen Andes. *Woman's Book of Strength: Empowering Guide to Mind/Body Fitness.* New York: Perigee Books, 1995. The author takes a mind–body approach to weight training, encouraging a focused workout with attention to form. She also offers some training programs for both free weights and gym equipment and includes a discussion of nutrition.

Thomas D. Fahey and Faye Hutchinson. *Weight Training for Women.* Mountain View, CA: Mayfield Publishing, 1992. This book takes the special needs of women's bodies into account when using weights and weight machines. It outlines programs for weight training.

Miriam F. Nelson, Ph.D. *Strong Women Stay Young.* New York: Bantam Books, 1997. The author looks at the encouraging research on strength training. Strength training not only reduces fat and builds muscle, but can also reverse bone loss and improve energy and balance. This book gives you ideas for using free weights and gym equipment. It includes a section on bone health and a means to chart your progress.

YOGA

Lorna Belle, R.N., and Eudora Seyfer, *Gentle Yoga*. Berkeley, CA: Celestial Arts, 1987. A yoga book for people who just want to take it easy as well as for people who are disabled in some way. This book was written by a woman who pioneered yoga for people in wheelchairs.

Paddy O'Brien. *Yoga for Women: A Complete Mind and Body Fitness*. San Francisco: Aquarian, 1991. Postures for different life transitions, including menopause.

Mary Stewart. *Yoga Over 50: The Way to Vitality, Health, and Energy in the Prime of Life*. New York: Simon and Schuster, 1994. A good beginning yoga book that is very well illustrated with photographs of real people in the prime of life.

Louise Taylor. *A Woman's Book of Yoga: A Journal for Health and Self-Discovery*. Rutland, VT: Tuttle, 1993. An illustrated journal that explains postures and addresses women's health issues from yoga's point of view. A beginner's book.

Audio/Video

Some of the agencies listed in Organizations and Services, such as *Health Action* (see Qi Gong), have excellent audiocassettes and videotapes available for sale or rental. Two particularly good catalogs for exercise and movement are listed below. There are so many exercise tapes on video that we can't even begin to suggest which is right for you. **Collage Video Specialties** (see listing below) is the place to start looking. You'll find catalogs for other good sources of tapes for exercise, yoga, t'ai chi, and other movement or mind–body programs in Chapter 5, "Breathe Easy"; Chapter 7, "The Holistic Kit and Caboodle"; and Chapter 8, "What's Up, Doc?"

Collage Video Specialties, Voice: (800) 433-6769 or (612) 571-5840. Internet: www.cybercise.com/collage. Collage carries health-related fitness videos, including yoga and t'ai chi as well as aerobics, strength training, and a wealth of others. The company also carries some exercise products and the book *The Complete Guide to Exercise Videos* (1997 edition)—descriptions of exercise videos (including some evaluation of safety) by a person who has actually seen the video. Call or access the web site to request a free catalog.

Living Arts, P.O. Box 2939, Venice, CA 90291. Voice: (800) 254-8464. Fax: (800) 582-6872. A great place for yoga supplies (blankets and other props) and instructional tapes.

VIDEO

Awakening and Mastering the Medicine Within You. 60 minutes. Available from Health Action. Roger Jahnke, qi gong instructor and practitioner of Chinese medicine, is featured in this video. Easy to follow directions make this well suited for both the beginner and someone familiar with qi gong.

Easy T'ai Chi with Strawberry Gatts. 60 minutes. Available from Sounds True (see Audio/Video, Chapter 5). Helps beginners learn the twenty-seven basic postures, individually and in flowing movement.

T'ai Chi Workout. 60 minutes. Available from The VideoFinders Collection (see Audio/Video, Chapter 8). The basic dynamics of t'ai chi, how to loosen your joints, and movements and mental techniques. Narrated by John Saxon and accompanied by beautiful nature footage.

Yoga Journal's Yoga Practice for Beginners. 72 minutes. Available from Living Arts (listed above). Instructor Patricia Walden presents easy-to-follow instruction in Hatha yoga that includes a full range of yoga poses and relaxation techniques designed for all levels of fitness.

55+ & Fit. Available from University of Iowa Audio Visual Center, 215 Seashore Hall Center, Iowa City, IA 52242. Voice: (800) 369-IOWA. Fax: (319) 335-2507. A stretch-and-tone video for people fifty-five and older.

Online

Most of the organizations in this chapter have home pages on the Internet. In addition, you can use a search engine to find a large—and growing—list of health, sports, fitness, and exercise sites. Both **Women's Wire** (www.women.com) and **Power Surge** (members.aol.com/dearest) have the latest on sports and fitness, as do the growing number of online sports magazines (find links to them in the general web sites below).

News Groups

Look under **alt.sports**, **rec.sports**, or **rec.misc** to find the sport that interests you. For recreation and outdoors, check out **phl.outdoors** or **pnet.rec.talk**.

Web Sites

Jump into fitness at **The Fitness Partner Connection Jumpsite!**, www.cdc. net/~primus/fpc/fpchome.html. You'll find whatever you're looking for here. A fitness library; training activities for everything from aerobics and bodybuilding to walking, running, swimming, volleyball, and others; plus articles and links to women's health and fitness, the human body, FAQs, online sports publications, and more things than we have room to describe.

At **The Yellow Pages of Swimming**, www.tcd.net/~jj/swimlinx.html, you'll find links for everything from Masters clubs and swimming pools across the United States to an index of swimming products and where to find them.

You'll find **Alexander Technique** at www.life.uiuc.edu/jeff.alextech.html. The **Feldenkrais Method Web Pages** are at www.usc.edu/hsc/neuroprotection.feldenkrais. **HealthWorld Online** at www.healthworld.com is a good place to find information and resources about qi gong and other mind–body practices.

4

ARE YOU WHAT YOU EAT?
Food and Supplements

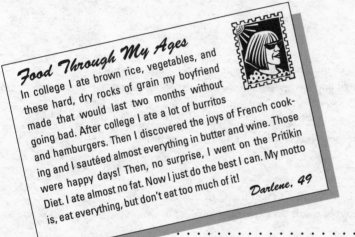

Food Through My Ages

In college I ate brown rice, vegetables, and these hard, dry rocks of grain my boyfriend made that would last two months without going bad. After college I ate a lot of burritos and hamburgers. Then I discovered the joys of French cooking and I sautéed almost everything in butter and wine. Those were happy days! Then, no surprise, I went on the Pritikin Diet. I ate almost no fat. Now I just do the best I can. My motto is, eat everything, but don't eat too much of it!

Darlene, 49

Food is basic to our survival. It's so important that most major religions concern themselves with prohibited and allowed foods. Our relationship to food is simple: If we don't get enough of the nutrients we need, we will not thrive. And if we don't get enough to eat, we don't survive.

It's probably safe to assume that if you're reading this book, you have enough food to keep you alive. Nonetheless, food is an enormous issue for women. Adolescent girls and young women are at risk for eating disorders such as anorexia and bulimia. Women of all ages, "just trying to drop that last five pounds," make commercial diet centers and diet foods a booming business. In our lifetime we've seen a lot of food fads come and go and come back again—from the brown rice and vegetables of macrobiotics, to the butter and cream sauces of the French Chef, to the tiny but beautiful portions of California cuisine and *cuisine minceur* (which a friend once described ruefully as "cuisine miniature"), to the television gourmets, galloping or frugal.

We're accustomed to starving ourselves and pigging out as the need arises, but in midlife this thoughtless behavior often comes to a screeching halt. The food we eat just doesn't treat us the same way anymore. Suddenly, we have trouble digesting foods we considered our friends, and that morning cup of coffee does *way* more than just wake us up in the morning. A food we've always loved may bring on a hot flash, or the doctor may tell us that the combi-

nourishment The food or other substances we need to sustain life.

nation of menopause, a steady diet of delicious high-fat foods, and a family risk for heart disease is a deadly combination. Or we realize that we're simply not burning up the calories at the same rate we used to.

Whatever has got you thinking about reevaluating the way you eat, hold on to that thought. You don't have go on a punishing diet, you don't have to give up that special treat, you don't have to "eat like an old lady." Midlife is the perfect time to begin eating with the awareness that when you put a variety of healthful (and delicious) foods into your body, you are supporting your continued good health. The old saying is true: You are what you eat. Eating your vegetables will not make you green and leafy, but it will help make you feel good so you can go out and think about something besides food!

 ## PACKING FOR THE JOURNEY

Why Should I Reevaluate My Diet?

What you eat has a direct effect on how you feel from day to day: on how clearly you think, on your emotional ups and downs, on your level of energy, and on the health of your body. When you eat the foods your body needs, you naturally feel better. What's more, you can modify your diet to help cope with many of the signs of hormonal imbalance. And food still works the same way it did when you were growing up: It helps build strong bones and healthy bodies. If you intend to live a long,

Midlife is a time to reconsider how we are nourishing ourselves on many levels. When it comes to eating, nourishment is more than just what we eat; it's how we eat. Take time to sit down and enjoy your meal. It sounds simple, but how often do you really do it? You don't have to be Martha Stewart, but do take time to create your own form of gracious dining. Especially if it's only for yourself, try to eat in a way that promotes relaxation and enjoyment—you'll help your digestion immeasurably! Set your table with care, serve your food thoughtfully, and eat with attention. Appreciate what you put in your body and give it the opportunity to do its job of supporting and sustaining you on your journey.

Every woman seems to have a menu she's used to cooking week to week and a well-worn path around the market. Changing your diet gives you a chance to branch out beyond the same five vegetables you're used to bringing home. Make food shopping a total body experience: Feast on the colors, smell the fruits to find which ones are ripe, pick up the foods and feel them for firmness, take them home, eat them, and listen to the crunch. Buy a mango instead of an orange, a yellow Finn potato instead of an Idaho, a red onion instead of a white onion, a shiitake mushroom instead of a button mushroom. Experiment. Enjoy. Eat!

healthy life (and we hope you do), you should know that the right diet can help protect you against heart disease, cancers, and other ills.

What Kind of Diet Is Best for Me?

It's easy to become obsessed with food. And the more questions you ask, the worse it gets, as we discovered in writing this chapter. One expert says eat less protein and more complex carbohydrates, while another says eat a lot of protein and not as many complex carbs. One nutritionist says vitamin supplements are a must, while another advises meeting your nutritional needs through food alone. One woman thrives on a vegetarian diet; another feels better with meat in her diet; still another grew up eating pasta every day and is not about to stop now; and yet another follows a diet based on an ancient system of energy medicine. As soon as we think we know something, research seems to prove it wrong. In the movie *Sleeper*, Woody Allen's character wakes from centuries of cryogenic sleep to find that much has changed since 1973: Brown rice is out, and red meat, fat, and cigarettes are the health foods of choice.

With all this confusion, how can you know what's right for *you*? The best way is to keep it simple, try not to get obsessed, and pay attention to the messages your body sends you. Every woman's nutritional needs are slightly different, as are her personal tastes in food. Your family history, culture, personal tastes and beliefs, health needs, and goals will all influence what you eat. There is some consensus on what constitutes a good diet for midlife, but you can customize that food pyramid with your own choices. For example, to keep and build muscles that will support your bones, you need protein: Whether you get it from chicken or chickpeas is a personal choice.

GUIDED TOUR:
Food and Supplements

Eating well is not only the best revenge, but is also the foundation of your continued good health and well-being. A good diet for women in midlife is rich in a variety of fresh fruits and vegetables and includes an adequate amount of good-quality protein. Make sure you're getting enough of the antioxidant vitamins (including vitamins A and C and beta-carotene), to boost immune function and protect against heart disease; calcium, to prevent bone loss; essential fatty acids (from cold-water fish or flaxseed oil); fiber, to aid digestion and decrease carcinogens; whole grains, to provide B vitamins and fiber; and six to eight glasses of water per day.

WESTERN MEDICINE

You may need to structure your diet according to your health needs. Talk to your health practitioner about what foods you should eat or avoid to optimize your health.

COMPLEMENTARY THERAPIES

Healing diets are part of several systems of complementary therapy, including Ayurveda and traditional Chinese medicine. These generally involve other lifestyle changes in addition to eating.

EXERCISE

Getting enough exercise will help you metabolize what you eat and will help keep your digestion working properly. Taking a walk after a meal is still a great idea.

MIND–BODY

Stress can affect how we digest food and even how much of the nutrients we eat get absorbed and used. Practices such as meditation, relaxation techniques, yoga, and t'ai chi can help reduce stress and keep your body in good condition.

Some ways of eating are carefully designed healing tools. Both the East and West have their own versions of healthful ways to eat.

In the East, Ayurveda and traditional Chinese medicine date back thousands of years. According to *A Woman's Best Medicine*, "One of the essential discoveries of Ayurveda, as well as other ancient traditional medical systems, such as the Chinese and Native American, is the realization that the mind and body are intimately connected and that consciousness is inseparably merged with both." The lifestyle shift these systems involve encourages exercise, healthful eating, meditation, and awareness of ourselves as more than just bodies.

The West's history of food fads and health-conscious dieting (beginning perhaps with Dr. Graham and his legacy, the graham cracker) has had one group of Americans calling another group of Americans "health nuts" for most of a century. Nonetheless, the efforts of Westerners concerned with trying to modify meat-heavy, pesticide- and preservative-rich diets have induced many people to eat healthier foods and the food industry to reevaluate its practices.

Many Americans now follow some form of vegetarian diet. Variations include lacto-ovo (dairy and eggs allowed), vegan (no animal products whatsoever), and macrobiotics (a simple diet of Japanese origin based on brown rice and cooked vegetables). Today, you can choose from a number of medical diet approaches. The protein-rich Atkins Diet and the almost-no-fat-whatsoever Pritikin Diet of the last couple decades have been replaced by more balanced approaches. More recently, the plans of Dr. Dean Ornish and Dr. John A. McDougall approach health through a combination of low-fat diet and exercise; Ornish, who

(continued)

What Foods Should I Limit in My Diet?

A few foods (or foodlike substances) just aren't good for you, at least in excess. You probably already know what they are. Here's why.

SALT   Table salt and other forms of sodium increase blood pressure in many people and deplete calcium from the bones—1,000 milligrams of sodium can cause you to lose 26 milligrams of calcium. Limit your salt or sodium intake to no more than 2,400 milligrams per day and preferably 1,800 milligrams per day. This is less than 1 teaspoon of salt. If you eat fresh foods, you won't have too much trouble keeping on top of this. If you eat processed foods, read the nutrition label (one can of Campbell's Home Style Chicken Noodle Soup has more than 2,000 milligrams of sodium). Use fresh flavorful foods and interesting herbs and spices, and you'll find you won't need as much salt to make the food taste good.

REFINED SUGAR   Refined sugar (this includes white sugar, confectioners' sugar, brown sugar, raw sugar, and corn syrup) contains no vitamins, minerals, or fiber that can aid metabolism. In fact, it can destabilize blood sugar levels, making you feel tired and depressed. Sugar can also rob your body of other nutrients in order to be digested and can contribute to weight gain. Try to get your sugar fix in its natural form, from fresh fruits and dried fruits.

CAFFEINE   As a society we seem to live on caffeine, as found in coffee, tea, and many sodas and, to a lesser degree, in chocolate. It wakes us up and makes us feel alert and happy. Unfortunately, it soon lets us down. Then we need more caffeine to perk us up again. It's fun, but clearly doesn't lead anywhere. Caffeine can also quicken the heart rate and contribute to palpitations and hot flashes, and it has a diuretic effect that can contribute to loss of calcium and other minerals.

ALCOHOL   The subject of alcohol usually arouses strong feelings. Alcohol is an important part of the cuisine and social structure of many cultures. As often as it has been vilified as the demon rum, it has been praised for health benefits (the French Paradox theory proposes that the French habit of drinking red wine every day contributes to a lower rate of heart disease). Alcohol has its good points and its bad points, and a lot depends on how your body metabolizes it and how much you drink—alcohol in moderation seems to offer some protection against cardiac problems, but alcohol in excess can rob your body of nutrients and impair calcium metabolism and bone structure. Drinking may also affect blood estrogen levels of women who are taking hormone replacement therapy. Research on this question is ongoing.

The latest federal Dietary Guidelines advise drinking alcohol in moderation—for women that's one drink a day (12 ounces of beer, 5 ounces or wine, or 1.5 ounces of 80-proof spirits). Alcohol overconsumption has also been linked to increased risk of breast cancer and impaired memory, and it can adversely affect blood sugar, leading to feelings of fatigue and

POINT OF INTEREST (continued)

developed his plan for heart patients, also includes a program of stress management. The Zone, a diet popularized by John Sears, stresses adequate protein along with carbohydrates and fats. For more information, see Resources.

TRAVEL TIP

Five Good Reasons to Eat Your Fruits and Vegetables

Fresh fruits and vegetables contain all kinds of good things for your body. If you eat a variety, you're bound to enjoy these benefits:

1. Phytochemicals that can decrease the toxicity of carcinogens.

2. Phytoestrogens that can help with hormonal imbalance.

3. Antioxidants that have antiviral properties and may reduce the risk of many types of cancer.

4. Bioflavonoids (found in the pith of citrus fruits and elsewhere) that help relieve symptoms of hormonal imbalance.

5. Fiber that aids digestion and helps lower cholesterol.

Nourishment
It feels like I've been feeding other people all my life. I'm tired. I can't even think of anything to make for dinner anymore. I feel like it's time to stop worrying about what everybody else is eating, and start feeding myself. I don't mean just food.   *Billie, 50*

Soy: Is She Really the Queen Bean?

Soy, the bean of the moment for women who are interested in controlling symptoms of declining hormones through natural means, is loaded with phytoestrogens, is a potent cholesterol-lowering agent, may reduce breast cancer risk, and is an excellent source of protein.

Should you eat soy? A lot of money is currently being poured into soybean research and the results seem encouraging. But, as always, remember that we are our own clinical trials—even in the case of adding more soy to our diet. Soy, like wheat and dairy products, is a common allergenic food and is often not easily tolerated. If you increase your soy consumption and notice any negative effects on your well-being or energy levels, this may not be the phytochemical for you.

How much soy is enough? In "Phytoestrogens and Breast Cancer," Y-Me says, "Certain experts believe that as little as one serving of soy per day (that's half a cup of tofu or a cup of soy milk) may reduce cancer risk." But to get the full range of benefits—as a help for symptoms of declining hormones, and for help retarding osteoporosis and preventing heart disease—you'll need 30 to 50 grams a day—not an easy prospect for most Americans. If you do decide to eat soy, include whole grains and fresh vegetables in your diet, and be aware that tofu has a relatively high fat content.

- Soy milk: one 8-ounce glass = 6 grams of soy protein. Try it over cereal or blended with fruit in a smoothie. It comes in flavors, too!
- Soy flour: 1 cup = 30 grams of soy protein. Combine it with other flours for baking.
- Tofu: 1/2 cup = 10 to 20 grams of soy protein. Soy curd adapts to many recipes easily. Cube it for stir frying, mash it and mix it like egg salad, or blend it with sauces for a creamy effect.

depression. Although it initially works to relax, alcohol may later wake you from a good night's sleep and may trigger hot flashes. Many women in midlife find that their bodies just can't handle alcohol the way they used to. Pay attention to how your body reacts when you drink.

SATURATED AND HYDROGENATED FAT Saturated fat (in animal foods and whole milk products) and hydrogenated fat (solid vegetable fats, like margarine and Crisco) can clog your arteries, contribute to high cholesterol, and generally make you feel heavy and sluggish. Hydrogenated fats are considered carcinogenic, and a high-fat diet has also been implicated as contributing to cancer rates. Yikes. Substitute a monounsaturated oil like olive oil, but remember, the goal is to decrease total intake of fat.

PROCESSED FOODS AND JUNK FOODS As a rule of thumb, it's a good idea to eat foods whose parts you can identify without reading a label. The processing in processed foods generally includes high amounts of sugar, salt, the bad kinds of fat, and preservatives. And you already know about those!

What Should I Try to Include in My Diet?

There's a wide world of food to choose from, and most of it will help you feel healthy and energized. Try to use the following guidelines in establishing your basic diet.

EAT A VARIETY OF FRESH FRUITS AND VEGETABLES Even if you take all the supplements in the store, you still won't get all the good things that come from eating fresh fruits and vegetables. Eat them every day, eat a variety of types and colors, and eat a lot. How much? The American Cancer Institute recommends eating five to seven servings of fruits and vegetables a day, and other sources (including the USDA food pyramid) recommend eating up to ten servings a day (a serving is about one-half cup).

EAT ADEQUATE PROTEIN Eating protein helps us maintain energy, build lean muscle mass, repair tissue, and promote healthy skin, hair, and nails. The amino acids in protein are also building blocks for antioxidants that our body makes. Yet the older we get, the less efficient our bodies are at using protein. So how much is enough? The Recommended Daily Allowance (RDA) for women over fifty is about 50 grams (equivalent to about 8 ounces) of lean protein over the course of a day. Pay attention to how you feel when you vary the amount of protein you eat. According to *Nutrition Action Newsletter*, 1 cup of cooked beans, peas, or lentils is about 13 to 17 grams of protein; 1 cup of plain nonfat yogurt is about 13 grams of protein; 1/4 pound of skinless cooked chicken breast is about 34 grams of protein; 3 ounces of tofu is 4 to 10 grams of protein.

USE MONOUNSATURATED FATS Despite what we sometimes hear, fats are not all bad. In fact, we need fats to survive. Monounsaturated fats, such as olive oil, seem to be better for the body than some other types of oils and fats. Studies show olive oil is helpful in lowering the rish of heart disease by lowering the bad cholesterol, LDL.

GET YOUR EFAS Essential fatty acids (EFAs), or omega-3 oils, are found in cold-water fish like salmon, halibut, mackerel, and sardines, and in walnuts and flaxseed oil. EFAs can help lower cholesterol and have been linked to reduced risk of heart disease. Some women use flaxseed oil to ease aches and pains in their

Eat Your Phytoestrogens

Isoflavones, a kind of phytoestrogen, are plant-derived estrogens. They are similar to the hormones our bodies make, but weaker. Because they are so similar, they attach to our estrogen receptor sites. Current research indicates that they may be able to provide some estrogenic activity when our own levels drop. They may also lock out the stronger estrogens our bodies produce and the potentially harmful xenoestrogens, by-products of industrial pollution (for more about xenoestrogens, see Chapter 13, "What Are My Chances?").

Studies suggest that phytoestrogens can alleviate hot flashes and night sweats. In Japan, where the diet is high in soy products, the main complaint of perimenopausal women is headaches, not hot flashes. There is some evidence that phytoestrogens may also reduce the risk of breast cancer, lower cholesterol, and slow bone loss. Researchers are currently looking into the effects of phytoestrogens on heart disease, various types of cancer, osteoporosis, and more. You can eat your phytoestrogens in soy products (see the Point of Interest "Soy: Is She Really the Queen Bean?"), potatoes, bean sprouts, sunflower seeds, carrots, and many other foods. If you want to learn more, call the American Institute for Cancer Research at (800) 843-8114 and ask for a free copy of "Taking a Closer Look at Phytochemicals."

joints. EFAs can also help improve dry skin and hair. When you can, substitute essential fatty acids and monounsaturated fats for other fats and oils in your diet.

EAT MORE FIBER   Fiber is the part of plant foods that is not absorbed and passes through the stomach and small intestine unaltered. Fiber performs a cleansing function by removing toxins from our system. Dietary fiber has been associated with lowering cholesterol levels and reducing the risk of intestinal cancer, and it also helps keep us regular. To make sure you're getting enough fiber in your diet, include some of the following high-fiber foods: oats, flaxmeal, beans, apples, carrots, celery, root vegetables, and beans.

USE WHOLE GRAINS AND LEGUMES   The recent emphasis on low-fat diets has meant that a lot of us end up eating too many carbohydrates—and often the wrong kind. Overloading on carbohydrates—even in the form of pasta, bread, rice, and oats—can actually lead to a craving for sugar. Your body eventually breaks down carbohydrates into sugar. Legumes (beans and peas) and whole grains, the more complex the better, take longer to digest and are less able to destabilize blood sugar levels. Whole grains contain more nutrients than their "white" counterparts. They are also a way to increase fiber in your diet and are associated with a lower risk of colon cancer.

DRINK PLENTY OF WATER   Our bodies need six to eight glasses of water a day. Drinking enough water minimizes the risk of getting urinary tract infections, aids in digestion, and helps flush toxins from our bodies. If you eat more dietary fiber or increase your exercise, your need for water will also increase. Remember: Coffee, tea, and sodas don't replace your body's need for water. In fact, these diuretics actually increase your need for water. Good-quality bottled water and water-filtration systems ensure that the water we drink is good water.

How Can I Tell If I Have a Food Sensitivity?

Food sensitivities are more prevalent than you may think. Common culprits include wheat, soy, and dairy foods. A simple way to discover if a food is right for you or if you have any food sensitivities is to keep a food diary. If you add a new food like soy, notice how you feel after you eat it. How's your energy level? Do you feel bloated or have headaches? If you suspect a food you are eating is causing you some problems (this often happens at midlife, when digestion sometimes gets a little sluggish), don't eat the food for one to two weeks. When you add it back, eat it alone first and see if you notice any sensitivities or change in your energy level. No one knows better than you how you feel.

Which Vitamins Are Important for Women at Midlife?

Pretty much all of them! Here is a selection for your consideration.

B-COMPLEX VITAMINS   This complex of vitamins—which includes niacin, pantothenic acid, thiamine, folic acid or folate, and B_1, B_3, B_6, B_{12}, and the rest—helps you turn food into energy, strengthens the immune system, and helps alleviates stress. Evidence indicates that people who don't have enough folate in their diet run a greater risk of heart disease and stroke. B vitamins are all over the food groups: in whole grains, in leafy greens, in seeds, and in meat, poultry, dairy products, and seafood.

VITAMIN C   Vitamin C is one of the many antioxidants that are touted as being so good for us these days. Vitamin C has long been praised for its antiviral properties (it may help stave off colds or help us recover faster, and it may be effective in cancer prevention). It's hard to avoid this vitamin, which fortifies a

TRAVEL TIP:
The Spices of Life

Spices add flavor to food, but they also do something more. Cinnamon, fennel, sage, and turmeric all contain phytohormones and can help prevent hot flashes.

TRAVEL TIP
Fruits and Vegetables to Go:
Good-for-You Snack Foods

Just Veggies are bits of dehydrated and/or freeze-dried corn, peas, carrots, bell pepper, and tomato. Just Fruit Crunchies are dehydrated apples, blueberries, pineapple, and raspberries. Both of these products are good healthful snacks with no salt or preservatives. Look for them in the grocery store, or see Resources to order. If you own a food dehydrator, you can make these yourself!

Paint Your Plate

Think "multicolored palette" when designing your next meal. Not only are colorful foods lovely to look at, but the compounds that make up the color are also loaded with nutrients that can help our bodies fight disease.

- Glorious Green: broccoli (vitamin C, calcium, chlorophyll, anticancer properties); spinach (vitamin C, magnesium, folate); kale (great source of calcium and vitamin A)

- Outrageous Orange: carrots (vitamins A and C), butternut squash, yams (vitamins A and C, copper, fiber, folate), cantaloupe (vitamins A and C and potassium); mangoes (vitamins C and E, bioflavonoids, boron)

- Robust Red: tomatoes, watermelon (lycopene, an antioxidant); strawberries, red bell peppers (vitamin C); cherries (phytohormones)

- Particularly Purple: eggplants, grapes (the more colorful the skin, the greater the levels of antioxidants, which inhibit LDL), blueberries (anthocyanin, an antioxidant); plums (bioflavonoids); boysenberries (vitamin C, calcium)

- Yes, Yes, Yellow: cornmeal (magnesium, phytohormones, vitamin E); yellow peppers (vitamin C, beta-carotene)

- Beautiful Brown: buckwheat or kasha, whole wheat pasta, (B-complex, magnesium); brown rice (phytohormones, B-complex), shiitake mushrooms (vitamin D), mushrooms (chromium)

- White on White: potatoes (phytohormones); onions and garlic (heart-protective qualities); tofu (calcium, magnesium, phytoestrogen, heart-protective qualities)

- Basic Black: black beans (folic acid)

number of fruit juices, cereals, and other foods. Food sources include citrus fruits, strawberries, red peppers, kale, broccoli, cherries, and oysters.

VITAMIN D   We need vitamin D to help us absorb calcium and prevent bone loss. Our bodies manufacture vitamin D from sunlight (fifteen minutes of sun a day in the summer), but as we get older our bodies get less efficient at doing this. Sunscreen also interferes with absorption. So don't count on the sun. You can also get your vitamin D from fortified milk, orange juice, cereal, shiitake mushrooms, and egg yolks.

VITAMIN E   Vitamin E is another antioxidant that seems to boost immune function and protect against heart disease. Are you getting enough? People on low-fat diets tend to avoid any form of fat, even fats the body needs. Unfortunately, they may be missing out on vitamin E because many food sources of this vitamin are high in fat—almonds, safflower oil, canola oil, olive oil, peanuts, peanut butter. If you are on a low-fat diet, try to get your fat from these healthful sources. Lower-fat sources include whole wheat bread, toasted wheat germ, spinach, and sweet potatoes. Some fortified breakfast cereals, such as Total and Product 19, have high amounts of vitamin E and little fat.

FOLIC ACID   Folic acid protects against heart disease and cancer and strengthens the immune system. You'll find it in many foods, including whole grains, beans (chickpeas, black beans, pinto beans, and many others), spinach, leeks, artichokes, avocados, cantaloupe, pistachio nuts, tuna, turkey, beef, and some fortified cereals.

What Are Some Important Minerals for Women at Midlife?

Our bodies need a balance of many minerals. A few minerals, however, are particularly meaningful for midlife needs.

CALCIUM   In midlife, when declining estrogen levels leave us vulnerable to osteoporosis, calcium is important for slowing bone loss. Even if you take supplements, it's a good idea to include calcium-rich foods in your daily diet. The calcium in food is accompanied by other important minerals and is more easily absorbed by your body. See Chapter 11, "Boning Up," for more on how to retard osteoporosis as well as a long list of calcium-rich foods.

MAGNESIUM   Recommended as a complement to calcium, magnesium may play a role in reducing the risk of heart disease and is important in building bones and relaxing muscles. Magnesium can help improve sleep and may even help curb chocolate cravings. Foods that contain magnesium include almonds, walnuts, bulgur wheat, beets, broccoli, figs, avocados, and eggs. You can absorb magnesium by soaking in an Epsom salts bath.

BORON   Not mentioned as often as calcium or magnesium, boron helps your body metabolize calcium, and it may help diminish hot flashes and sleep disturbances connected with menopause. If you're taking hormone replacement therapy, it may enhance the effects of estrogen. You only need a tiny amount of boron (2 to 3 milligrams a day)—too much

Colorful Roasted Pepper and Black Bean Burrito

This simple and flavor-packed recipe includes many nutrients and lots of color. Serves four.

Tortillas: Use at least one corn tortilla (preferably made without lard) per person. Steam in a steamer (they'll be very soft) or heat briefly in the oven wrapped in aluminum foil. *(A good source of calcium.)*

Peppers: Roast red and yellow peppers (as many as you like—4 or 5 are sufficient for four people) over the burner or in the broiler until the skin blackens. Let the peppers in a closed brown paper bag for about fifteen minutes to loosen the skin. Then scrape off the skin with a knife or your fingers, remove the seeds, and slice into strips. *(A good source of Vitamin C.)*

Salsa: Dice 2 medium or large fresh tomatoes and 1 small or ½ large red onion. Combine in a small bowl with 1 tablespoon chopped fresh cilantro, about 1 tablespoon lemon juice, and salt to taste. If you like it spicy, mince a jalapeño or serrano pepper and add that. Avocado, used in guacamole, is full of good things but very high in fat. Chop ¼ to ½ avocado and add it to the salsa. *(Tomatoes are a great source of vitamin C and are anticancer agents. Avocados are loaded with potassium, vitamin A, and glutathione, a powerful antioxidant.)*

The beans: Use a 16-ounce can of black beans for four people. Rinse and drain. Heat (or use at room temperature) and bring to the table in a bowl. *(A good source of protein and folic acid.)*

Extras (if desired): A few tablespoons of chopped fresh cilantro, chopped red onion, seeded and chopped fresh serrano peppers, pickled jalapeño peppers, some grated Monterey Jack cheese. Use your imagination!

(continued)

boron can actually take calcium from your bones. If you're eating a variety of foods, you can't miss eating boron. It's found in kasha (buckwheat), whole rye, soybeans, carrots, onions, potatoes, apricots, pears, bananas, shrimp, almonds, and many other foods.

What Is Organic Food?

Organic foods are grown without chemical fertilizers or pesticides. Meats, eggs, and dairy products that are free of hormones and antibiotics and that come from animals raised on organic feed may also be called organic. To be certified organic, a farm must meet these standards and pass inspection by an independent third party. For many years organic foods were available only in health food stores, but now they are widely available. You can find organic foods in supermarkets and in open-air farmers' markets. Eating organic foods whenever possible leaves us less exposed to toxins that could be damaging to our health and that of mother earth.

Should I Take Supplements?

Supplementation is a hot topic. Do we get all the nutrients we need from the food we eat, or do we need to take supplements? Even the experts don't agree on this issue.

In the best of worlds, we would all eat the freshest, most nutrient-rich food possible, containing all of the nutrients (approximately forty-five) our bodies need. But in real life, we're often pushed for time and rely on convenience foods to keep us going. Even if we do eat mostly fresh food, nutrient content varies depending on the soil in which the food was grown. And some nutrients, such as vitamin E, are available mostly in high-fat foods.

Don't go wild with supplements. Real vitamin and mineral deficiencies are not common, and you don't want to overload your system—some vitamins and minerals are toxic in high doses. Also, you can't live on vitamins alone. Foods contain many protective compounds that are not duplicated in supplements, and foods also exercise our digestive tract to keep it working right. Remember, if you're taking supplements, you still have to eat!

You may want to supplement if: You're taking medications, you drink coffee, you drink a lot of alcohol, you smoke or are exposed to cigarette smoke, you don't exercise, your diet is high in simple carbohydrates (white bread, white rice) and junk foods (high in sodium and fat) and low in fruits and vegetables, you are under stress and recovering from illness. If you're interested in supplements, it might be worth your while to talk to a nutritionist or dietitian.

How Can I Find a Dietitian?

If you're struggling with your diet, feel you may have some food sensitivities, or just want some guidance in developing your own food plan, you might consider consulting a nutritionist or registered dietitian. Look for someone with experience, particularly with any issue that particularly concerns you. Try to find someone who designs diets for the individual rather than someone who prescribes the same general diet for everyone, and look for someone who wants to determine your personal needs before designing that diet. Ask about education, and ask for referrals from other clients. For more information, call the National Center of Nutrition and Dietetics: (800) 366-1655. The recorded announcement will refer you to prerecorded messages about nutrition or tell you how to order a free booklet and other products. Call (900) 225-5267 to get a customized consultation with a registered dietitian. This call costs $1.95 for the first minute and 95 cents

EAT IT! (continued)

Burrito: Steam as many corn tortillas as you like and bring them to the table on a plate covered with a clean towel to keep them warm. Put the peppers, salsa, guacamole, and beans on the table and let all put together their own burrito.

free radicals Harmful oxygen molecules that may result from the action of pollution, sunlight, and the normal aging process; they can damage cells. Free radicals are implicated in both heart disease and cancer.

antioxidants Vitamins E and C, beta-carotene, selenium, and other nutrients that help neutralize free radicals and help protect cells from damage.

EAT IT!
Six-Fruit Stew

This dish from Melene's Swedish heritage is a real treat served warm on a cold winter day. You can use any fruits you like—experiment! For added richness, when you use dried fruit, try adding 1/3 cup red wine at the end of cooking and let it reduce.

2 apples, peeled, cored, and chopped into bite-size pieces *(fiber)*

2 pears, peeled, cored, and chopped into bite-size pieces *(potassium)*

1/2 cup dried cherries or 1 can pie cherries (without sugar) *(phytohormones, vitamin A)*

1/2 cup chopped dried Mission figs *(calcium, anticancer properties)*

1/2 cup mixed golden and black raisins *(calcium)*

1/2 cup dried prunes *(fiber)*

1 piece ginger (2 inches long), peeled and finely chopped *(anticancer properties)*

1 or 2 cinnamon sticks *(phytohormones)*

3 or 4 whole cloves *(anti-inflammatory)*

Combine all ingredients in a heavy-bottomed pot and just cover with water. Bring to a boil, lower heat, and simmer until tender, about 20 minutes. Allow to cool slightly, and serve warm with nonfat plain yogurt.

per additional minute. You can also ask for telephone numbers of three registered dietitians in your area based on your zip code.

Are Spicy Foods Harmful?

Contrary to popular myth, spicy foods do not cause ulcers. They do contain an amazing array of healthful helpers.

GARLIC   This ancient medicine contains vitamins A and C, potassium, phosphorus, selenium, sulfur, and amino acids in each potent bulb. It can improve blood pressure and lower cholesterol levels; has antibiotic, anticancer, and antifungal properties; strengthens the immune system; may balance high blood sugar; and has at least ten different antioxidants. If you're worried about garlic odor, neutralize it by eating a handful of fresh parsley.

GINGER   This fragrant root has many wonderful properties: It stimulates digestion, helps with upset stomach and nausea, and is also considered to be an anti-inflammatory and painkiller. Use the fresh root, candied ginger root, ginger syrups, or dried ginger. Steep ginger root in hot water to make tea, or use powdered ginger in capsule form (but be aware that the different forms have slightly different properties).

CHILE PEPPERS   These little pistols are loaded with vitamin C. They also contain capsaicin, which makes them hot and seems to offer protection against heart disease, blood clots, and stroke. Capsaicin is also used in topical treatments for arthritis pain. For some women, spicy foods can bring on hot flashes. If this is you, you'll probably want to cut back on chile peppers for a while.

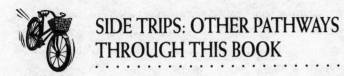

SIDE TRIPS: OTHER PATHWAYS THROUGH THIS BOOK

CHAPTER 2: WHY IS THIS HAPPENING TO ME? You can eat your way through menopause—a pleasant thought! Look here to see what you may have to contend with.

CHAPTER 3: KEEP ON MOVING Diet and exercise are partners in your continued good health. Look here to learn more about all kinds of movement and exercise programs to build bone density, promote balance, and aid cardiovascular health.

CHAPTER 7: THE HOLISTIC KIT AND CABOODLE Diet is an integral part of a number of healing systems. Look here for an overview.

CHAPTER 11: BONING UP Eating calcium-rich foods can help retard osteoporosis. This chapter explores other avenues of good bone health.

CHAPTER 12: AND THE BEAT GOES ON Eating a low-fat diet is one part of preventing heart disease. Look here to learn more about what you can do to protect yourself from this disease that kills more women every year than any other disease.

CHAPTER 13: WHAT ARE MY CHANCES? A number of fruits and vegetables have anticancer properties that may help protect you against breast cancer. Look here to learn more about this disease.

RESOURCES

Organizations and Services

American Dietetic Association (ADA), 216 W. Jackson Blvd., Chicago, IL 60606-6995. Voice: (800) 877-1600. Fax: (312) 899-4899. Internet: www.eatright.org. ADA publishes an annual catalog that features an extensive collection of educational material, books, and tapes dealing with nutrition. The material is related to particular ailments and nutritional needs as well as general nutrition and food supplements. Consumer nutrition information and position papers are available at the ADA web site (see Online).

Center for Science in the Public Interest, 1875 Connecticut Ave. N.W., Suite 300, Washington, DC 20009-5728. Voice: (202) 332-9110. Fax: (202) 265-4954. E-mail circ@essential.org. This nutrition advocacy group periodically publishes information about the nutritive content of fast foods, pizza, Chinese restaurant food, and other staples of the American diet. Call to find out about the group's many projects—the voice mail service is very helpful. The group also publishes the always interesting *Nutrition Action Newsletter* (see Periodicals).

Eating Disorder Awareness & Prevention, 603 Stewart St., Suite 803, Seattle, WA 98101. Voice: (206) 382-3587. This nonprofit organization conducts education and awareness programs and provides some free information.

Food and Drug Administration, 5600 Fishers Lane, Rockville, MD 20857. Voice: (800) 532-4440. This federal agency offers access to phone services and information, including nutrition and FDA-approved food products.

Kushi Institute of the Berkshires, Box 7, Becket, MA 01223. Voice: (800) 97-KUSHI or (413) 623-5742. Fax: (413) 623-8117. E-mail: Kushi@macrobiotics.org. Internet: www.macrobiotics.org. The Institute, located in the middle of 600 acres, offers weekend, week-long, and month-long residential courses in macrobiotics. It also offers a weekend seminar for women that deals with all aspects of women's health.

Society for Nutrition Education, 2850 Metro Drive, Suite 416, Minneapolis, MN 55425-1412. Voice: (612) 854-0035. Fax: (612) 854 7869. E-mail: Lansi001@ gold.tc.umn.edu. This organization offers educational material about nutrition for consumers in both Spanish and English. The video *No Better Gift* is available in Spanish, but only for orders in multiples of four.

The Vegetarian Resource Group, P.O. Box 1463, Baltimore, MD 21203. Voice: (410) 366-VEGE. This action group works to bring vegetarian choices to the menus of hospitals, universities, and schools; it has developed a packet of quality recipes for institutions. The group offers vegetarian teaching materials, including software, as well as recipe books. This membership organization also publishes a newsletter, *Vegetarian Journal.*

Hotlines

The Garlic Information Center: (800) 330-5922. Call to get information about garlic. A free brochure is available. A service of Cornell University.

National Center of Nutrition and Dietetics: (800) 366-1655. This bilingual service offers free referrals to dietitians in your area. You can get advice from a registered dietitian at (900) 225-5267. Cost is $1.95 for the first minute and 95 cents for every minute thereafter.

Soybean Council: (800) 769-4636. Call the help line, "Talk Soy," for lots of information on soy, including recipes.

Catalogs and Products

Gold Mine Natural Food Co., 3419 Hancock St., San Diego, CA 92110. Voice: (800) 475-FOOD. Fax: (619) 296 9756. Call for a catalog that describes the array of products—macrobiotic, organic, and earth-wise foods and other items.

Just Tomatoes, P.O. Box 807, Westley, CA 95387. Voice: (800) 537-1985. Fax: (800) 537-1986. This company has a selection of great-tasting bits of dehydrated or freeze-dried foods in snack-sized packages and larger. Just Veggies is a mix of corn, peas, carrots, bell pepper, and tomato. Just Fruit Crunchies, a mix of apples, blueberries, pineapple, and raspberries, satisfies a sweet tooth *and* qualifies as one or more of your daily fruit servings.

L & H Vitamins, 3710 Crescent St., Long Island City, NY 11101. Voice: (800) 221-1152. Fax: (718) 361-1437. This international company sells vitamins at a 20 to 40 percent discount.

Mountain Ark Trading Company, 799 Old Leicester Highway, Asheville, NC 28806. Voice: (800) 643-8909. Fax: (704) 252-9479. Internet: www.mountainark.com. This is a mail-order catalog for quality natural foods, cooking supplies, natural body care products, herbal remedies, and books—including cookbooks. The company also offers a short course in whole foods and their use.

Nutritious Foods. Voice: (800) 445-3350. This company makes Take Care, the soy protein powder used in a study of plant estrogens and osteoporosis at the University of Illinois–Urbana. The powder dissolves quickly into any liquid you want and comes in plain, vanilla, strawberry, and chocolate. The women in the study ate one or two ounces a day and saw an increase in bone density in their spines. Call for information or to order.

Queen and Company Health Communications, Inc., P.O. Box 49308, Colorado Springs, CO 80949-9308. Voice: (719) 598-4968. Fax: (719) 548-1785. Sam Queen is a nutritionist who specializes in interpreting blood chemistries and connecting them with diet. Mr. Queen offers a consultation service that includes nutritional recommendations. The organization also has printed educational material, books, research reports, and supplements. Call for a catalog.

Vitamin Express, 1428 Irving St., San Franciso, CA 94122. Voice: (800) 500-0733. Internet: www.vitaminexpress.com. This is a neighborhood vitamin shop that does national and international shipping. The prices reflect an effort to pass savings on to customers.

Vitamin Shoppe, 4700 Westside Ave., North Bergen, NJ 07047. Voice: (800) 223-1216. This mail-order vitamin shop offers discounts. Call for a catalog.

Women to Women, 1 Pleasant St., Yarmouth, ME 04096. Voice: (207) 846-6163. This women's medical clinic, run by Dr. Christiane Northrup and three other practitioners, sells some supplements formulated for women. Ask for a price list.

Periodicals

FDA Consumer Magazine, U.S. Food and Drug Administration, HFI-40, Rockville, MD 20857. Voice: (800) 532-4440. This newsletter contains a wealth of information on FDA-related health issues: food safety, nutrition, drugs, medical devices, cosmetics, and more. The FDA also has information on how to read food labels.

Health, P.O. Box 56863, Boulder, CO 80322-6863. Voice: (800) 274-2522. This glossy magazine is available on newsstands as well as by subscription. Each issue is packed with interesting articles and news flashes about food and nutrition as well as other health subjects. It's intelligent and fun to read, and it has great graphics and layout.

Health Realities, Queen and Company, Health Communications, P.O. Box 49308, Colorado Springs, CO 80949-9308. Voice: (719) 598-4968. Fax: (719) 548-1785. This newsletter reports on the latest nutrition news. It's geared to the professional or well-read student of nutrition.

Natural Health, P.O. Box 7440, Red Oak, IA 51591-0440. Voice: (800) 526-8440. This hefty magazine is for readers interested in whole foods, herbs, and alternative health care. Each issue contains a number of articles and regular columns on food and nutrition. It's available in natural food stores, on the newsstand, and by subscription. Andrew Weil and Christiane Northrup have columns here.

Nutrition Action Newsletter, Center for Science in the Public Interest, 1875 Connecticut Ave. N.W., Suite 300, Washington, DC 20009. Voice: (202) 332-9110. Fax: (202) 265-4954. E-mail: circ@essential.org. This newsletter is published by the group that issues reports on the high-fat content of pizza, Chinese food, and other staples of the American diet. The newsletter accepts no advertising and is supported by readers. It provides information about food products, nutritional research, and making wise food choices. It also includes information on nutrition policy. Published ten times a year.

Soy Connection, Missouri Soy Board, 10525 N.W. Ambassador Drive, Suite 202, Kansas City, MO 64153. Voice: (800) TALK-SOY. This newsletter about soy and its uses will keep you up to date on the latest information and research.

Books

American Dietetic Association. *The Complete Food and Nutrition Guide.* Minnetonka, MN: Chronimed Publishing, 1996. All the basics about the food you eat, including fat grams and food additives. This book also discusses ways to lose weight.

Robert A Barnett. *Tonic: More Than 100 Recipes That Improve the Body and the Mind.* New York: Harper Perennial, 1997. Tonics have restorative powers, and not all the tonics in this book are liquid. The author looks at foods like apples, yogurt, cranberries, and more and describes their properties, research, and uses; interesting recipes are included as well.

Robert Crayhon. *Nutrition Made Simple: A Comprehensive Guide to the Latest Findings in Optimal Nutrition.* New York: M. Evans Company, 1996. This book explains the basics of nutrition in a quick, biting, and easy-to-read style. Crayhon is in favor of supplements and discusses them in detail.

Ann Louise Gettleman, M.S., with Lynne Dodson. *Super Nutrition for Women: A Food Wise Guide for Health, Beauty, Energy, and Immunity.* New York: Bantam Books, 1991. Gettleman, the former director of nutrition at Pritikin Longevity Center in Santa Monica, addresses eating and its relationship to hormone function and the immune system. She also looks at the dangers of eating sugar and skipping meals.

Elson Hass, M.D. *Staying Healthy with Nutrition.* Berkeley, CA: Celestial Arts, 1992. This book covers a lot of territory. It reviews diets around the world; discusses the building blocks of nutrition, special diets, and supplement programs; and has a section on building your own diet.

Colin Ingram. *The Drinking Water Book: A Complete Guide to Safe Drinking Water.* Berkeley, CA: Ten Speed Press, 1994. This very thorough book on safe drinking water discusses filters, identification of pollutants, and bottled water.

Gayla J. Kirschmann and John D. Kirschmann. *Nutrition Almanac.* 4th ed. New York: McGraw Hill, 1996. This complete nutritional guide provides you with the quick answers to questions about nutrients and helps you plan a down-to-earth, user-friendly nutritional program. It includes a section on the disease-fighting properties of various foods and many lists of foods and the nutrients they contain.

Mark Messina, Ph.D., and Virginia Messina, R.D., with Ken Setchell, Ph.D. *The Simple Soybean and Your Health.* Garden City Park, NY: Avery Publishing Group, 1994. This book explores the nutritional advantages of the soybean and research related to disease prevention. It also includes recipes and meal plans.

Michael T. Murray, N.D. *Encyclopedia of Nutritional Supplements: The Essential Guide to Improving Your Health Naturally.* Rocklin, CA: Prima Publishing, 1996. You'll find everything you ever wanted to know about vitamins, minerals, EFAs, bioflavonoids, and more in this compendium of facts, explanations, and recommendations. Clear and complete.

Paul Pitchford. *Healing with Whole Foods.* Berkeley, CA: North Atlantic Books, 1993. This book approaches diet through the lens of Eastern medicine and traditions of healing.

Prevention magazine and Alice Feinstein, ed. *Prevention's Healing with Vitamins.* Emmaus, PA: Rodale Press, 1996. This big book takes a look at many different illnesses. It suggests lifestyle changes as well as supplements.

Isadore Rosenfeld, M.D. *Doctor, What Should I Eat? Nutrition Prescriptions for Ailments in Which Diet Can Really Make a Difference.* New York: Random House, 1995. If you are interested in how to prevent and cure illnesses through the food you eat, this is a good place to start. It's based on scientific research, well organized, and easy to read.

Debra Waterhouse, *Like Mother, Like Daughter: How Women are Influenced by Their Mother's Relationship with Food and How to Break the Pattern.* New York: Hyperion, 1997. The title tells it all. A well-researched, easy-to-read, no-blame book that tries to free women from focusing on diet and redirect them to being conscious of health.

Sherry Wilson Saltenfuss, M.S., and Thomas J. Saltenfuss, M.D. *Women's Guide to Vitamins and Minerals.* Chicago: Contemporary Books, 1995. This book discusses vitamins and women's health concerns. It offers guidelines for supplements and also includes exercise and nutrition.

COOKBOOKS

Lissa De Angelis and Molly Siple, *Recipes for Change: Gourmet Wholefood Cooking for Health and Vitality at Menopause.* New York: Dutton, 1996. If you're interested in eating your way through the ups and downs of midlife, this is the book for you. The authors share their knowledge about midlife nutrition with lots of facts, tips, and tidbits. Recipes are healthful, interesting, and tasty, and they list the nutrients you'll get from the meal. It's fun to read, informative, and delicious.

Elson M. Hass, M.D. *A Diet for All Seasons.* Berkeley, CA: Celestial Arts, 1995. Hass addresses diet and individual needs and how to change your diet. He includes sections on avoiding fats, detoxifying, rejuvenation diets, and more. This book, based on Eastern medicine, includes recipes for each of the seasons.

Beth Hensperger. *Baking Bread: Old and New Traditions.* San Francisco: Chronicle Books, 1992. This book takes you through the steps of bread baking and has lots of recipes for bread and some recipes for spreads. Mouth-watering photographs.

Marcia Kelly. *Heavenly Feasts: Memorable Meals from Monasteries, Abbeys, and Retreats.* New York: Bell Tower, 1996. This book is a delight not only for the taste buds but for the aesthetic in all of us as well. There are thirty-nine menus—from Mennonites, Benedictines, and Buddhists, to name a few—with descriptions of the place and people. It's not particularly low fat, but it will nourish you on another level!

Dean Ornish. *Everyday Cooking with Dean Ornish: 150 Easy Low Fat, High Energy Recipes.* New York: HarperCollins, 1996. Ornish again stresses that changes in diet and lifestyle can make a difference in the quality of your life. This book contains slimmed-down versions of favorite comfort foods like French toast and lasagna.

Dolores Riccio. *Superfoods for Women: 300 Recipes That Fulfill Your Special Nutritional Needs.* New York: Time Warner, 1996. The author explains the importance for women of a number of nutrients—fiber, vitamin B, cruciferous vegetables, yogurt, tofu, fish, herbs, spices, teas. Each food topic is accompanied by recipes that use these foods.

Laurel Robertson, Carol Flinders, and Brian Ruppenthal. *The New Laurel's Kitchen, A Handbook for Vegetarian Cookery and Nutrition.* Berkeley, CA: Ten Speed Press, 1986. This is a classic: a good basic vegetarian cookbook with easy-to-follow recipes. It also contains a chapter on special concerns, such as "Nutrition in Later Years," and "Diet Against Disease." There is also a very good section on nutrients, including a chart of the nutrient composition of foods.

Alice Waters. *Chez Panisse Vegetables.* New York: HarperCollins, 1996. The illustrations in this book are so lovely you will want to rip out the pages and frame them. The recipes are good too! Each chapter is devoted to a single vegetable, from amaranth greens to zucchini, illustrated with a colored woodcut. Waters tells you all there is to know about the nature and preparation of each, and follows up with recipes that use the vegetable in all sorts of ways.

Audio/Video

Some of the agencies listed in Organizations and Services, above, have excellent audiocassettes and videotapes available for sale or rental. **Layna Berman** (listing follows) is a good source for a variety of nutrition tapes, as is **Tree Farms Communications**. You'll find this and other good catalogs for tapes on healthful eating in Chapter 7, "The Holistic Kit and Caboodle," and Chapter 8, "What's Up, Doc?"

   Layna Berman, P.O. Box 2714, Petaluma, CA 94953. (707) 769-1458. Layna Berman is a "health integration specialist." She hosts a talk show on KPFA in Berkeley, California, on which she interviews authors and nutritionists of all beliefs, from conservative to way out on the edge. Call or write to get a list of her taped interviews, available for purchase at a small charge.

Online

You'll find all sorts of food discussions online, from restaurant and recipe recommendations to diet plans. Explore the variety

NEWS GROUPS

Discuss food, nutrition, or diet at **alt.support.diet, alt.support.food-allergies, rec.food.veg** (for vegetarians), and **sci.med.nutrition.**

WEB SITES

The International Food Information Council, at ificinfo.health.org, has a wealth of brochures and articles online, including reports on antioxidants and aging, women's health, and cancer and diet, as well as other nutrition information. The **American Dietetic Association**'s site at www.eatright.org has FAQs, nutrition books, resources, member services, and more, including access to the *Journal of the American Dietetic Association*.

Get the latest food and nutrition information from the **U.S. Department of Agriculture**, including the Dietary Guidelines for Americans, at its site: www.nalusda.gov/fnic. To calculate your "ideal weight" and nutritional needs, find out the nutritional breakdown of everything from fast foods to grocery store items, and get recipes and diet tips, go to the interactive **Cyberdiet** site, www.CyberDiet.com.

Vegetarians can explore the **Vegetarian Pages** at www.veg.org/veg or gang together at the **Vegetarians Unite!** site at www.vegweb.com. Both have recipes, nutrition and health information, and networking. For more on soy, see the **Soy Council** page at www.in.net/soy.

5

BREATHE EASY
Stress Relief

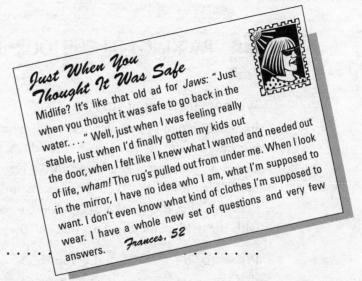

Just When You Thought It Was Safe

Midlife? It's like that old ad for *Jaws*: "Just when you thought it was safe to go back in the water...." Well, just when I was feeling really stable, just when I'd finally gotten my kids out the door, when I felt like I knew what I wanted and needed out of life, *wham!* The rug's pulled out from under me. When I look in the mirror, I have no idea who I am, what I'm supposed to want. I don't even know what kind of clothes I'm supposed to wear. I have a whole new set of questions and very few answers. *Frances, 52*

In a perfect world, stress would not exist. Right? Not necessarily. Stress exists for a reason: Pushing against resistance helps us grow. Physical stress on bones, for example, helps make them dense and strong. Emotional stress can act like a warning bell, letting us know that something in our lives needs our attention. Times of transition, such as midlife, are inherently stressful.

For many women, midlife stress is on a par with adolescent stress. Like teenagers, we have to cope with changing bodies and changing identities, even acne. Never knowing where and when you're going to be hit by a hot flash, waking up drenched, missing your period for two months and then getting it with a vengeance every two weeks—all this can take a toll. Bouncing hormones can leave you feeling unbalanced and disoriented. During this time you may also come up against some life issues that are inherently stressful—becoming aware of the lack of status that often goes along with growing older, losing friends and family members to illness or death, caring for aging parents and adolescent children. Meanwhile, you still have to get on with life—buying groceries, going to work, doing laundry . . . you need a break and you need it now!

Fortunately, help is at hand. You can't avoid stress, but you can learn ways to relieve stress. In *Alta Bates Connection*, cardiologist Jack Edelen puts it this way: "The only time you don't have stress is when you're dead. The challenge is learning how to cope with stress."

 ## PACKING FOR THE JOURNEY

What Are the Signs of Stress?

Ironically, when you're carrying a really heavy load of stress, you may not be aware of it. You know that you've been popping antacids like there's no tomorrow, you know you've been arguing with your partner more than usual, and you can't leave the house without a piece of chocolate, but it may take days or even weeks to connect these feelings with stress. Here are the signs that can tip you off.

PHYSICAL SIGNS OF STRESS   Your body may give you the first signs that you're under stress. You may experience any of the following: increased heart rate, changes in breathing, muscle tension, tension headaches, stomach or gastrointestinal problems, cold hands or feet, sweaty palms, hives, skin eruptions, increased perspiration, fatigue, and shakiness.

MENTAL AND EMOTIONAL SIGNS OF STRESS   Emotional signs of stress are easy to blame on other things. They include difficulty concentrating, anxiety, nervousness, moodiness, depression, self-deprecatory thoughts, irritability, and anger.

BEHAVIORAL SIGNS OF STRESS   Stress can show itself in how we behave with others and in our personal habits. These signs include increased arguing, increased crying, social withdrawal, sleep changes,

GUIDED TOUR: *Relaxation*

Hormonal imbalance and life changes can make midlife pretty stressful, even without added demands. Prolonged stress takes a toll, physically and emotionally. You can't avoid stress altogether, but you can learn how to soothe your frazzled nerves.

WESTERN MEDICINE

Chronic stress can lead to health problems, including high blood pressure, heart disease, and stroke. If you've been under stress for a while, get a check-up.

COMPLEMENTARY THERAPIES

Stress reduction is a basic component of virtually all complementary therapies, which strive to balance the whole system and prevent disease. Homeopathy, herbalism, Chinese herbal medicine, naturopathy, chiropractic, and aromatherapy all offer help for stress.

EXERCISE

Regular aerobic exercise releases tension, improves mood, and counteracts the physical effects of stress. Gentle stretching exercises help you slow down.

MIND–BODY

Most movement and body awareness techniques are geared toward stress reduction. Try yoga, Pilates, Rosen work, Feldenkrais, Alexander technique, t'ai chi, qi gong. Meditation, relaxation response, progressive relaxation, biofeedback, Shiatsu, reflexology, massage, and other techniques are great for easing tension.

NUTRITION

Stress can rob your body of nutrients. A good diet for stress includes a variety of fresh fruits and vegetables and whole grains. Avoid stimulants and depressants—products that contain caffeine, alcohol, or sugar. Eat regularly to keep your blood sugar stable.

SUPPORT

If your stress is simply more than you can bear, a counselor may be able to help you identify triggers and work on coping strategies. Joining a support group is a good way to find out you're not alone.

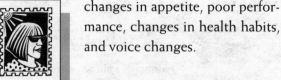

changes in appetite, poor performance, changes in health habits, and voice changes.

What Does Prolonged Stress Do to the Body?

A constant load of stress can really wear you down—just take a look at the list of signs of stress! This kind of pressure is real. According to clinical psychologist and stress expert Kenneth Pelletier in *Mind as Healer, Mind as Slayer,* "Prolonged stress can create physical damage." Stress can deplete your body of nutrients (particularly vitamin B_6, zinc, and magnesium); it can depress the immune system (leaving you open to disease); and it is a major contributor to high blood pressure, heart attack, and stroke. A chronic load of stress can also lead to depression.

stress response (fight or flight) The body's response to danger, real or perceived: Adrenaline and cortisol start pumping through our system, blood vessels dilate, blood rushes to protect the vital organs and extremities become cold, the stomach feels tied up in knots, the heart beats faster; we begin to sweat, and our muscles tense.

How Can I Use Stress to Make Some Positive Changes?

Think of stress as a signal that something needs attention. Transform your attitude: Look at stress not as an intolerable burden but as an opportunity for change, and you'll see a big difference in how you feel about your life, even before you get out from under. Here are some ideas on how to begin:

DO A REALITY CHECK   What's the source of your stress? You may feel as if your life is just one big unraveling ball of anxiety; but when you break it down, you may be able to identify individual problems you can solve one at a time.

LET GO OF WHAT YOU CAN'T CONTROL   Some things are out of your hands. Reflect on them, but don't use your energy worrying about them. For example, you can't control how other people act or the passage of time.

GIVE UP SOME OF YOUR RESPONSIBILITIES If you're doing too much, ask friends and family to help you with the load. See if you can find at least one job that someone else can do.

FIND SUPPORT Feeling isolated can be very stressful. Share what you're going through with friends and family. Support groups can also be a wonderful source of help and comfort.

How Can I Dissolve Stress Without Really Trying?

Taking care of ourselves doesn't have to mean 100 percent intensity on the issues. Sometimes the best thing to do is—nothing. Take a deep breath, then take another one, and then take another one. . . . Here are some more ideas:

PET YOUR PET According to zoologist James Serpell, author of *In the Company of Animals*, pet owners report fewer minor health problems, think less about problems, and tend to be happier with their lives. One study found that you can lower your blood pressure simply by petting a cat or a dog. If you have allergies, watching fish swim around a tank will do the same thing.

TAKE A BREAK Get up from whatever you're doing—right now. Walk around the block, sit in the sun. Stop working and loosen your shoulders. Water your plants. Take a five-minute break, watch a movie (preferably a comedy!), go for a run, learn a new skill, paint a picture, read a book.

TAKE A BREATH Breathing is the basis of life. When we're relaxed, we breathe easily. When we're tense, we tend to hold our breath or constrict the chest muscles, making breathing more difficult. Paying attention to your breathing is a great way to release tension and

Low-Stress Eating

When you're under stress and out of time, it's easy to grab a candy bar, a cup of coffee, or a fast-food lunch—or skip a meal altogether. Unfortunately, this will play havoc with your blood sugar and make you feel even more irritable and fatigued. Even if you're running late, try to eat regularly (carry healthy snacks with you in case of emergency), and eat foods that will help keep you on an even keel. The important nutrients for stress, according to nutritionist Robert Crayhon, are protein, vitamin B-complex, antioxidant vitamins C and E, essential fatty acids, and magnesium. For more on eating well, see Chapter 4, "Are You What You Eat?"

- Eat regularly to maintain blood sugar levels.
- Eat complex carbohydrates to increase energy and serotonin levels (for a feeling of well-being), including whole wheat products and pasta, perhaps the ultimate comfort food.
- Keep protein servings small (3 ounces of protein is considered to be one serving).
- Eat a variety of fresh fruits and vegetables— bananas, potatoes, and onions are particularly calming when you're under stress.
- Eat foods high in vitamin B-complex, such as whole grains, legumes, dark green vegetables, fish, and poultry.
- Eat foods high in vitamin C, such as peppers, broccoli, citrus fruits, strawberries, and papayas.
- Eat foods high in vitamin E, such as whole grains, sweet potatoes, avocados, mangoes, almonds, eggs, and olive oil.
- Eat foods that contain essential fatty acids: flaxseed oil; cold-water fish (mackerel, salmon, sardines); dark, leafy greens.
- Eat foods that contain magnesium: whole grains, dried beans, spinach, figs, shrimp, egg yolks.
- Sweeten your food with honey, which is said to have a calming effect.

quiet your anxious mind. Many mind–body practices include attention to breathing, and some of the books listed under Resources (in this chapter, and in Chapter 7, "The Holistic Kit and Caboodle") include instructions on breathing techniques. Here's an easy way to begin: Exhale, squeezing the air out of your lungs. You'll inhale naturally, filling your lungs. Now pay attention to your breathing. Breathe in a slow, relaxed way, and try to make the inhalations and exhalations the same length. Don't force your breath, or try to fill your lungs. Eventually, you may feel as if you are "being breathed." Enjoy!

GET SOME SLEEP You'll deal with stress much more effectively if you've had enough sleep (we don't think as well when we lose sleep). If you can't get at least eight hours at night, try to take a short nap during the day. Even twenty minutes will help.

TALK TO FAMILY AND FRIENDS You may have unwittingly taken on more than your share of responsibilities. Talk to supportive family members and friends for ideas about how you can lighten your load.

TALK POSITIVELY TO YOURSELF If your mind is filled with thoughts of self-doubt, self-blame, or fear of the future, it's no wonder you're stressed out and not sleeping! Focus instead on acknowledging what is going well in your life and give yourself credit for it. Remind yourself that, for the most part, the things we most fear never happen. Allow yourself to be hopeful instead of fearful.

PULL YOUR HAIR When stress makes you want to tear your hair out, try this ancient

Chinese stress-reduction technique: Pull your hair gently, a small segment at a time, tugging at your scalp for thirty seconds. Move on until you've relaxed your entire scalp.

GET A MASSAGE   Few things are more calming than a good hands-on massage. No matter what you choose—a Swedish massage, acupressure, Shiatsu, or any of the many varieties—you can work out the knots and feel yourself melt. According to the American Massage Therapy Association, the best massage for stress is a foot massage—not only does it feel good, but it also lowers levels of cortisol and norepinephrine, the so-called stress hormones.

LIMIT CAFFEINE   Some people are unaffected by caffeine, but for others it can bring on palpitations, anxiety, and headaches. If you're already under some kind of stress, you don't need to add to it. If you're taking the low-dose birth control pill, you may have an increased reaction to caffeine.

WORK IN THE GARDEN   Gardening works on stress from all sides. It's exercise, it smells good, it creates awareness, it takes your mind off of all the details of life, you're creating beauty, and you can reflect on the cycles of nature. . . . And if you're growing vegetables, you're eating right too!

Can Exercise Help Relieve Stress?

Regular physical activity decreases tension and anxiety, increases feelings of well-being, and enables you to do more work. And you don't need a long, hard workout to dissipate stress. Regular, moderate exercise is one of the

Birthday at the Spa

For the last few years, I've spent my birthday at the spa of a nearby hotel. For under $100 (it makes a lovely gift!) I get to pretend I'm a hotel guest. Not only do I get all the spa stuff, like the hot tub and massage, I get to enjoy warm, clean towels, a shower someone else has to clean, and complementary fresh fruit, herbal tea, and water with cucumber and lemon slices. I can't imagine a more pleasant way to begin my personal year.   *Toni, 50*

TRAVEL TIP
Make an Eye Pillow

If you've never relaxed with an eye pillow over your eyes, you've missed out on one of life's great experiences. This is a wonderful way to take a relaxing ten-minute break or to help you fall asleep. Eye pillows are long silk rectangles filled with flax seeds (and dry lavender, if you like). The gentle, comforting weight of the flax seeds helps eye muscles rest, and the lavender and soft silk are soothing. You can make one yourself. Here's how:

1. Cut a square of soft silk, about 7 by 7 inches (it can be larger or smaller, depending on your preference).

2. Stitch together all four sides, leaving a small opening. Turn the pillow right-side out, fill with flax seed and lavender, and stitch up.

Don't overfill the bag—you want it soft and floppy enough to form to your face. Try it out and relax.

best and fastest routes to feeling more hopeful and less burdened. See Chapter 3, "Keep on Moving," for details.

What Does Complementary Medicine Offer for Stress?

You've hit the jackpot here. Most healing systems have built-in stress reducers.

ACUPUNCTURE   An acupuncture "tune-up" can bring you closer to balance by relieving stress and promoting energy. You can de-stress with an acupuncture session that is designed to lower anxiety by stimulating endorphins, the brain chemicals that make us feel good. If thinking about needles makes you nervous, try acupressure or a Shiatsu massage.

AROMATHERAPY   According to herbalist Jeanne Rose, these are the four best essential oils to relieve anxiety: spearmint and rosemary verbenon (to be relaxed and alert), and ylang-ylang and lavender (to be relaxed and drowsy). Sniff from the bottle (we each keep a bottle of lavender on our desk at all times!) or relax in a lavender-scented bath.

BACH FLOWER REMEDIES   Rescue Remedy seems to be everyone's favorite flower remedy for most stressful situations, from falling down to recovering from surgery. Try Aspen for anxiety, Elm if you're feeling overwhelmed.

HERBS AND BOTANICALS   Valerian is the herb of choice for calming anxiety. You may also want to drink a cup of stinging nettle tea (it won't sting you this way) to calm your anxious feelings.

Relax at work? It seems like a contradiction in terms. But what if someone brought a massage chair to the office, invited you to sit down, and began working out those knots? TouchPro Resources, an organization that trains and certifies people to do chair massage, will provide you or your employer with names of nationally certified practitioners in your state. For information, call (888) 777-7817.

Can Mind–Body Practices Help Prevent Stress?

Nowhere is the connection between mind and body so clear as when we are under stress. Just an anxious thought can cause muscles to tighten and heart rate to increase; worrying about the future or dwelling on the past is sure to create some degree of stress. Being present in the moment can make you feel as if time is slowing down and it can allow new solutions to enter the suddenly open spaces of your mind. When you seriously need to take stress out of your life, consider mind–body methods. Biofeedback and meditation are two excellent techniques. Movement practices, such as yoga, qi gong, t'ai chi, Alexander technique, and Rosen work, are also aimed at integrating mind, body, and spirit and creating awareness of the present moment. For more on movement, see Chapter 3, "Keep on Moving."

What Is Biofeedback?

Can we regulate the responses of our autonomic nervous system? That's what practitioners of yoga and other techniques claim, and the proof is in biofeedback. In this learning process, you're hooked up to instruments that give you information—feedback—about your biological processes, such as blood pressure, heart rate, brain waves, and body temperature. Through trial and error, you can learn to regulate these processes by breathing techniques, by relaxing certain muscles, by thinking calm thoughts, and so on. You'll soon find what works for you. As a stress-reduction technique, biofeedback is an eye-opener. When you see what stress is doing to your body and you also learn what you are able to do to bring your body's responses to a livable rate, you can't help but relax.

What Is Meditation?

Meditation has been practiced in many societies and virtually all religions for hundreds and even thousands of years as a way to quiet the mind and

You may not be able to laugh *all* your troubles away, but you can definitely lighten your load:

- According to Loma Linda University researcher Lee Berk, laughter can significantly increase measures of immune function, from T cells that battle infection to levels of gamma interferon.
- Research by psychologist Peter Derks at the College of William and Mary shows that laughter involves the entire cerebral cortex. He postulates that stimulating the brain's pleasure centers boosts the immune system.
- Laughter has been shown to relax muscles and lower blood pressure.
- You don't even have to be happy. Researchers have found that simply forming your lips into the *shape* of a smile begins a response that will make you feel happier.

A Scented Bath

This is my favorite way to relax: I go to my garden, pick a handful of lavender and a handful of rosemary. Then I put the herbs in a muslin bag, crush it gently, and toss it into a warm bath. The rosemary clears my mind, the lavender calms me down, and the scent is fabulous.

Jessie, 53

Traveling alone can help you develop your survival skills and increase your ability to trust yourself. It may not be easy, and you may have some scary moments; but in the end it's almost sure to be worth the effort. Here are some tips to get you started, adapted from Jay Ben-Lesser's *Foxy Old Woman's Guide to Traveling Alone.*

Read to develop comfort and knowledge: Start reading the travel section of your local newspaper. Reading travel stories by other women will also help you gain confidence, comfort, and knowledge.

Practice going it alone: Gradually build comfort in being by yourself—go to the theater alone, take yourself out to a good dinner. Make it easy on yourself: Pick a show or restaurant that won't make you feel too conspicuous or fearful.

Practice being adventuresome and assertive: Eventually, work up to taking yourself out to better restaurants or productions. Ask for what you want—a better table or a menu variation—without feeling as though you really don't deserve it.

By the time you're ready to take your trip, you won't have to spend time worrying about how you're ever going to manage on your own because you'll already know. Now you can just relax and enjoy. Bon voyage!

body. Today, an amazing variety of people and organizations, from the most conservative to the cutting edge, recommend meditation and meditation-based techniques as the number-one way to relax. According to the American Heart Association, a daily twenty-minute Transcendental Meditation session can lower blood pressure.

VARIETIES OF TECHNIQUES You can meditate in a number of ways—with walking meditation and sitting meditation, with eyes open or eyes closed, with Transcendental Meditation or the relaxation response, with techniques from the Buddhist, Christian, or Jewish traditions. All these types of meditation have one thing in common: They are a way to quiet the mind, connect with the spirit, and learn to live in the present rather than dwell in the past or future. As we quiet the mind, the body also becomes quiet; heart rate drops, breathing slows, muscles relax, blood pressure drops, and we are open to a feeling of well-being. People meditate for many reasons—to live rich, full lives despite chronic pain, to go more deeply into spiritual beliefs, to become participants in their own well-being, to cultivate skills of self-nurturing. And in so doing, stress is dissolved without effort. Midlife is an especially good time to take a deep breath, clear your mind, and allow your life to flow.

LEARNING TO MEDITATE The best meditation technique for you is the one that you can best make work in your life. Whether you practice for five minutes a day, twenty, or more, taking the time out will serve you well. It is possible to learn to meditate by yourself, but most teachers of meditation agree that the best way to learn is in a group. Teachers and other group members can give clear instructions and help with problems and questions—How can I keep my foot from falling asleep? What if my mind just won't shut up? That guy coughing in the corner is really distracting. An added bonus is the opportunity to join a community of like-minded people. It's relatively easy to find a meditation class. Check your local hospital's stress-management clinic, the YMCA, a local Buddhist meditation center, the

Traveling with Women

I love traveling with my family, but traveling with women is something really special. In my experience, women are much more inclined to cut each other some slack, not to be so tied down to schedule, really supportive of inexperience, willing just to let things happen.

Grace, 47

Jewish Community Center, or your local church. See Resources for sources of meditation books and tapes.

Are There Any Vacation Spots on the Midlife Journey?

You bet. The midlife journey isn't *all* slogging through the mud. Nothing clears your head like taking a vacation. Just getting away, even for a day, can give you a new perspective on life. And vacations can cost as much or as little as you can afford. Wherever you go, make it a real vacation and leave home *at* home: Don't take the cell phone or the laptop!

DAY TRIPS   A day may not seem like much, but there's a lot to be said for the therapeutic effects of a change of scenery. The possibilities are endless: Go for a drive, take a hike in the country, go camping, walk on the beach, go fishing, go skiing, take a day-long bike trip, spend the night at a spa, visit a friend in another city, pretend you're a tourist and explore your own city, take the train or fly somewhere you've never been.

RELAX AT A SPA   If you'd like to relax and spend some money at the same time (that is, if spending money doesn't stress you out even more!) consider spending a day or two at a spa. Spas have everything you need for relaxation—sauna, hot tub, steam room, massage. Some spas have mud baths, seaweed wraps, manicures, and more. Plus, being treated like a welcome guest and pampered

TRAVEL TIP
An Apple a Day in Another Way

The scent of green apples can increase alpha wave activity, reduce anxiety, and relieve headaches.

too is a great way to rejuvenate. To find a spa near you, look in the yellow pages or check nearby hotels. If you're out of town, try Spa Finders (see Resources).

SEEK PEACE OF MIND   Daily life at the end of the twentieth century is increasingly noisy and rushed. We are exposed to electronic overload and so much information that it is hard to find time and space to experience quiet. If your spirit needs a break, consider a retreat at a spiritual center, convent, or monastery. You do not have to be a practicing Buddhist or Catholic to benefit from these peaceful places, which welcome guests of all beliefs. They offer simple living, quiet times, sitting meditation, and more. Let stress fall away, absorb the silence (once you get used to it), and find thoughts and ideas ready to come forth. Here you can experience serenity and nurture reflection. Recharge your spirit, find yourself, listen to yourself, appreciate yourself. Surprisingly, many retreat centers are very reasonably priced. For books on finding spiritual retreat centers, see the Resources in Chapter 17, "The Inner Journey."

TAKE A WOMEN-ONLY VACATION   Consider taking a "women-only" vacation. Women who travel with another woman or a group of women often return with a sense of greater competence and personal power. These trips can provide an opportunity to learn many new skills, experience independence, and develop a sense of camaraderie with other women through sharing new challenges. Plan a trip with a friend, or check out tour organizations that cater to vacations for women only. See Resources for ideas.

TAKE A MIDLIFE JOURNEY   Taking a journey that coincides with the midlife transition is an increasingly popular option for a number of women. This kind of trip is a conscious attempt to parallel the ritual stages of midlife: separation, unknowing, and return. Don't overplan this kind of trip. Leave room in your time of unknowing to discover the unexpected and to connect with yourself in a new

TRAVEL TIP
Sink into Restorative Yoga

Hatha yoga practice is energizing yet calming, a wonderful thing for both mind and body. Restorative yoga, developed by hatha yoga master B. K. S. Iyengar, is aimed at relieving stress. According to yoga instructor and author Judith Lasater in *Relax and Renew,* "The antidote to stress is relaxation. To relax is to *rest deeply.*" These practices, in which you do each pose while your body is fully supported by "props" such as bolsters and pillows, make you feel deeply rested almost immediately. See Resources for more information.

way. This can be an exciting and profound opportunity to honor, acknowledge, and process the physical, emotional, and spiritual changes of midlife.

SIDE TRIPS: OTHER PATHWAYS THROUGH THIS BOOK

CHAPTER 3: KEEP ON MOVING Exercise is a great stress reducer. Look here to learn more about what constitutes a good exercise program.

CHAPTER 4: ARE YOU WHAT YOU EAT? Eating the right foods and avoiding the wrong foods can help you deal with stress and stay healthy. Look here for information.

CHAPTER 15: EVERYBODY NEEDS ME NOW If you're a caregiver, stress is almost inevitable. Look here for some ideas on how to take some of the stress out of caregiving.

CHAPTER 16: GETTING HELP Sometimes even a little stress is too much. Look here for information on getting the emotional help you need to deal with your situation.

CHAPTER 17: THE INNER JOURNEY A satisfying spiritual life can help put things in perspective. Look here to explore this deepening process.

RESOURCES

Organizations and Services

American Institute of Stress, 124 Park Ave., Yonkers, NY 10703. Voice: (914) 963-1200 or (800) 24-RELAX. E-mail: stress124@earthlink.net. Internet: www.stress.org. A resource and clearinghouse for information on stress-related matters. The AIS evaluates stress-reduction techniques and stress-management programs currently being offered to industry and the public. It publishes a monthly newsletter, *The Newsletter of The American Institute of Stress*, with information, reviews, and events related to stress and cancer, stress and heart disease, women and stress, stress and children, job stress, and more. For a fee, the Institute will also put together packets of information on aspects of stress and stress-reduction techniques.

American Massage Therapy Association, 820 Davis St., Suite 100, Evanston, IL 60201. Voice: (847) 864-0123. Fax: (847) 864-1178. This is a nonprofit association of professional massage therapists who practice a variety of massage techniques. To find someone for your specific needs or health concerns, contact the national office. You'll be put in touch with your local chapter (there's one in every state), which in turn will give you some referrals.

Biofeedback Certification Institute of America, 10200 W. 44th Ave., Suite 304, Wheat Ridge, CO 80033. Send a stamped, self-addressed business-size envelope to receive printed material on biofeedback and a list of practitioners in your area.

Academy for Guided Imagery, P.O. Box 2070, Mill Valley, CA 94942. Voice: (800) 726-2070. Fax: (415) 389-9324. Call for a directory of imagery practitioners, a catalog of books and tapes, and general information about the technique.

The Mind/Body Medical Institute, Deaconess Hospital, 1 Deaconess Road, Boston, MA 02215. Voice: (617) 632-9525. Fax: (617) 632-7383. Internet: www.med. harvard.edu/programs/mindbody. Dr. Herbert Benson, author of *The Relaxation Response*, operates this clinic, which offers programs on stress reduction and related topics. You can also order a series of stress-response audiotapes or call to find out about local affiliates of the Mind/Body Medical Institute, which offer programs on stress reduction, pain, and more.

Rolf Institute, 205 Canyon Blvd., Boulder, CO 80306. Voice: (800) 530-8875. Fax: (303) 449-5978. (303) 449-5903. E-mail: rolfinst@aol.com. Internet: www.rolf.org. Call to ask for a referral to a trained Rolfer in your area.

The Shealy Institute, 1328 East Evergreen St., Springfield, MO 65803-4400. Voice: (417) 865-5940. Fax: (417) 865-6111. This institute offers a comprehensive health care program for people suffering from stress, pain, and depression. The program is multidimensional and includes exercise, nutrition, and relaxation components.

Stress Management Research Associates, 9725 Louedd, Houston, TX 77070. Voice: (281) 469-6395. Fax: (281) 469-6976. Call or write for free printed information on stress reduction. This group also sells a series of relaxation tapes.

TouchPro Resources. Voice: (888) 777-7817. Call to find out about certified chair massage practitioners in your state. You sit in a chair and rest your weary body while they go to work. They are available to come to your place of work, or even to massage the necks and shoulders of your support group. For information on workshops and seminars, call (800) 999-5026.

WOMEN-ONLY TRAVEL

Call of the Wild, 2519 Cedar St., Berkeley, CA 94708. Voice: (510) 849-9292. E-mail: trips@callwild.com. Women-only wilderness backpacking, hiking, and camping trips—featuring great food—in the American West, Alaska, and Hawaii. Trips are designed for different levels of ability, and some use animals or vehicles to haul the equipment. Owner Carol Latimer, author of *Wilderness Cuisine,* has more than twenty years of experience as a wilderness guide and outfitter. Pre-trip classes teach women practical skills to demystify the wilderness.

Camping Women, 7623 Southbreeze Drive, Sacramento, CA 95828. Voice: (916) 689-9326. This organization offers outdoor experiences for women interested in camping, backpacking, hiking, canoeing, and white-water rafting. The group's objectives include providing opportunities for women to experience an outdoor program in a supportive atmosphere, helping women become comfortable in the outdoors, and developing women's camping and leadership skills.

Hawk, I'm Your Sister, P.O. Box 9109, Santa Fe, NM 87504. Voice: (505) 984-2268. Beverly Antaeus, a midlife woman herself, leads women's wilderness journeys, including canoeing, in the United States, Russia, and Peru.

Olivia Travel, 4400 Market St., Oakland, CA 94608. Voice: (800) 631-6277. E-mail: Olivia@eor.com. Internet: oliviatravel.com/. This women-only travel business is a leader in its field. Olivia offers many trips for lesbians, including cruises in many parts of the world and trips to Club Med.

Outdoor Vacations for Women Over Forty, P.O. Box 200, Groton, MA 01450. Voice: (508) 448-3331. Fax: (508) 448-3514. E-mail: ov40fun@aol.com. This company has been leading outdoor vacations for women over forty for fourteen years. Hiking, rafting, canoeing, skiing, snorkeling, sea kayaking, canal boating, sailing, biking. Trips are in the United States and abroad.

Rainbow Adventures, 15033 Kelly Canyon Road, Bozeman, MT 59715. Voice: (800) 804-8686. E-mail: rainbowadv@aol.com. Worldwide adventure travel—kayaking, canoeing, sailing, hiking, walking, fly-fishing, and more—for women thirty and up. Travel groups average about ten women ranging in age from thirty to seventy-five years of age.

RVing Women, P.O. Box 1940-MV, Apache Junction, AZ 85217 Voice: (602) 983-4678. Fax: (602) 982-6125. This organization has a membership of about four thousand. It offers rallies, events across the country, and a support system for women who travel in their RVs alone. A newsletter is published six times a year. The member directory allows women to network.

Sheri Griffin Expeditions, Box 1324, Moab, UT 84532. Voice: (800) 332-2439. Fax: (801) 259-2226. E-mail: classriver@aol.com. This company offers some women-only rafting trips and will do private charter trips in the United States.

Woodswomen, 25 W. Diamond Lake Road, Minneapolis, MN 55419. Voice: (800) 279-0555. Fax: (612) 822-3814. This nonprofit women-only travel company is celebrating twenty years of offering trips all over the world. It offers both adventure travel and vacations for women, and publishes *Woodswomen's News*, a quarterly that lists the company's trips and adventure travel.

Hotlines

American Institute of Stress: (800) 24-RELAX. Ask about information packets on stress-related topics that interest you.

Headache Hotline: (800) 843-2256. Call for information on headaches—causes and treatment, a list of physicians in your area who are experienced in treating headaches, and information about the newsletter on headaches (subscription only).

Spa Finders: (800) 255-7727. Consultants at this full-service reservation agency for spas located around the world will help you pick one that suits your needs. Ask about the annual catalog of spas and free quarterly newsletter.

Products and Catalogs

Christine Columbus, P.O. Box 2168, Lake Oswego, OR 97035-0643. Voice: (800) 280-4775. This mail-order catalog is devoted to women travelers. It offers a complete assortment of travel essentials for comfort, safety, and convenience.

Living Arts, P.O. Box 2939, Venice, CA 90291. Voice: (800) 254-8464. Fax: (800) 582-6872. A great catalog for all things soothing: meditation tapes, healing music, silk eye pillows filled with flax seed and lavender, meditation pillows, yoga blankets, Chinese teapots, and more.

Periodicals

Maiden Voyages Magazine, 109 Minna St., Suite 240, San Francisco, CA 94105. Voice: (510) 528-8425. Fax: (510) 528-5163. E-mail : info@maiden-voyages.com. Internet: maiden-voyages.com. This quarterly magazine is for women who love to travel or dream about travel. *Maiden Voyages* starts from the premise that "journeys taken by women are different from those taken by men. Women are as absorbed with point of view and the transformative process of the journey as they are with the destination." Filled with information by and for the female traveler, the magazine also includes a calendar that lists travel by and for women and tips for solo travel.

Massage Magazine, 1315 W. Mallon Ave., Spokane, WA 99201. Voice: (800) 533-4263. This magazine contains a lot of information for professionals, but you can also learn a lot about the latest news and techniques of massage. It has a very good resource section.

The Women's Traveller, P.O. Box 422458, San Francisco, CA 94142. Voice: (415) 255-0404. This annual guide caters primarily to lesbian women traveling in the United States and Canada—where to stay, maps to help you get there, bookstores, services, and much more.

Books

Herbert Benson and Eileen Stuart. *The Wellness Book.* Secaucus, NJ: Carol Publishing Group, 1993. This comprehensive book addresses preventive measures to ensure health and also gives ideas for treatment of stress-related illnesses. Stuart and Benson, who developed the relaxation response, include mind–body techniques.

Larry Blumenfeld, ed. *The Big Book of Relaxation: Simple Techniques to Control the Excess Stress in Your Life.* Roslyn, NY: The Relaxation Company, 1994. This book looks at meditation, yoga, food for relaxation, aromatherapy, music, creative visualization, and more. Well-known practitioners contribute chapters on their fields of expertise. It also contains a good collection of resources.

Alice D. Domor, Ph.D., and Henry Dreher. *Healing Mind, Healthy Women: Using the Mind-Body Connection to Manage Stress and Take Control of Your Life.* New York: Henry Holt, 1996. Dr. Domor, from the Harvard Medical School of Behavioral Sciences, offers therapeutic methods to protect and enhance life. She also discusses methods to help women with health problems, including menopause, endometriosis, and breast cancer.

Alix Kirsta. *The Book of Stress Survival: Identifying and Reducing Stress in Your Life.* New York: Simon and Schuster, 1986. This book has a questionnaire to help you figure out how to address stress. It gives a lot of helpful tips on stress-proofing your life.

Mirka Knaster. *Discovering The Body's Wisdom.* New York: Bantam Books, 1996. This book talks about all kinds of mind–body practices, from acupressure to zero balancing. The author explains the theory of each practice and offers exercises to help the reader experience it. The book also contains some consumer tips.

Susan M. Lark, M.D. *Anxiety and Stress: A Self-Help Program.* Los Altos, CA: Westchester Publishing, 1993. This self-help stress-management book covers all the bases, from conventional medicine to complementary techniques.

Judith Lasater, Ph.D., P.T. *Relax and Renew: Restful Yoga for Stressful Times.* Berkeley, CA: Rodmell Press, 1995. Lasater, a respected Iyengar method yoga teacher, has put together a wonderful program of simple restorative yoga poses designed to restore energy while stretching and toning your body. Chapter 14, "Opening to Menopause," is devoted to poses that the author says "should help you feel calmer, less fatigued, and less battered by your perimenopausal experiences."

Kathleen McDonald. *How to Meditate: A Practical Guide.* Boston: Wisdom, 1984. This book, written by a Tibetan Buddhist nun and meditation teacher, is a good introduction to meditation.

TRAVEL

Jay Ben-Lesser, *A Foxy Old Woman's Guide to Traveling Alone, Around Town, and Around the World*. Freedom, CA: Crossing Press, 1995. Lots of good tips for getting yourself acclimated to traveling alone before you begin your journey.

Bernard Burt. *Fodor's Healthy Escapes—Spas, Fitness Resorts, and Cruises*. Fodor Travel Publications, 1995. Describes spas, fitness resorts, and cruises, and what they offer in the United States, Mexico, Canada, and the Caribbean. A great way to explore the world of spas.

Judith Gilford. *The Packing Book*. Berkeley, CA: Ten Speed Press, 1994. If you always want to take your entire wardrobe on vacation with you, even though you know you'll wind up wearing the same three things, this is the book for you. Learn how to decide what to bring and how to pack, unpack, and repack easily and quickly. It really works.

Jean Gould, ed. *Season of Adventure, Traveling Tales and Outdoor Journeys of Women Over 50*. Seattle: Seal Press, 1996. An inspirational collection that illuminates the fact that the spirit of adventure doesn't wane with age but that women gain a sense of increased courage and sense of self. The stories illustrate women's ability to capture with keen awareness the landscapes and cultures of new places.

Natania Jansy and Miranda Davies, eds. *More Women Travel: Adventures and Advice from More Than 60 Countries. A Rough Guide Special*. London: Rough Guides, 1995. This book addresses the pleasures, concerns, and pitfalls of women traveling alone, and discusses different culture and customs as they apply to women. This book includes solo treks in the Himalayas and Malaysia; backpacking in Canada and India; and working in Japan and Greece.

Ellen Lederman. *Vacations That Can Change Your Life: Adventures, Retreats and Workshops for the Mind, Body, and Spirit*. Naperville, IL: Sourcebooks, 1996. This book is a resource for many transformative vacations. Visiting a holistic center or taking a spiritual vacation, a social action workshop, or a learning vacation are just a sample of what you'll find in this book.

Mary Morris, ed. *Maiden Voyages: Writings of Women Travelers*. New York: Random House, 1993. This book is a collection of writings by women travelers and travel writers. It offers reflections on a gender as illuminated by unfamiliar surroundings and experiences.

Thalia Zepatos, *Adventures in Good Company: The Complete Guide to Women's Tours and Outdoor Trips*. Portland: The Eight Mountain Press, 1995. This well-known travel editor describes 100 companies worldwide that offer adventure travel and vacations for women.

Thalia Zepatos. *A Journey of One's Own: Uncommon Advice for the Independent Woman Traveler*, 2d ed. Portland: The Eight Mountain Press, 1996. Zepatos focuses on women's tours and outdoor trips with a blend of advice, practical information, and stories of her adventures and how travel has made her a confident person willing to take risks. The book includes a directory of tour organizers.

Zoe. *Women Going Places: A Woman's Complete Guide to International Travel.* London: Women Going Places Production, 1996. This book gives a very thorough list of accommodations and facilities for lesbians and women only, but no descriptions.

Audio/Video

A wealth of audiocassettes and videotapes is available on various strategies of relaxation and meditation. Some of the agencies listed in Organizations and Services have tapes for sale or rent. **The Mind/Body Medical Institute,** for example, has a number of relaxation response tapes made by Herbert Benson, M.D., and other physicians. Check the catalogs listed here and in Chapter 7, "The Holistic Kit and Caboodle," and Chapter 17, "The Inner Journey," to see which ones intrigue you.

Sounds True, 735 Walnut St., Boulder, CO 80302. Voice: (800) 333-9185. A good source for meditation and relaxation audio- and videotapes. This source carries Deepak Chopra, Jack Kornfeld, Jon Kabat-Zinn, Thich Nhat Han, and many more.

AUDIO

Letting Go of Stress. Emmett Miller, M.D. Available from Audio Editions, P.O. Box 6930, Auburn, CA 95604-6930. Voice: (800) 528-2737. Miller, a noted hypnotherapist, instructs in techniques for easing the tension in daily life.

Mindfulness Meditation in Everyday Life. Dr. Jon Kabat-Zinn. 2 hours. Available from Sound Horizons (see Audio/Video, Chapter 7). Kabat-Zinn is the director of the Stress Reduction Clinic at the University of Massachusetts Medical Center. This tape includes natural ways to meditate and to reduce stress by learning to be more self-aware and fully present in the moment.

Spectrum Suite. Steven Halpern. Available from Inner Peace Music, P.O. Box 2644, San Anselmo, CA 94979. Voice: (800) 909-0707. This is peaceful music that claims to align and attune the chakras.

VIDEOTAPES

The Inner Art of Meditation. Jack Kornfeld. 90 minutes. Available from Sounds True. A how-to video course in meditation: Awareness of Breath, Working with Body Sensations, Awareness of Thought and Feelings, and The Practice of Lovingkindness. Kornfeld is a well-known therapist, author, and meditation instructor who lived as a Buddhist monk for six years.

The Joy of Stress with Loretta La Roche. Available from The VideoFinders Collection (see Audio/Video, Chapter 8). Loretta La Roche, a stress-management expert, explains how you can use humor and laughter to de-stress your life and even improve your health.

Online

Relaxing while sitting in front of the computer is a neat trick, but at least you can find out how to de-stress when you get up from your chair. For stress-related links, see the Online section in Chapter 3, "Keep on Moving," Chapter 7, "The Holistic Kit and Caboodle," Chapter 8, "What's Up, Doc?," and Chapter 16, "Getting Help." Search the Internet for the words *stress* and *stress management*. Most online health and women's magazines, such as **Women's Wire** (www.women.com) have articles or columns about stress reduction. For travel-related links, search for the keywords *travel* and *women's travel*.

MAILING LISTS

The **insight** list is a discussion of Buddhist meditation, although you do not have to be a Buddhist to participate. For subscription information, contact Majordomo@world. std.com.

NEWS GROUPS

For meditation talk, try **alt.meditation**. For stress-reducing scents, try **alt.aromatherapy**, and for relaxing herbs check out **alt.folklore.herbs**. And for information about massage, try **alt.backrub**.

WEB SITES

To get you off to a good start, how about a nice, relaxing massage? For answers to all your massage questions and links to other relaxing sites, try the **alt.backrubs** FAQ, at www.ii.uib.no/~kjartan/backrubsfaq.

Maiden Voyages Adventure & Tour Guide Directory, maiden-voyages.com/ ventures.html, is an online directory of companies owned by women, run for women, or "geared toward a woman's sensibility" that provide tour opportunities and traveling goods and services. It's prepared by *Maiden Voyages* magazine.

6

LOOKING GOOD
Appearance

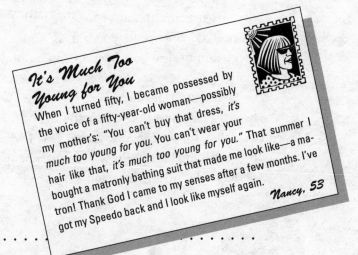

Beauty, it is safe to say, is in the eye of the beholder. But when that's your own eye beholding your changing self, it can become much more problematic. In our society beauty is often equated with youth, and when we meet midlife, we know that we are no longer young. Aging is a taboo subject and aging women are particularly invisible— most women entertainers begin plastic surgery procedures early on. For many of us, continuing to look good and feel comfortable with the image we project to others is important. It's also important to feel at home in our own changing bodies.

As is abundantly clear to every woman in midlife, youth is fleeting. We will live the second half of our lives as older women. Coming to terms with the fact that we age and letting our experiences, wisdom, and strengths be the basis for feeling good about ourselves can be the foundation for inner beauty and a sense of peace. Our attitude about ourselves as we age will in many ways be important in *how* we age.

Looking good begins with accepting who we are. Realistically, we are not going to conform to our culture's idea of perfection, which is fleeting for everyone. Several hours spent in a women's locker room will let you know in no uncertain terms that every woman's body is different. Several days or months spent in this sort of observation will tell you that every woman's body is hers and hers alone, and you'll begin to see that each has its own unique beauty.

When you look at yourself in the mirror, really look at the face and body you see in front of you—look with awareness. See yourself as you are now, not as you wish you still were or as you fear you may be some day. Treat yourself and your body with respect, and try to be as kind in your comments to yourself as you would be to a friend. When you begin to deal with your changing body, do it with awareness and gentleness.

There's no right or wrong way here. We can choose to enhance a healthy face and body with the many products and procedures now available. Or we can take good care of what we have and grow to love it more. Dress it up, dress it down, change its image. Seek your own perfect solution and have fun with it.

 PACKING FOR THE JOURNEY
. . . .

TRAVEL TIP
Collagen-Age Gals

Collagen, the substance that firms up the skin and plumps up the lips, is another thing that changes in midlife. According to *Recipes for Change,* eating potatoes, tropical fruits, and cashews, which contain vitamin C, B$_6$, and copper, can aid our bodies in manufacturing collagen.

What Causes Skin Changes in Midlife?

The skin is the body's first line of defense, and it's out there taking abuse from the environment all of our lives. Most skin changes can be blamed on environmental wear and tear. So even without hormonal changes, it's bound to show some wear and tear after a while. Here are some factors that can change your skin:

GUIDED TOUR: *Looking Good*

As our bodies change in midlife, so does body image. Understanding your looks in the present tense can help you feel good about yourself. You can't turn back time, but you can repair some damage to skin and hair. If you treat your body with respect—and give it plenty of exercise, plenty of rest, and good nutrition—your appearance will reflect the care.

WESTERN MEDICINE

For skin: A dermatologist can help you evaluate your skin. Petroleum jelly and AHA creams can help retain moisture; sunscreens, AHA creams, Retin-A, Renova, skin peels, dermabrasion, and similar procedures may help mitigate sun damage; plastic surgery and laser treatments may help firm skin.

COMPLEMENTARY THERAPIES

For skin: Improve your skin health and tone with an acupuncture facelift, aromatherapy, massage, meditation, and other stress-reduction techniques.

EXERCISE

For skin and hair: A regular program of exercise promotes blood flow to the skin, which keeps it healthy. (Don't forget that your scalp is part of your skin!) *For weight control:* Regular exercise combined with a healthful diet is effective in weight reduction and maintenance.

MIND–BODY

For skin: Yoga, t'ai chi, and similar techniques promote grace and balance and reduce stress, which makes you look better and improves circulation. Regular relaxation or meditation practice will also help your facial muscles to relax. *For weight:* Some women notice a change in weight distribution from regular practice.

NUTRITION

For hair, skin, and weight: A healthful diet low in fat and high in fiber and nutrients ensures the inner glow that radiates through your skin; a balanced diet combined with regular exercise is effective in weight reduction and maintenance.

AGING As we get older, our skin feels drier because epidermal cells (the cells on the surface of the skin) are replaced more slowly. The skin loses elasticity because two important components of the epidermis, elastin and collagen, weaken over time, and there are also changes in subcutaneous fat. Lips begin to lose fullness, and skin may seem thinner (actually, the thickness is just more variable than it used to be). Many women report that their skin is more sensitive. And the pull of gravity, which has been working on us invisibly for many years, contributes to sagging jawlines.

photoaging Skin damage—lines, blotchy "age" spots, leathery skin—and other changes attributed to aging that are really caused by years of exposure to the sun's ultraviolet rays.

HORMONAL CHANGE Hormonal changes around menopause may contribute to adult female acne—it's ba-ack! Even though estrogen clearly has some effect on the structure of the skin, apparently it's not enough. It does seem to help the skin retain moisture (as it helps with moisture in other parts of the body), but it is not advertised as a product that can keep your skin youthful.

SUN DAMAGE (PHOTOAGING) Sun damage is cumulative—the tanning you did in your twenties is going to come back to haunt you now! Excess sun exposure (too much ultraviolet A and B rays) hastens the loss of collagen and elastin. Over the years, repeated tanning and burning gives skin a leathery look and feel. Overexposure to the sun can also lead to lines and wrinkles, freckling, and those brown splotches we refer to as age spots or liver spots. Although the tendency to wrinkle is inherited to some degree, sun damage can cause wrinkles. Most important, too much of the sun's warming rays can damage the skin's DNA and may lead to skin cancer.

Why Me?

What's with this *acne* all of a sudden? I know it's just changing, but it really feels like my body's turning against me. *Sheryl, 48*

FREE RADICALS One area of controversy involves free radicals, unstable chemicals that are said to form when the skin is exposed to excessive pollutants, sunlight, poor diet, and certain toxins. (No, they're not activists left over from the 1960s.) In some cases, free radicals can rearrange the genetic code in DNA, leading some people to suspect that free radicals cause wrinkles and other signs of aging. Antioxidants such as vitamins A, C, and E are thought to be able to "mop up" free radicals, alter immune response to carcinogens, and absorb UV radiation. Whatever the ultimate outcome of this debate, it *never* hurts to eat your fruits and vegetables!

SMOKING If you love your skin, don't smoke. Smoking dries your skin and adds lines to your face, making you appear years older than you actually are.

Do All Skin Types Age at the Same Rate?

No. The sun breaks down lighter skin much faster than darker skin. This is because darker skin has more melanin (that's what gives it the color) and is generally thicker. Lighter skin tends to be drier and thinner. A dark-skinned African American woman, for example, will show fewer effects from the sun than will her lighter-skinned sister, and a red-headed, fair-skinned woman will show the effects of photoaging much sooner. No matter how light or dark your skin is, however, you are still susceptible to the harmful effects of ultraviolet rays (this means tanning salons, too!).

Reflections

The other day I told my mother how great she looked, how I appreciated her attitude and her style, and just her life in general—she's seventy-three, and she really knows how to live. And I was surprised at how much it meant to her, and how seldom she hears these things reflected back to her. I realized how important it is for us to acknowledge each other as we get older. Compliments aren't rationed!   *Evelyn, 48*

POINT OF INTEREST
The Return of Acne

Many women in midlife awaken one day to find themselves beset by the scourge of their adolescence: acne. Even women who never had acne in youth may experience what dermatologists call "adult female acne." The causes are not certain, although hormonal changes and stress are both thought to play a part. Here are some things you can do help yourself (acne can be stubborn, so be patient):

1. See a dermatologist to rule out other causes. Acne rosacea, for example, can look like adult female acne, but it's treated differently. For stubborn cases, your doctor may prescribe antibiotics or topical creams. (You may want to use a humidifier, especially in winter—these creams can be drying.)

2. If your acne is mild, try calendula cream, or soothe your skin with moistened mint tea bags (you can drink the tea too).

3. Make some lifestyle changes. Get more exercise to relieve tension, take time out, destress any way you can.

4. Try complementary therapies. Acupuncture and traditional Chinese medicine offer treatments for problem skin, including advice on how to eat.

Ten Simple Things You Can Do for Your Skin

Until someone finds a way to stop the aging process dead in its tracks, here are a few simple things you can do to minimize the effects of aging on your appearance:

1. Get adequate rest. Stress and fatigue show up in your face even more as you get older.

2. Stop smoking. Smoke wrinkles skin faster than almost anything else.

3. Exercise regularly. Exercise increases circulation and blood flow to the skin. Nothing looks healthier and says "I feel good about myself" than the post-exercise glow.

4. Eat a variety of fresh fruits and vegetables. A healthful diet means healthier skin and hair, and an adequate supply of antioxidants (vitamins A, C, E, and beta-carotene) may help ward off the effects of free radicals.

5. Limit your alcohol intake. Alcohol is dehydrating, and excess alcohol may cause spider veins in your cheeks.

6. Stay hydrated. Drink at least six to eight glasses of water a day. Hydrated skin is plumper and healthier looking.

7. Use a good sunscreen daily. Sunscreen (SPF 15 or higher) helps prevent premature aging of the skin and is especially important when you are using Retin-A or Renova.

8. Moisturize. Adequately moisturize and hydrate your skin daily, both with creams and a facial mist.

9. Relax. Stress makes you scrunch up your face.

10. Make peace with yourself. It's your face: You earned it, and no one else has it. Appreciate the way only you can look.

Can I Mitigate Sun Damage?

All is not lost! Consistent use of sunscreen will protect your skin now and may prevent future damage. As far as repairing the damage that's been done, tretinoin (the active ingredient in Retin-A and Renova) can erase age spots (keratoses). According to the American Academy of Dermatology, retinoic acid and alpha hydroxy acids both show promise in reversing sun damage, although neither has been approved by the FDA for this use.

According to skin-care expert Zia Wesley-Hosford in *Fifty and Fabulous*, "Regardless of what state your skin is in or how old you look, real improvements can be made . . . with proper treatment, which includes working from the inside out with good nutrition, supplemental vitamins, and exercise; and working from the outside in with daily skin care, appropriate use of cosmetics, and various nonsurgical skin and body treatments." This holistic approach to skin care makes sense to us—a rested, relaxed, well-nourished person who is paying attention to the needs of body and spirit can't help but reflect that self-valuing behavior in her face!

Can Skin Creams Help Repair Skin Damage?

To varying degrees, yes. Here's a brief tour of the creams that are available as of this writing.

ALPHA HYDROXY ACID (AHA) Alpha hydroxy acid (AHA) creams and gels are derived from foods such as grapes, milk, and citrus. You can find them in virtually every supermarket, drugstore, discount beauty store, and cosmetics counter. AHAs seem to be a safe, natural way to exfoliate the skin. You may not be able to get all your facial lines to disappear, but over a period of months your skin will look healthier, become moister, and even reflect light better. If you stay within the 3 to 5 percent range of AHA products, side effects are minimal. However, effectiveness of AHA varies with concentration of the cream and condition of your skin, and concentrations can be as high as 10 percent in over-the-counter creams. AHAs can cause stinging and redness and also irritate your eyes—so be careful. You can pay any price for AHAs, from $6.95 at discount chains to $125 at cosmetics counters. A lot of $10.50 creams work just as well as the expensive ones. Try one of these first, and remember: You need only one AHA product.

RETIN-A   Retin-A is an acid derivative of vitamin A that has tretinoin as its active ingredient. It helps to retard the effects of chronic sun exposure, such as age spots and premature wrinkling. There is also good evidence that Retin-A can decrease the frequency of precancerous spots (actinic keratosis). Retin-A must be prescribed by a physician. It is relatively inexpensive but requires a lifetime commitment—if you stop using it, your skin will return to its original condition. Many people who use Retin-A find it drying and irritating. Retin-A lowers the threshold for sunburn, so use a very heavy moisturizer and at least an SPF 15 sunscreen.

RENOVA   Renova is another prescription cream that has FDA approval as a wrinkle warrior. It increases cell turnover and collagen production and reduces the keratoses. Like Retin-A, it has tretinoin as its active ingredient, but has a creamier emollient base. Renova also increases your skin's sensitivity to sun, so be sure to use sunscreen.

VITAMIN C CREAMS   This is the latest in the quest for smoother skin. Scientists have done preliminary research on a liquid vitamin C,

Cellex-C, which can penetrate the skin and prevent the damage done by free radicals as well as speed collagen growth. These are promising results, but there is more research to be done. Cellex-C is available at certain salons and stores. Check Resources for ordering information.

Creams Aren't Helping. What About Cosmetic Procedures?

Several nonsurgical and surgical cosmetic procedures can help your skin. Consult a dermatologist to determine the best treatment for your skin.

COSMETIC PEELS This procedure repairs uneven pigment and sun damage along with fine lines. An acid of varying strengths is used to remove the top layers of the skin. This procedure is better for light-skinned women because there tends to be less risk of pigment alteration.

DERMABRASION This procedure repairs deeper imperfections and scars with the use of a high-speed rotary tool, something like a sander. Like chemical peels, it is better for light-skinned women.

COLLAGEN INJECTIONS Bovine collagen is used to temporarily get rid of wrinkles. The emphasis is on *temporary*: The effect of plumpness diminishes in three to nine months. You will need to be tested for allergic reaction.

FAT INJECTIONS You really have to want this one. The doctor removes fat from fat places on your body (like the buttocks and belly). The fat is then cleaned of blood and other fluids, and injected into lines and wrinkles. This procedure must be done once a month for a year to be effective, but because it is your own fat there is no danger of allergic reaction.

LASER RESURFACING The goal here is to remove the sun-damaged, age-spotted, and wrinkled outer layers of the skin. This new laser procedure consists of short bursts of energy that vaporize surface skin cells and don't

POINT OF INTEREST
Getting a Facial

Why get a facial? To relax, feel pampered, and be nice to your skin. A good esthetician (that's what they're called) can get your skin cleaner than you ever dreamed possible. All kinds of facials are available, and you will want to pick one that suits your needs.

Choose an esthetician the same way you'd choose a doctor. Recommendations from friends are a great way to start. Make sure the person you choose is licensed and experienced. If you are using Retin-A or anything else that makes your skin particularly sensitive, be sure to share this information. Here are some cleansing activities you may experience during a basic facial:

- Gentle exfoliation of dead skin
- Steaming to open pores
- Gently unclogging pores
- Head and neck massage to relax muscles and help blood circulation
- Facial mask to tone skin

harm the deeper layers, which then regenerate new, smoother skin. This is a fairly new procedure, and the risks and benefits are still being evaluated. Make sure your surgeon has been trained in this technique, and ask how many surgeries he or she has performed.

Admirable Women
When I think of women I admire—Katherine Hepburn, Jessica Tandy, Angela Lansbury, Audrey Hepburn, Georgia O'Keeffe—you never notice their makeup, you just remember them: Simple, elegant, natural. *Bea, 52*

PLASTIC SURGERY The ultimate surgical procedure, plastic surgery can tighten skin, remove puffy bags from under eyes, and remove the excess skin over the eyes that can sometimes interfere with vision. Some procedures are now done with a laser rather than a scalpel. Check with a qualified plastic surgeon to learn more.

Can Eating the Right Foods Help My Skin?

If you eat a balanced diet that includes a variety of fresh fruits and vegetables, you'll find it's hard not to get the vitamins and minerals your skin needs. And don't forget to drink plenty of water to keep your skin hydrated. For more on specific foods, see Chapter 4, "Are You What You Eat?"

VITAMINS The antioxidant vitamins (including A, C, and E) that are good topically may also benefit your skin from the inside out, possibly helping protect against skin cancer and photoaging. Vitamin C also helps the skin make collagen.

MINERALS Magnesium and zinc are skin-friendly minerals. And don't forget the bone-builder, calcium: Your skull is bone too, and if your skull shrinks, your skin will sag.

BAD FATS Hydrogenated fats are terrible for the skin, and a diet high in any type of fat, especially saturated fats, can also add to your risk of getting skin cancer. Avoid margarine

TRAVEL TIP
That Crawly Feeling

Who makes up these names? *Formication* (from the root word for "ants") is actually an appropriate name for the sensation of itching, crawling skin that occasionally occurs in midlife. At the very least, it's annoying. And at the worst, it can cause a dry, scaly looking skin that can scab if you scratch it. If this is a problem for you, soothe the sensation with cold compresses and moisturize with a cream that contains calendula.

According to El Cerrito, California, dermatologist Camilla McCalmont, M.D., when it comes to moisturizing, the choice is fairly simple: "There are two basic ways to moisturize skin: the old-fashioned, greasy way or the newfangled AHA way. Greasy moisturizers work by sealing in moisture. Plain petroleum jelly is the prototype for this type of moisturizer, and is, by itself, an excellent moisturizer." Despite its availability and low cost, however, most women don't like the esthetics of petroleum jelly, which is greasy, can clog pores, and takes work to remove.

Alpha hydroxy acids give skin a cleaner feel because they work by taking away the top dry layers of skin cells. "The younger cells underneath hold water better," says McCalmont, "giving the skin a softer, moister feel." What's in between? Other moisturizer bases include vegetable oil, silicon, gel, and liposome. Experiment to find the one that's right for you.

and fried foods, and check package labels to make sure you're not buying food that contains hydrogenated fats.

GOOD FATS Your skin oil is monounsaturated, so eating monounsaturated oils like olive oil and almond oil makes good sense. Essential fatty acids, found in salmon, tuna, flaxseed oil, and other sources, are also very important for skin.

Can Complementary Therapies Help My Skin?

A number of complementary treatments can help improve the health of skin—from the inside *and* the outside.

FACIAL MASSAGE A gentle facial massage will increase the flow of blood to the face and bring oxygen to your skin. Try acupressure or Shiatsu for a change of pace.

AROMATHERAPY A wide range of botanicals can help improve your skin, including rose and cypress for broken capillaries, clary sage and geranium for dry, aging skin, and bergamot and lavender for acne.

HERBAL THERAPY In *The Herbal Menopause Book*, Amanda McQuade Crawford suggests drinking teas made from the following herbs to tone skin gently, "from the inside out": sarsaparilla (*Smilax ornata*), horsetail (*Equsetum arvense*), and yellow dock root (*Rumex crispus*).

ACUPUNCTURE "FACELIFT" An acupuncturist can improve muscle tone, increase blood flow to the face, and help rid the skin of toxins in a facial rejuvenation technique that's thousands of years old. It requires successive sessions over a period of months, but is said to be effective even between treatments.

MEDITATION Stress is behind many skin problems, including fine lines and adult acne. Daily periods of meditation or other stress-reduction techniques can clear your skin as well as your mind.

What's Happening to My Hair?

Both men and women lose hair as they age, and women in midlife begin to notice thinning hair in the pubic area as well as on the head. Although some hair loss is associated with declining estrogen levels,

hair thinning appears to be more a factor of age; a heredity component is also involved, as in male pattern baldness.

Hair also changes color and texture: Gray hair is usually coarser, drier, and less flexible than the hair it is replacing.

Recent research suggests that prematurely gray women—about 50 percent gray before age forty—may be predisposed to osteoporosis. According to one study, their risk is four times greater. If this is you, check Chapter 11, "Boning Up," for tips on retarding and preventing bone loss.

What Can I Do About Facial Hair?

Getting older also means that hair begins to grow where we don't want it: the upper lip, chin, and sometimes around the nipples. This is due to plunging estrogen levels, which may not be high enough to offset the effects of the male hormone testosterone. Here's how to remove unwanted facial hair:

TWEEZE IT   If it's just a few stubborn hairs growing out of your chin, pull them out yourself with tweezers.

WAX IT   To get rid of mustache hair completely (this will not work on coarse chin hair), try waxing. It's really not as bad as it sounds! You can do it yourself, or have it done professionally by a licensed esthetician. A word of warning: If you're fair-skinned,

The Six Most Aging Looks for Hair

1. Too permed.
2. Too colored.
3. Too much height on top.
4. Too "done" (Tammy Faye Bakker).
5. Anything "cute" (Rose Marie and that darn bow).
6. "L.A. mall hair" (spiral perm with too much highlight).

thin-skinned, or using a product like Retin-A that makes your skin particularly sensitive, consult with a dermatologist before waxing.

TRY ELECTROLYSIS For really stubborn hair problems, consult a licensed electrolysist. This procedure is time-consuming and uncomfortable, but it is permanent.

What Can I Eat to Make My Hair Healthy?

The health of your hair begins with what you put in your body. A healthful diet will reflect itself in the health of your hair. Your hair is protein, so make sure you eat enough good-quality protein to support its health. The same vitamins that are beneficial for your skin also contribute to the health of your hair, particularly vitamin A and the B-complex vitamins (in particular folic acid, B_{12}, and pantothenic acid).

Is Weight Gain Inevitable in Midlife?

Weight gain is a big complaint of women reaching midlife. But does weight gain have to be part of growing older? There is some debate on this. Certainly, it depends on your body type and metabolism. Some women are thin and stay thin throughout their lives, some women who never had trouble maintaining their weight find themselves gaining in midlife, and some women have a lifelong struggle maintaining their weight.

With perimenopause come body changes: Fat deposits itself differently (on the back, waist, and stomach in addition to the hips and thighs); breasts get larger and lose elasticity. The proportion of lean muscle in our body decreases. Some of this has to do with the fact that we tend to exercise less as we get older, but much of this is

Remember Your Hands
One summer day when I was driving home from vacation I suddenly looked at my hands and realized they were getting a tremendous amount of sun. Now I always keep a tube of SPF 15 sunblock in my purse and in the glove compartment of my car. And most of the time I remember to use it!   *Marlene, 39*

related to (what else?) hormones. One theory is that we gain weight because our body is trying to hang on to its estrogen, which is stored in fat tissue.

Why would it want to do that? Weight does seem to have some protective qualities as we age. Thinner women, for example, are more at risk for osteoporosis. On the other hand, obese women are more at risk for diabetes, heart disease, breast and other cancers, and stroke. Maintaining a reasonable weight for your height and build is not just a question of vanity, but is also important for your good health.

What Can I Do to Maintain My Weight?

The increased ratio of fat to lean tissue in midlife means that both exercise and diet are increasingly important to maintaining your weight. Fat requires fewer calories to maintain than muscle, and our metabolic rate declines as we get older. So we need to do *more* exercise as we get older, not less! (See Chapter 3, "Keep on Moving," for more information.) A diet rich in high-fiber foods, fruits and vegetables, and lower in high-fat foods (like red meat, whole dairy products, and junk foods) will not only give you the nutrients and energy you need to live your daily life, it will help you keep off pounds you don't want or need.

My Hair! My Makeup! Aarrgh!

Most of us have an image of ourselves as we were in our twenties or thirties. When the image we see in the mirror no longer reflects this younger self, we panic. How do we dress this older woman? How do we do our hair? Do we need less makeup or more? These questions may seem frivolous, but for many women they are the basic questions of how to face the world every day. As we age, skin, hair, and body tone change. The colors we look good in change. Makeup needs to change. Adjusting to change doesn't mean abandoning yourself, but refining and redefining your personal style.

What Are Some Makeup Tips for Midlife?

You can make a number of small changes and adjustments in the way you conceive of your makeup to keep your look fresh and alive. In general, says hair cutter and consultant Lee Ringlaro, "avoid iridescent anything—lipstick, eye shadow, blush. Lipstick collects in lines and only shows them up more. Intense eye shadows, blusher, and lipstick are for the very young. Past a certain age they can look garish and a little sad." Here are some more ideas.

MAKEUP   Keep makeup to a minimum. A heavy foundation will work its way into the creases and amplify wrinkles. Powder cuts down on light reflection, so avoid it. If you must use powder, use it very lightly—you want fresh, shining skin, not dull, powdery skin. *Things to try*: After you apply moisturizer, mix a tiny amount of foundation and moisturizer together in your hand, then apply to your face—you will find the makeup has a softer look to it. Skin looks more natural with a bit of shine.

EYE SHADOW   Always use matte eye shadows in natural colors—gray-browns or taupe for all eye colors. Never match your eye shadow to your eye color or to your clothes—you want people to notice your eyes, not your eye shadow. *Things to try*: As you get more lines around your eye area, apply foundation mixed with moisturizer to your eyelid (lightly, leaving off the eye shadow). Then, next to your eyelashes, smudge eye-liner pencil in gray or light brown or taupe—this gives a softer look that is more flattering to your eyes. If you have heavily lined eyes or a heavily overhanging lid, leave off all eye shadow and

1. Use a gentle shampoo.

2. Use a lighter-weight conditioner during the week and a deeper conditioner once a week, once a month, or once every six months—whenever your hair needs it.

3. Get a good haircut. This means one that suits your hair and your lifestyle, not your friend's hair or your fantasy of what your hair *should* be.

4. Work with your hair, don't fight it. The secret of a good haircut is to let your hair do what it does naturally. If it curls, let it be curly. If it's straight, let it be straight. Here's the test: If you can go for a walk in the rain, and your hair looks as good after the walk as it did before, you've got it!

5. Regardless of what your mother may have told you, there is no rule that says older women must have short hair!

eye pencil and apply a smidgen of petroleum jelly on the lids for a little shine. Your eyes will have a wonderful, healthy glow.

LIPSTICK   Lips have a tendency to get smaller with age, and many of us will have small lines around the mouth. Dark lipstick not only makes lips look smaller, but when it feathers into these areas it is also very noticeable. Medium to soft colors, such as peach, soft rose, pink-brown, blush, and natural, are shades everyone can wear. *Things to try*: Outline lips with a nude or natural lip pencil. Fill in with one of the shades above. The lip pencil will help the feathering—the more natural your lips look, the less you have to worry about your lipstick.

BLUSHER   Blusher should look as if nature did it, not your local cosmetics counter. Look for colors with names like Barely Peach, Bare Blush, Next to Natural. Apply color to the apple of the cheek and make sure you blend. Check for lines, then blend again. *Things to try*: Use a tiny bit of lipstick rubbed lightly with fingertips across cheeks.

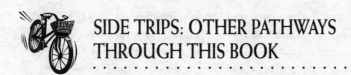

SIDE TRIPS: OTHER PATHWAYS THROUGH THIS BOOK

CHAPTER 2: WHY IS THIS HAPPENING TO ME?   Many women notice skin and hair changes around the time of menopause, and there are other changes as well. Look here to understand what's going on with your body.

CHAPTER 3: KEEP ON MOVING   Exercise is great for everything, including the health of your skin and hair and your ability to maintain a healthy weight. Look here for ideas about exercise programs.

CHAPTER 4: ARE YOU WHAT YOU EAT?   Beauty, as they say, starts from the inside. Look here for nutritional roads to good hair, skin, and weight.

CHAPTER 7: THE HOLISTIC KIT AND CABOODLE   Many ancient (and still viable) health care systems are very nurturing to hair and skin. Look here to find other avenues to explore.

RESEARCH

RESOURCES

Organizations and Services

American Academy of Dermatology, 930 N. Meacham Road, Schaumburg, IL 60173. Voice: (847) 330-0230. This group has public information and educational material, plus referrals to dermatologists in your area. You can request a catalog that includes educational information, posters, and videos, all for sale.

American Academy of Facial Plastic Surgeons, 1110 Vermont Ave. N.W., Suite 220, Washington DC, 20005. Voice: (202) 842-4500. Contact this organization for a referral list of facial plastic surgeons in your area.

American Society for Dermatologic Surgery, 930 N. Meacham Road, Schaumburg, IL 60173. Voice: (800) 441-2737. Fax: (708) 330-0050. A good source of consumer information regarding dermatological procedures. Ask for a referral list of surgeons in your area.

National Institute of Aging, National Institutes of Health, Information Center, P.O. Box 8057, Gaithersburg, MD 20898-8057. Voice: (800) 222-2225. Fax: (310) 589-3014. E-mail: niainfo@access.digex.net. Internet: www.nih.gov/nia. Ask for free printed material on skin care and aging.

Office of Cosmetics and Colors, Food and Drug Administration, 200 C St. S.W., Washington, DC 20204. Voice: (800) 205-4061. This is a voluntary regulatory program for producers of cosmetics. Its database records complaints and allergic reactions to products and suggests steps to take if allergic reactions occur.

Skin Cancer Foundation, 245 Fifth Ave., Suite 1403, New York, NY 10016. Voice: (800) SKIN-490. Fax: (212) 725-5751. Ask for complimentary information on skin cancer, types and detection.

Hotlines

American Hair Loss Council: (800) 274-8717. Call for information on hair loss.

American Society for Dermatological Surgery: (800) 441-2737. Call for information about any dermatology procedure.

Cellex-C: (800) 423-5539. Call to find out where you can purchase Cellex-C in your area or how you can receive free information on the product.

FDA Cosmetic Complaint Line: (800) 205-4061. Call this consumer information line with questions about cosmetic products or adverse reactions to any FDA-approved cosmetic product.

Plastic Surgery Information Service: (800) 635-0635. Call to get a list of board-certified plastic surgeons in your area or to check on board certification of a particular surgeon.

Products and Catalogs

Avena Botanicals, 219 Mill St., Rockport, ME 04856. Voice: (207) 594-0694. This woman-owned-and-operated herbal business offers herbal body-care products.

The Body Shop of the USA, Box 1409, Wake Forest, NC 27588-1409. The Body Shop has a wide variety of beauty and self-care products made of natural and organic ingredients. No animal testing.

Jeanne Rose Aromatherapy, 219 Carl St., San Francisco, CA 94117-3804. Voice: (415) 564-6785. Fax: (415) 564-6799. Herbalist Jeanne Rose's catalog includes books, hydrosols, and aromatherapy kits. You can also request information on classes, intensives, and certification.

Paula's Choice, 5418 S. Brandon, Seattle, WA 98118. Voice: (800) 831-4088. E-mail: paulab@accessone.com. Paula Begoun, who researched commercially available cosmetics for a number of years, has produced her own line of reasonably priced, fragrance-free cosmetics.

The Raj, Maharishi Ayur-Ved Health Center, 1734 Jasmine Ave., Fairfield, IA 52556. Voice: (800) 248-9050. Contact the Raj for their catalog of Ayurvedic and herbal skin and hair products.

Shepherd's Garden Seeds, 30 Irene St., Torrington, CT 06790. Voice: (860) 482-3638. Fax: (860) 482-0532. A seed catalog for gardeners that offers great botanicals. The "Complete Skin Care Seed Collection" contains seeds for growing herbs to use in making your own cosmetics and step-by-step instructions on how to make a cucumber facial mask, calendula shampoo, and lavender skin toner.

Snow Mountain Botanicals, P.O. Box 337, Potter Valley, CA 95469. Voice/Fax: (707) 743-2642 or (707) 743-2037. E-mail: harnish@pacific.net or msherb@pacific.net. This company grows its own herbs in the foothills of the California coastal range and buys wild herbs when necessary. The range of herbal extracts for women includes Valarian Compound for sleep and nerve restoration and Gotu Kola Compound for brain and memory. The company also prepares a healing skin salve made with calendula and other herbs.

Transitions for Health, 621 S.W. Alder, Suite 900, Portland, OR 97205. Voice: (800) 888-6814. Fax: (800) 944-0168. Send for a catalog from this woman-owned company, or call toll free to ask questions about the products. Products range from ProGest cream to remedies for memory, PMS, and stress, to vitamins, herbs, and skin-care products.

Periodicals

Cosmetics Counter Update, Beginning Press, 5418 S. Brandon, Seattle, WA 98118. Voice: (206) 722-7200 or (800) 831-4088. E-mail: paulab@accessone.com. This bimonthly newsletter reviews new cosmetic products, fashion trends, shampoos, and conditioners. Send for a free introductory copy. You can also subscribe to the newsletter by e-mail. It is less expensive but not formatted—your choice!

Skin Basics, Zia Cosmetics, 410 Townsend St., San Francisco, CA 94107. Voice: (800) 334-7546. This newsletter reviews other skin-care products and offers some great information on everything from thigh creams to cosmetic laser surgery. You can call to get a copy in the mail or pick one up at your local health food store.

Books

Philip B. *Blended Beauty: Botanical Secrets for Body and Soul.* Berkeley, CA: Ten Speed Press, 1995. All kinds of body-care products you can make at home using ingredients you probably already have in your kitchen. The recipes are clear and easy to follow, and each tells you exactly what it's used for and how long it will keep.

Paula Begoun. *Don't Go to the Cosmetics Counter Without Me.* 3d ed. Seattle: Beginning Press, 1996. If you get confused by the array of cosmetics that are available, this is the book for you. Begoun has been studying cosmetics for a number of years, and in this latest edition she reviews more than 10,000 products (no wonder you're so confused!) and discusses the latest in skin-care information.

Paula Begoun. *Don't Go Shopping for Hair Care Products Without Me.* Seattle: Beginning Press, 1995. Begoun reviews the latest in hair-care products. She describes the ingredients and points out the ones that are likely to cause allergies.

Wilma F. Bergfeld, M.D., F.A.C.P, with Shelagh Ryan Masline. *A Woman Doctor's Guide to Skin Care: Essential Facts and Up-to-the-Minute Information on Keeping Skin Healthy at Any Age.* New York: Hyperion, 1995. This book address how to clean and moisturize your skin and how to care for hair and nails. It also contains a test to determine skin type so you can better select products. The section that helps you determine when it is time to see a dermatologist is valuable.

Body Shop Team. *The Body Shop Book.* New York: Penguin, 1994. This book tells you all about taking care of your body's appearance. It includes a section on aging along with the where, why, and how-to of skin, hair, and body care. You'll also find beauty recipes to make at home.

Bobbi Brown. *Beauty: The Ultimate Beauty Resource.* New York: HarperCollins, 1997. Bobbi Brown's emphasis is on a natural look. This book gives basic techniques and information on makeup for different occasions, from a job interview to a gala opening. She includes chapters on makeup for women in their forties and fifties, for African American, Asian, and Hispanic women, for women undergoing chemotherapy, and more.

Jessica B. Haris. *The World Beauty Book, How We Can All Look and Feel Wonderful Using the Natural Beauty Secrets of Women of Color.* San Francisco: HarperSanFrancisco, 1995. This book contains a collection of stories, recipes, and beauty secrets from women of color around the world.

Michelle Dominique Leigh. *The New Beauty.* Tokyo: Kodansha International, 1995. East-West teachings in the beauty of body and soul, with a multicultural and botanical emphasis. Includes recipes for inner and outer beauty.

Zia Wesley-Hosford. *Fifty and Fabulous: Zia's Definitive Guide to Anti-Aging—Naturally!* Rocklin, CA: Prima Publishing, 1995. This book tells you everything you ever wanted to know about how to take good care of your skin and, not incidentally, the rest of your body. You'll find information on skin-care products that are kind to your skin, nutritional advice, rejuvenating facial exercises, and more, all from a holistic approach.

Audio/Video

Tapes on appearance are not nearly as plentiful as tapes on health and fitness. Don't forget to look at tapes on nutrition (Chapter 4), stress relief (Chapter 5), and exercise (Chapter 3). Here are two tapes to help your face.

VIDEOS

The 15-Minute Acupressure Face Lift. Meredith MacRae and Catherine Politte. Available from the VideoFinders Collection (see Audio/Video, Chapter 8). How to reduce facial tension with a simple program of facial exercises. Also includes interviews with a dermatologist, acupuncturist, and esthetician.

Ultimate Face: Exercise and Yoga for Your Face. Available from The Learning Lane (see Audio/Video, Chapter 8). Yoga exercises, nutrition, and stress-management techniques for facial rejuvenation from holistic fitness physician Jean Rosenbaum, M.D.

Online

Ahh, beauty. For weight issues, take a look at some of the links in Chapter 3, "Keep on Moving," and Chapter 4, "Are You What You Eat?" For general information on looking good, including hair and skin tips, search for the keyword *beauty.* You'll also find regular columns on these subjects in online magazines such as **Women's Wire** at www.women.com.

NEWS GROUPS

To discuss skin, try **alt.skincare.** For help with weight loss, take a look at **alt.support.diet.**

WEB SITES

For specific information on skin, search for the words *dermatology, skin, skin cancer,* and so on. One place to begin is the American Academy of Dermatology's **Dermatology Home Page** at www.add.org. It has a number of informative brochures online. Don't miss the **Dermatology in the Cinema** page, itsa.ucsf.edu/~vcr/Actors.html. You'll find the **Plastic Surgery Home Page**, sponsored by the American Society of Plastic and Reconstructive Surgeons (ASPRS) and the Plastic Surgery Educational Foundation (PSEF), at www.plasticsurgery.org. Go to the **FDA** site, www.fda.gov, to find out about what cosmetic products are subject to pending approval, which have been approved, and for what purpose.

7

THE HOLISTIC KIT AND CABOODLE
Complementary Medicine

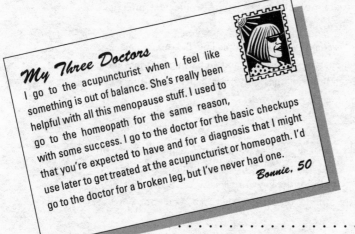

My Three Doctors

I go to the acupuncturist when I feel like something is out of balance. She's really been helpful with all this menopause stuff. I used to go to the homeopath for the same reason, with some success. I go to the doctor for the basic checkups that you're expected to have and for a diagnosis that I might use later to get treated at the acupuncturist or homeopath. I'd go to the doctor for a broken leg, but I've never had one.

Bonnie, 50

In 1993 the *New England Journal of Medicine* made this startling statement: "It is likely that virtually all medical doctors see patients who routinely use unconventional therapies." Even the National Institutes of Health has an Office of Alternative Medicine. Its director, Wayne Jonas, M.D., puts conventional Western medicine into the context of world healing techniques: "While the average half-life of a new drug introduced in the conventional community is about twenty years, homeopathy has been around essentially unchanged for 200 years; acupuncture for more than 2,000 years; prayer, spirituality, and shamanism for at least 20,000 years; and, if one believes reports of monkeys using plants to regulate their menstrual cycles, herbalism has probably been around for more than 200,000 years."

Today we are beginning to see complementary therapies being accepted by the Western medical community: Holistic medicine, preventive medicine, and wellness clinics led the way; medical schools are offering classes in complementary medicine; and some insurance companies now cover acupuncture, chiropractic, and other alternative therapies.

 ## PACKING FOR THE JOURNEY

What Is Complementary Medicine?

Complementary medicine is a general term for healing systems other than traditional Western medicine. It encompasses a wide range of treatment techniques, many of which have been around for hundreds and even thousands of years: Ayurveda from India, a diversity of traditional practices from China, Native American healing techniques from this continent. Other terms you may be more familiar with include *wellness* (working to keep people healthy instead of treating symptoms of illness), *holistic medicine* (treating the whole person, including emotional and spiritual aspects as well as physical), and *alternative medicine* (techniques used as an alternative to modern Western medicine). We use the term *complementary* because these therapies can complement—work alongside—Western medical practice, as well as be used on their own or in combination.

> We don't have to deal with early or late menopausal symptoms by default. It's our fault if we decide on a course of nonaction once we've decided we don't want the "action" of hormone replacement therapy. The options are out there. Some have benefits that have withstood the test of "orthodox" medical analysis. Others have been used for generations—even millennia—and have withstood the test of time. . . . Let's seek out the alternatives!
>
> DR. JUDITH REICHMAN, *I'm Too Young to Get Old*

Can I Explore Alternatives and Work with My Regular Doctor at the Same Time?

Not too long ago, the division between Western medicine and other systems was sharp. But as more people seek alternative treatment and as concepts of holistic medicine, wellness, and prevention become part of the mainstream, this attitude is changing. Several top medical schools, including the University of California, San Francisco, School of Medicine, are incorporating classes on alternative therapies into the curriculum, and some insurers now cover chiropractic, acupuncture, and other complementary therapies. In popular culture, Dr. Andrew Weil, author of *Spontaneous Healing*, and Dr. Christiane Northrup, author of *Women's Body, Women's Mind*, are examples of this sort of integration.

universal life force   Also known as *qi* or *chi* in China, *ki* in Japan, and *prana* in India, it is defined by *Harper's Encyclopedia of Mystical and Paranormal Experience* as "a vital force or energy that transcends time and space, permeates all things in the universe, and upon which all things depend for health and life."

Make sure you keep your doctor informed about what else you are doing, especially if you are taking some form of medication or are grappling with a particular medical problem. Not every alternative is appropriate for every person or circumstance. If your doctor is not open to your explorations, you may want to find a doctor with whom you are more compatible.

How Can I Find a Doctor Interested in Complementary Medicine?

The first and best way is to ask your friends to recommend someone. If you have a medical school in your community, ask there. If you are a health plan member, ask if any of the doctors there are interested (a friend who belongs to a large HMO discovered that her primary care physician was also a licensed acupuncturist). Write to the American Holistic Medical Association for a list of members in your area (see Resources).

My Cat and the Life Force

The nature of the life force was really brought home to me last week when my cat almost died of a systemic infection. She was so sick, all she could do was lie on the bed. Her fur, which is normally cream colored, was flat and brown and lifeless, and her eyes were very dark. She didn't even seem to reflect light anymore. Then, as she got better, she seemed to fluff up and lighten up as I watched. It was so striking. By the time she was all well, she practically seemed to be radiating light from the inside.   *Lily, 41*

What Is Aromatherapy?

Few medicinal experiences are as downright pleasant as aromatherapy: inhaling the aromatic essence of flowering plants and herbs to energize, calm, or otherwise smooth the waters of body and soul. Used topically, many essential oils

GUIDED TOUR:
Complementary Medicine

Complementary medicine includes a wide range of healing systems that share some common goals and beliefs: that mind, body, and spirit are integrated, that the body has the wisdom to heal itself with the right help, and that prevention is more effective than intervention. Virtually all work to help people strive for wellness and balance.

WESTERN MEDICINE

Increasingly, Western medicine is integrating treatment approaches of complementary therapies, as evidenced by the trend toward preventive medicine and wellness. If you are interested in complementary medicine, look for a doctor who is open to these ideas and willing to work with you.

COMPLEMENTARY THERAPIES

Some of the many systems of complementary medicine include Ayurveda, Chinese traditional medicine (including acupuncture and acupressure), herbal and botanical remedies, homeopathy, aromatherapy, Bach flower essences, naturopathy, chiropractic, reflexology, reiki, and others.

MIND–BODY

Movement techniques based in spiritual practice, such as yoga, t'ai, chi, and qi gong, as well as modern practices such as Rosen work, also have healing, prevention, and wellness as goals.

NUTRITION

Food and diet are integral to some healing systems, especially Ayurveda and traditional Chinese medicine. Part of a prescription for healing may include dietary change.

Choosing a Complementary Practitioner

Choose a complementary practitioner the same way you choose a conventional medical doctor: Look for a competent person with whom you can communicate. (For more on the basics of choosing a health care practitioner, see Chapter 8.) Here are some other considerations.

Licensing: Many alternative therapists—including naturopaths, acupuncturists, chiropractors, and homeopaths—must be trained and certified or licensed in their techniques. If you are choosing one of these, check accreditation through the licensing organization. You can also ask for a list of practitioners in your area. See Resources.

Personal recommendations: Some practitioners don't fall into neat categories. Healers, for example, have a natural talent for healing, but no organization gives them an official stamp of approval. Make sure they will be helpful rather than harmful! Ask friends and people you trust. Use your intuition as well.

Trust your instincts: Complementary medicine has its share of charlatans. Be sure to question yourself after a session. How do you feel about this person? Do you feel confident that you are being treated as an equal participant in your care, or are you being manipulated? Does this person want to prevent you from exploring other alternatives, or is he or she open to your explorations? In *Without Estrogen,* Dee Ito gives very good advice: "Be suspicious of anyone in any discipline who practices mumbo-jumbo medicine. Effective alternative therapies are rational, and the people who practice them do not have secrets about what they do. They should be willing to tell you what they are doing and why they are doing it. They should demystify, not complicate, the experience of healing."

have medicinal properties. Aromatherapy can trace its roots back 6,000 years to the ancient Egyptians, up through the Greeks, and through Western history. You can find a trained aromatherapist (see Resources) or experiment on your own. The essential oils are sold in most natural food stores or body shops. Put a few drops of oil in a bath, mix a few drops with a neutral carrier oil or cream and rub it on your skin, or use a diffuser to allow the aroma to permeate the air. If you doubt the potent effects of aroma, take a moment to think about warm cinnamon rolls.

BENEFITS   Essential oils can be used to stimulate energy, promote feelings of well-being, calm stress, and so on. They are also used to treat skin conditions, and many, such as tea tree oil and peppermint oil, have antiseptic and medicinal properties.

USE YOUR COMMON SENSE   Used correctly, most essential oils are simply wonderful, and harmful side effects are few and far between. The concentrated oils can be strong, however, so mix them with a carrier oil or cream—don't put them directly on your skin. Don't ingest any oil without first consulting a doctor. As with any naturally derived product, some people may be allergic to certain scents (eucalyptus oil, popular in hot tubs, has been known to cause breathing problems).

What Is Acupressure?

Acupressure is a massage technique based on the principle of traditional Chinese medicine (see below). The acupressurist will first use her fingers to read your "pulses" and determine the flow of *chi* through your body, and then she'll go to work stimulating the appropriate points on the meridian (energy channels). She uses finger pressure and massage on the energy points, rather than needles, to move the *chi*.

BENEFITS   Because it involves a form of massage, acupressure can be very soothing as well as refreshing and can be used to treat headache, back pain, anxiety, fatigue, cramps, and much more. Some people enjoy regular acupressure "tune-ups" to balance their systems. Shiatsu, jin shin, acu-yoga, and qi gong are related techniques.

USE YOUR COMMON SENSE   Acupressure is gentle and is considered a fairly safe technique. Pregnant women and people with skin conditions are sometimes warned to be careful about acupressure. Practitioners have completed a training program, but are not licensed.

What Is Acupuncture?

Acupuncture is a technique of traditional Chinese medicine (see below) that restores and promotes health by inserting fine, sterile needles at various points on the body's meridians (energy channels) to unblock or stimulate energy. Many people who haven't tried acupuncture are put off by the idea of needles, but the needles are very thin and don't penetrate very far into the skin. Most people say they feel hardly anything at all when the needles are inserted. Most acupuncturists today use individually wrapped, disposable, one-use-only needles, to dispel worries of spreading blood-borne diseases.

BENEFITS   Acupuncture is used to treat a wide variety of ailments, with such success that some insurers will now pay for the treatment. It is best known as a form of pain relief and, in China, has been used instead of anesthetic during some operations. It's also effective for insomnia, menopausal and other hormonal

POINT OF INTEREST
Uncommon Medicine/Common Ideas

Each healing system is unique, yet most share a common philosophy of health based on prevention and wellness.

Body/mind/spirit: Complementary therapies assume that mind, body, and spirit work together. Each part affects the other, so everything we are and do—our emotions, our beliefs, our thoughts, our ways of dealing with stress, our diets, and so on—are inseparable parts of a whole. This means that the physical body is not the only route to healing.

Wisdom of the body: The body has the wisdom to heal itself, especially with the right kind of help. This belief means that the person being healed is actively involved in effecting the healing, not only through medicines but also through lifestyle changes.

Preventive medicine: Complementary therapies work with the body's wisdom—strengthening, supporting, and balancing the life force within the individual. They seek to heal the underlying cause of recurring disease, rather than just the symptoms, and to keep the body strong enough to resist illness. In general, treatments tend to be less toxic, less invasive, and have fewer side effects than do those of conventional medicine.

Is Complementary Medicine for You?

Is complementary medicine a path you want to take? Here are some questions to help you gather your thoughts. If you answer "yes" to most of these questions, you will probably be able to reap the benefits of complementary therapies. If you answer "no" to most of them, you may not. If you had a mix of answers, you show an interest in exploring new paths. Go ahead and research the complementary therapies that interest you, but don't abandon your regular doctor.

1. Are you open to new ideas?
2. Are you willing to experiment?
3. Are you willing to participate in your healing process?
4. Are you willing to give the treatment time to work?
5. Are you willing to pay attention to how your body feels and adjust remedies or herbal formulas and dosages to find what is most suitable for your needs?
6. Are you willing to try another type of treatment if the first doesn't work?
7. Are you comfortable with the technique being used (do you have a problem with needles, with being touched, with taking nonprescription drugs)?

imbalances, asthma, allergies, chronic fatigue syndrome, digestive problems, pain, stress reduction, and much more.

USE YOUR COMMON SENSE Acupuncture should not be used to treat acute conditions, hemorrhages, broken bones, or undiagnosed pain. Practitioners have individual styles, so make sure your practitioner's style suits you. Practitioners are licensed.

What Is Ayurveda?

This traditional healing system was practiced in India as early as the fifth century B.C. and is mentioned in the ancient Indian scriptures, the *vedas*. Ayurveda holds that each person is a unique blend of physical, emotional, and spiritual traits called *doshas*; it seeks to keep these traits in balance with the life force, or *prana*. Ayurvedic practitioners diagnose people through a lengthy analysis in terms of three types, *vatta*, *pitta*, and *kapha*. Treatment usually consists of an individual mix of diet, herbs, exercise, sleep, and environmental and lifestyle changes aimed at bringing balance. Currently, Deepak Chopra is the foremost popularizer of Ayurveda in the West.

BENEFITS Ayurveda can be a healthy lifestyle choice that corrects a number of imbalances and thus aids problems associated with digestion, stress, allergies, insomnia, and other chronic ailments. It's a good preventive system that works best over the long term.

USE YOUR COMMON SENSE Ayurveda is a complex system, a philosophy, and a way of life that can be difficult for Westerners to assimilate. Because Ayurveda is not recognized in the United States, practitioners are licensed under other specialties, such as homeopathy or chiropractic. Be sure you are dealing with a reputable practitioner. In an article in

Natural Health, David Lonsdorf, administrative director of Maharishi Ayur-Veda Medical Center in Washington, DC, advises, "The more advanced a disease, and the more serious it is, the more likely you will need modern medicine's approach in order to buy Ayurveda some time to change lifestyle and build healing ability."

What Are Bach Flower Remedies?

Developed by homeopathic physician Dr. Edward Bach in the 1930s, these thirty-eight remedies use the spiritual properties of flowers to treat the emotional states that underlie disease. The remedies are made by placing flower buds in water and allowing sunlight to extract the essence.

BENEFITS Flower essences are great for smoothing out emotional states, such as fear and anxiety. Rescue Remedy is a very popular remedy for emotional trauma and is used for everything from soothing nerves after a fall to speeding recovery from surgery.

USE YOUR COMMON SENSE As with homeopathic remedies, these are microdoses. Flower essences are said to be safe.

What Is Chiropractic?

Chiropractic works on the musculoskelatal system to bring it into alignment with the nervous system. Chiropractors originally sought to cure most illness by manipulating the spine, looking for "subluxations" or misalignments that made the body more susceptible to disease. Today, many chiropractors also incorporate a number or other alternative healing techniques. Directional Non-force Technique, or "soft" chiropractic, features gentle alignments performed by a series of measurements and light thrusts, allowing for a healthy flow of energy and healing that continues after treatment. Licensed chiropractors are required to take the same premed courses as medical doctors, so their knowledge base is quite broad.

BENEFITS Chiropractic is most suited to treating skeletal and muscular problems, especially back and neck pain. But chiropractors

TRAVEL TIP
When to Consult Your
Western Health Practitioner

When your symptoms are severe or unusual (bleeding, vomiting, extended periods of weakness, stomach pains, and so on), consult your doctor for standard medical tests to rule out serious or life-threatening illness. If you have a bone fracture or severe sprain, get yourself to the doctor for evaluation.

also treat a number of other problems, including those associated with hormonal imbalance.

USE YOUR COMMON SENSE   Make sure you're in the hands of a qualified practitioner. Improper manipulations have been known to cause harm, from strains and sprains to strokes and paraplegia. Chiropractors are licensed.

What Are Herbal and Botanical Remedies?

Human beings have been treating their ailments with plants (roots, leaves, flowers, bark, and berries) for as long as we know. A number of the drugs we rely on today—notably digitalis and quinine—are plant derived. Many of the complementary therapies incorporate plants in treatment: not only the ancient traditional systems of Ayurveda and Chinese medicine, but also homeopathy, naturopathy, aromatherapy, flower remedies, and others. In addition, there are trained herbalists who are knowledgeable in the medicinal properties of plants. Herbal and botanical preparations take many forms: You can boil up a batch of herbs and drink them as tea or take them neatly in capsules; you can use them as ointments, salves, or suppositories; you can chew them or sniff them or hold a few drops under your tongue.

BENEFITS   Botanicals can help a wide range of ills: Feverfew seems effective in preventing migraines; ginger helps nausea; slippery elm bark helps sore throats; echinacea seems to help prevent or mitigate colds; evening primrose capsules help some women reduce the frequency of hot flashes; a tea made of oatstraw and nettle is a way to get calcium; hawthorn has long been used for heart problems.

USE YOUR COMMON SENSE   "Natural" does not necessarily mean "safe." Herbs can help, but they can also be dangerous and even deadly. Herbs sold over the counter are not necessarily FDA-approved; it's often impossible to be certain what dosage you're getting. The strength of herbs can vary depending on how the herbs are prepared. Even two plants grown in different gardens can have different medicinal strengths. Herbal preparations that contain multiple ingredients can play havoc with your system, and you may never know which ingredient caused the problem. The FDA has identified the following herbs as potentially harmful when used in excess or in an improper manner (dangers include kidney damage and stroke): chaparral, comfrey, ephedra (also called ma huang), germander, jin bu huan, lobelia, magnolia, stephania, and yohimbine. If you're concerned about adverse reactions, consult a health care provider who prescribes herbs.

What Is Homeopathy?

Popularized by German physician Samuel Hahnemann in the late eighteenth century, this system is based on the idea that "like cures like"—the same substance that causes a symptom can be used to cure it—and that microdoses of a remedy are more effective than concentrated doses. Homeopaths ask a lot of questions about all aspects of a patient's problem and lifestyle to select exactly the right remedy—out of the 1,200 there are to choose from! Because there are so many remedies, symptoms are described in detail: You don't just have a hacking cough, you have a "very dry violent cough sounding like a saw being driven through a board." Homeopathy seeks to strengthen the entire system; sometimes cures are effected quickly, but sometimes they require a lot of experimentation.

BENEFITS   Homeopaths treat pretty much everything, from allergies and hormonal imbalances to early bronchitis and colitis. Remedies can be used in tandem with other treatments (consult your homeopath for guidance).

USE YOUR COMMON SENSE   Because the doses are minute to the point of invisibility, homeopathic remedies are generally considered safe. You may sometimes experience a healing crisis (a worsening of symptoms) before getting better. If you have a broken bone, severe infection, internal injuries, or an acute illness that is not responding to treatment, consult your Western medical practitioner. You can treat with remedies purchased over the counter at natural food stores, but cures tend to be so specific that it's more efficient to consult a licensed homeopath.

No matter how hard we try to avoid it, sometimes we get sick. Western medicine works hard to get us well, so if it doesn't happen right away, we may blame the doctor or take it as a personal failure. But a long tradition of complementary medicine asks us to use this down time to reflect, to learn from illness and pain. In *A Match to the Heart,* Gretel Ehrlich recounts this story:

"Takashi, the farmer-monk from Japan who visited me at the beach house, said, 'You have always been so strong. Now it is time to learn about being weak. This is necessary for you.'

"How could I grow strong by becoming weak, I asked. I was being purposefully naive. What he was asking for was balance. Health cannot be accomplished any other way."

What Is Hypnotherapy?

Hypnosis is a way to relax, turn off the conscious mind, and enter a trance state where you are more amenable to suggestion. Although hypnotherapy has been around for many years and is in fairly common use, how it works remains a mystery. Nonetheless, self-hypnosis, hypnosis with a trained hypnotherapist, visualization, and guided imagery work are variations that are frequently used for relaxation, healing, pain control, weight control, addiction treatment, anxiety relief, and other emotional work. Hypnotherapists are licensed.

BENEFITS   The various forms of hypnosis are good ways to learn to relax and to access your creative potential. You can also use hypnosis to achieve positive results without the use of drugs.

USE YOUR COMMON SENSE   Remember, you are in control. If you have fears that the hypnotherapist will be invasive, hypnosis will probably not work for you. You might be more amenable to self-hypnosis, guided imagery, and visualization techniques, which you can easily learn from books or tapes. If you do consult a hypnotherapist, make sure he or she is licensed and recommended by someone you trust.

What Is Naturopathy?

Naturopathy is an eclectic approach—naturopaths use aspects of traditional Chinese medicine, homeopathy, botanicals, and many other complementary systems to put together individual healing plans for patients. Some naturopaths specialize in a particular area, but most are like general practitioners. Naturopaths are licensed after completing a four-year graduate-level federally accredited naturopathic medical school. They take the same basic science classes required for M.D.s, and they also study holistic and nontoxic approaches that stress prevention. Not all naturopaths are doctors, but some doctors are also naturopaths. In some states naturopaths are licensed as primary care physicians, and some insurance companies cover naturopathic services.

BENEFITS   Naturopaths are knowledgeable in many treatment approaches. Frequently, they have the time and inclination to give you the more personal treatment that you don't get from Western medical doctors, who are often rushed and under pressure to turn over patients.

They may also see a route toward health that your regular physician overlooked, and the best ones will know their limitations.

USE YOUR COMMON SENSE Be sure you find a licensed naturopath—anyone can claim to be one—and preferably one who has graduated from one of the two accredited naturopathic universities, Bastyr University or the National College of Naturopathic Medicine (see Resources). A few naturopaths do chelation therapy, which the American Heart Association has found to be harmful.

What Is Reflexology?

Reflexology is based on the idea that points in the hands and feet reflect specific organs of the body. Reflexologists gently massage these areas to promote health and healing in the related physical areas.

BENEFITS Few things feel better than a foot massage, and it's amazing how a foot massage (done by you or a reflexologist) can relax and invigorate your entire body and improve your mood. Asthma, headaches, migraines, stomach upset, and stress can be relieved by a reflexology massage.

USE YOUR COMMON SENSE Reflexology is one of the more benign complementary therapies—it's darn near impossible to do harm. *The Encyclopedia of Alternative Health Care* does include one warning: "Stimulating circulation of energy may accelerate the spread of infection and other conditions compromised by increased circulation."

What Is Reiki?

This technique of transferring healing energy (*rei* means "boundless and universal," *ki* means "life force") was developed and named by a Japanese theologian who based it on ancient Tibetan practices. Practitioners transfer healing energy through their hands to the patient (there are also long-distance techniques, where the person being healed does not have to be in the room).

BENEFITS Reiki sessions can be calming or energizing. (Or they can be both—these are not necessarily exclusive states!) Reiki makes no claims past stress reduction, but anecdotal evidence points to speeded-up healing times. It's a good adjunct therapy for other treatments.

USE YOUR COMMON SENSE   Reiki has no harmful effects associated with it. Don't use it to treat something that could be handled easily by another kind of health practitioner.

What Is Traditional Chinese Medicine?

Traditional Chinese medicine has been practiced for at least 3,000 years. Like Ayurveda, this form of health care is also a spiritual pursuit that encompasses all aspects of life. Practitioners work with the flow of *qi* energy (life force), balancing yin and yang, and harmonizing the five elements. They look for the flow of qi and for areas where it's blocked, and they try to find the root of the problem. They can treat symptoms before they become a named disease. Treatment usually involves herbal preparations (more than 4,000 herbs are used in this practice) and acupuncture (see listing, above).

alternative medicine   Defined by the Office of Alternative Medicine, National Institutes of Health, as "an unrelated group of non-orthodox therapeutic practices, often with explanatory systems that do not follow conventional bio-medical explanations."

In China the postmenopausal years are known as a woman's "second spring," and women who use acupuncture and Chinese medicine to smooth the menopausal journey report a good degree of success. See the discussions of acupuncture and acupressure in this chapter for more details on these aspects.

BENEFITS   Traditional Chinese medicine is very strong on prevention because practitioners look for changes in the pulses that may indicate the beginnings of the disease process before it manifests in the body. Acupuncture treats a wide range of complaints, from immune system problems to headaches and bronchitis.

USE YOUR COMMON SENSE   Herbal medicines are complex and specific: Don't try to prescribe herbal medications for yourself. Usually, they are prescribed in combination with acupuncture treatments. Always consult a qualified practitioner of Chinese medicine.

What Complementary Therapies Can Ease Menopausal Symptoms?

If you're around complementary medicine for even a moment, especially if you're looking for help with signs of menopause, you'll soon hear about two Chinese remedies, dong quai and ginseng, and two popular herbs, *Gingko biloba* and black cohosh.

DONG QUAI This root of *Angelica sinensis* is a traditional Chinese medicine used for improving circulation; it also serves as a general tonic for women. It is rich in phytoestrogens and is considered non-toxic. It is currently under study for use by Kaiser-Permanente, the largest HMO in California. Dong quai is a well-known tonic for women experiencing menstrual problems and problems associated with menopause such as lack of energy, hot flashes, and hormonal imbalance. It has been called "the women's ginseng."

GINSENG This slow-growing root (*Panax ginseng* or *Panax quinquefolium*) has been used medicinally in Asia for thousands of years. Its reputed benefits include improvements in appetite (both culinary and sexual), memory, and energy, although clinical tests have not been able to prove or disprove the claims. The Chinese do use ginseng to treat menopausal problems as do a number of complementary therapists, citing its estrogenic activity as effective in preventing hot flashes. However, according to Dr. Andrew Weil, this estrogenic activity may "argue against its use by women with hormonal imbalances or those who have estrogen-dependent diseases like uterine fibroids, fibrocystic breast disease, and breast cancer." Another caution: Ginseng can raise blood pressure.

Gingko Biloba The lovely leaves of the gingko tree are said to have some powerful properties: improved circulation and improved memory and concentration (which makes it especially popular among midlife women). According to one source, it's "one of the most popular drugs in Europe." Ginkgo may also have antioxidant properties and be effective in lowering blood pressure and cholesterol. Stay away from very high doses (40 milligrams is a standard dose), which can cause diarrhea, nausea, and vomiting.

BLACK COHOSH The ground-up root of *Cimicifuga racemosa*, black cohosh is a common herbal remedy (like ginkgo, popular in Europe) for balancing hormones, PMS, and other symptoms. According to Herb Mindell's *Herb Bible*, "Native Americans used this herb to

POINT OF INTEREST
Treat Yourself with Care

You can buy all sorts of preparations in natural food stores. How can you be sure of what you're getting? Here are a few points to remember:

1. Not all supplements contain the same amount of the active ingredient. Amounts and quality can vary widely.

2. Pay attention to how you are feeling. Just because it's natural doesn't mean it's good for you.

3. Keep track of your progress. If you are using wild yam progesterone cream to treat menopausal symptoms, keep track of how you feel as you are using it. Does it seem to be working? What happens when you use more or less of it?

treat an assortment of 'female complaints.'" It's usually sold in capsule form.

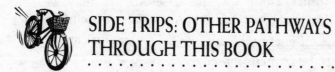

SIDE TRIPS: OTHER PATHWAYS THROUGH THIS BOOK

CHAPTER 2: WHY IS THIS HAPPENING TO ME?   Some systems of complementary medicine have been treating hormonal imbalance for thousands of years. Look here to find alternative ways to cope with hot flashes and sleep problems.

CHAPTER 5: BREATHE EASY   Seeking calmness and releasing tension is basic to most alternative therapies. Look here to see why this is such a good idea, and how you can do it.

CHAPTER 8: WHAT'S UP, DOC?   Western medicine has a role to play in your health care, especially when it comes to acute disease and injuries. Look here to learn how to find a doctor you can work with.

CHAPTER 17: THE INNER JOURNEY   Many systems of complementary medicine are spiritually based, and virtually all acknowledge the importance of the spiritual dimension in daily life. Look here to learn more about the spiritual aspects of the midlife journey.

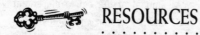

RESOURCES

Organizations and Services

American Holistic Medical Association, 4101 Lake Boone Trail, Suite 201, Raleigh, NC 27607. Voice: (919) 787-5181. Fax: (919) 787-4916. If you're looking for a holistic doctor in your area, send $5 to receive a directory listing of AHMA members in each state. Listings include a brief explanation of each practitioner's specialty and practice. The AHMA also publishes a magazine, *Holistic Medicine.*

Gladys Taylor McGarey Foundation, 7350 E. Stetson Drive, Suite 208, Scottsdale, AZ 85251. Voice: (602) 946-4544. Fax: (602) 946-6902. The stated goals of this organization are "to advance human understanding of body, mind, spirit, and emotion relationship; to encourage wellness and wholeness through the combination of the best of conventional and holistic medical practices, and to serve as a model for research, education, and application of integrative healing practices." The intriguing newsletter, *HealthLinks*, comes with membership.

Office of Alternative Medicine Clearinghouse, National Institutes of Health, P.O. Box 8218, Silver Spring, MD 20907-8218. Voice: (888) 644-6226. Fax-back Service: (301) 402-2466. Call to speak to an information specialist or for information about ongoing OAM studies on alternative therapies. The OAM has free information packets and a newsletter, *Complementary and Alternative Medicine at the NIH.* The fax-back service will fax you information.

Wellspring for Women, 900 28th St., Suite 201, Boulder, CO 80303. Voice: (303) 443-0321. Fax: (303) 443-3881. This group offers phone consultations with a nurse practitioner who will answer questions about herbal remedies and natural hormones and put you in touch with a practitioner in your area.

Wise Woman Center, P.O. Box 64, Woodstock, NY 12498. Voice: (914) 246-8081. This is herbalist Susun Weed's center. It offers one-, two-, and three-day workshops such as Spring Equinox Herbal Intensive and Pathways of Peace and also sells Weed's books and tapes.

Women to Women, 1 Pleasant St., Yarmouth, ME 04096. Voice: (207) 846-6163. Fax: (207) 846-6167. This medical clinic for women, co-founded by holistic physician Dr. Christiane Northrup and three other practitioners, addresses the specific health concerns of women. Dr. Northrup has produced audio- and videotapes, a newsletter, and the book *Women's Bodies, Women's Wisdom.*

World Research Foundation, 20501 Ventura Blvd., Suite 100, Woodland Hills, CA 91364. Voice: (818) 999-5483. Fax: (818) 227-6484. Second address: 41 Bell Rock Plaza, Suite C, Sedona, AZ 86351. Voice: (520) 284-3300. Fax: (520) 284-3530. This foundation offers tapes, books, and research reports on alternative health care. The organization will compile a report on a particular subject for a fee.

ACUPUNCTURE/TRADITIONAL CHINESE MEDICINE

American Association of Oriental Medicine, 433 Front St., Catasauqua, PA 18032. Voice: (610) 433-2448. Fax: (610) 264-2768. E-mail: AAOM1@aol.com. Internet: www.aaom.org. This is the place to go to find out *anything* you want to know about Eastern medicine and acupuncture, including information about schools, doctors, techniques, and types of treatment. This group offers a nationwide referral network if you're looking for a practitioner in your area and will refer only people who pass the board examination of the National Certification Commission for Acupuncturists (requiring between 2,000 and 4,000 hours of schooling and practice), or doctors who are licensed in their state. Also available are a number of books and publications, including a manual on carpal tunnel treatment with laser pen, an education options catalog, and more.

National Certification Commission for Acupuncture and Oriental Medicine, P.O. Box 97075, Washington, DC 20090-7075. Voice: (202) 232-1404. Fax: (202) 462-6157. Membership in this organization requires taking a minimum two-year training course at an accredited school or a four-year apprenticeship, plus passing a written and practical exam. Call to ask for informational brochures or a directory listing certified acupuncturists or Chinese herbalists in your area.

AROMATHERAPY

Pacific Institute of Aromatherapy, P.O. Box 6723, San Rafael, CA 94903. Voice: (415) 459-3998. This organization gives seminars nationally and offers a home-study course in aromatherapy. Call or write for more information.

AYURVEDA

The Chopra Center for Well-Being, 7630 Fay Ave., La Jolla CA 92037. Voice: (888) 424-6772. This is the center for all things Deepak Chopra. Call for a referral list to Ayurvedic doctors or centers in your area. The center also offers three-day and seven-day programs, healing and meditation courses, and products for sale.

Maharishi Ayur-Veda. Voice: (800) 255-8332. Call this number for referrals to Maharishi-Ayurved-trained doctors or health centers in your area.

BACH FLOWER ESSENCES

Nelson Bach USA Ltd., Wilmington Technology Park, 100 Research Dr., Wilmington, MA 01887. Voice: (800) 319-9151. Consumers: (800) 334-0843 for education hotline. This society sponsors educational programs all across the country. It has three levels of training, including an internationally recognized practitioner training course that involves on-site and home-study training. Call with questions about how to use Bach flower essences and to receive an informational packet about the organization and courses.

CHIROPRACTIC

American Chiropractic Association, 1701 Clarendon Blvd., Arlington, VA 22209. Voice: (800) 986-4636. E-mail: amerchio@aol.com. Internet: www.amerchio. org/aca. This nonprofit professional association is the largest organization representing doctors of chiropractic (D.C.s) in the United States. The group will give a limited number of referrals to doctors in your area.

Directional Non-Force Technique (DNFT), 256 S. Robertson, Suite 1636, Beverly Hills, CA 90211. Voice: (310) 657-2338. Fax: (310) 657-2279. Internet: www. nonforce.com. This group has a very efficient voice mail service you can use to find a referral to DNFT doctors in your area. You can also request information on scientific research.

National Directory of Chiropractic, P.O. Box 10056, Olathe, KS 66051. Voice: (800) 888-7914. This organization publishes a directory of almost 40,000 practicing chiropractors across the United States. Listings include names, addresses, phone numbers, and the techniques they use. It also places directories in chiropractic colleges across the United States.

HERBAL MEDICINE

American Herbalists Guild, P.O. Box 746555, Arvada, CO 80006. Voice: (303) 423-8800. Fax: (303) 423-8828. E-mail: ahgoffice@earthlink.net. Call or write this membership organization for referrals to professional herbalists in your area. It also publishes a directory of herbal education programs across the United States and *The Herbalist,* a newsletter for members (membership is for interested people as well as professionals).

HOMEOPATHY

National Center for Homeopathy, 801 N. Fairfax St., Suite 306, Alexandria, VA 22314. Voice: (703) 548-7790. Fax: (703) 548-7792. E-mail: nchinfo@igc.apc.org. Internet: www.healthy.net/nch. For a small fee, this nonprofit membership organization will send you an informational packet that includes homeopathic pharmacies and resources in the United States and Canada and a nationwide directory of licensed practitioners and study groups. Licensed practitioners must also be health care providers, such as M.D.s, R.N.s, or D.C.s, and the directory will tell you what their specialty is and how often they use homeopathy in their practice. The center also publishes *Homeopathy Today,* a newsletter for members, and offers a two-week training program to members and nonmembers.

HYPNOTHERAPY

American Society of Clinical Hypnosis, 2200 E. Devon Ave., Suite 291, Des Plaines, IL 60018. Voice: (847) 297-3317. Fax: (847) 267-7309. Send a stamped, self-addressed, business-size envelope to receive a list of practitioners in your state. They're broken down by city, and some list their specialty. Listed clinical hypnotists must be ASCH Members for three years and have additional training in order to be certified. You can also ask about information on workshops around the country.

International Medical and Dental Hypnotherapy Association, International Referral Service, 4110 Edgeland, Royal Oak, MI 48073-2285. Voice: (800) 257-5467. Fax: (248) 549-5594. E-mail: aspencer@infinityinst.com. Internet: www.infinityinst. com. This organization has referrals to certified hypnotherapists who work with health care practitioners to help reduce panic and fear in patients or prepare patients mentally for a successful procedure. Contact the association for a list of practitioners in your area.

NATUROPATHY

American Association of Naturopathic Physicians, 2366 Eastlake Ave. East, Suite 322, Seattle, WA 98102. Voice: (206) 323-7610. Naturopaths are currently licensed in eleven states, but there are qualified naturopaths all over the United States. Contact this association to order a directory of qualified naturopaths in your state.

YOGA

B. K. S. Iyengar Yoga National Association of the United States, 1676 Hilton Head Court, #2288, El Cajon, CA 92019. Voice: (800) 889-9642. This is the national headquarters. Call to find a yoga teacher in your area, for information about membership and programs, or to order hard-to-find books

HOTLINES

American College for Advancement in Medicine: (800) 532-3688. Call to find out how to get an information packet about doctors who practice complementary medicine and referrals to practitioners in your area.

Office of Alternative Medicine Clearinghouse: (888) 644-6226. Call for free information about research on alternative therapies

Products and Catalogs

Bach USA: (800) 314-BACH. Call for a catalog of Bach flower essence products.

The Chopra Center for Well-Being: (800) 757-8897. This group has two catalogs: one for Ayurvedic products, including body products, tapes, and books, and one for Dr. Chopra's education programs.

East Earth Trade Winds, P.O. Box 493151, Redding, CA 96049-3151. Voice: (800) 258-6878. E-mail: eetw@snowcrest.net. Call for a catalog of Chinese herbs, bulk Chinese herbs, Chinese patent medicines, jade medicine products, and books on Chinese medicine.

Ellon USA, Inc., 644 Merrick Road, Lynbrook, NY 11563. Voice: (800) 4-BE-CALM. Call for a catalog of flower essence products.

Essence Aromatherapy, P.O. Box 2119, Durango, CO 81302. Voice: (800) 283-0244. Call for a catalog of aromatherapy products, including candles, bath and body oil, and bath salts and body scrubs.

Flower Essence Society, P.O. Box 1769, Nevada City, CA 95959. Voice: (916) 265-9163. Fax: (916) 265-6467. E-mail: fes@nccm.net. Internet: www.floweressence. com. Call for information on products and catalog.

Hands-On Health Care Catalog, 1533 Shattuck Ave., Berkeley, CA 94709. Voice: (800) 442-2232. This catalog, published by the Acupressure Institute, offers acupressure books and instructional videos, visualization audiotapes, healing music, and more.

Homeopathic Educational Services, 2124 Kittridge St., Berkeley, CA 94704. For inquiries or catalog: (510) 649-0294. Fax: (510) 649-1955. Voice: (800) 359-9051. Internet: www.homeopathic.com. Call for a catalog of homeopathic books and remedies, tapes, software, and home-study courses.

Homeopathy Overnight, Inc., 4111 Simon Road, Youngstown, OH 44512. Voice: (800) ARNICA-30. The name says it all: Have remedies prepared by several leading homeopathic pharmacies delivered to your home the next day. Call for a catalog.

Mountain Rose Herbs, P.O. Box 2000, Redway, CA 95560. Voice: (800) 879-3337. Fax: (707) 923-7867. Internet: botanical.com/mtrose. For $1 you'll receive a forty-eight-page catalog of herbal products and more: organic herbs, tinctures, lotions, teas, books, body and bath products, bulk essential oils, clays, beeswax, bottles, droppers, medicinal herb seeds, and more. This catalog has a special section, "Changing Woman," that includes menopause teas, ProGest, and books about menopause, including Amanda McQuade Crawford's *The Herbal Menopause Book*.

Self-Care, P.O. Box 182290, Chattanooga, TN 37422. Voice: (800) 345-3371. This catalog offers a wide variety of self-care products, including skin care, fitness, relaxation, weight control, allergy relief, nutrition, and personal care.

Transitions for Health, 621 S.W. Alder, Suite 900, Portland, OR 97205. Voice: (800) 888-6814. Internet: www.progest.com. Call for a free catalog of natural health care products for midlife women, specifically for menopause. The company's products include transdermal creams, capsules, vitamins, tinctures, and other preparations.

Periodicals

Brain/Mind Bulletin, P.O. Box 421069, Los Angeles, CA 90042. Voice: (800) 553-6463. This monthly newsletter reports on intriguing breakthroughs in consciousness research, brain science, and the human potential field.

Dr. Weil's Self Healing, Thorne Communications, Inc., 42 Pleasant St., Watertown, MA 02172. Voice: (617) 926-0200. This interesting newsletter offers advice, tips, and remedies from the eclectic Dr. Andrew Weil, all based on natural remedies.

Health Wisdom for Women: Intelligent, Sensitive Solutions to Your Health Concerns, 7811 Montrose Road, Potomac, MD 20854. Voice: (800) 777-5005. This newsletter for women by Christiane Northrup, M.D., the author of *Women's Bodies, Women's Wisdom*, is not geared specifically to women in midlife. But her integrative approach, combining Western medicine and a complementary approach to illness and health, makes this a helpful newsletter.

HerbalGram, American Botanical Council, P.O. Box 201660, Austin, TX 78720. Voice: (512) 331-8868. This is the journal of the American Botanical Council and the Herb Research Foundation. A very credible publication with research articles and many resources.

Meno Times: Alternative Choices to Menopause and Osteoporosis, c/o The Menopause Center, P.O. Box 6558, San Rafael, CA 94903. Voice: (415) 459-5430. E-mail: Mtimes@nbn.com. The latest news on complementary approaches to menopause and osteoporosis. Features many in-depth articles and interviews with well-known practitioners.

Natural Health Magazine, P.O. Box 7440, Red Oak, IA 51591-0440. Voice: (800) 526-8440. This magazine offers a variety of natural health articles as well as book reviews, interviews, and sources for products.

New Age Journal, 42 Pleasant St., Watertown, MA 02172. Voice: (617) 926-0200. E-mail: editor@newage.com. This magazine claims to have "The Best Tools and Ideas for Body and Soul." It includes articles on many different aspects of New Age health, fitness, and spirituality and reviews of books, products, and organizations.

Total Health, 165 North 100 East, Suite 2, St. George, UT 84770. Voice: (800) 788-7806. This magazine has a column by nutritionist Robert Crayhon and features articles on herbs and exercise as well as other current health information.

Townsend Letter for Doctors and Patients, The Examiner of Medical Alternatives, 911 Tyler St., Port Townsend, WA 98368-6541. Voice: (360) 385-6021. Fax: (360) 385-0699. This publication describes itself as "An Informal Newsletter for Doctors and Patients." It includes many articles relating to contemporary medicine from a wide range of health care practitioners, and it has a monthly column titled "Women's Health Updates." It contains many articles submitted by health practitioners and patients about complementary medicine.

Yoga Journal, California Yoga Teachers Association, 2054 University Ave., Berkeley, CA 94704. Voice: (800) 334-8152. *The Yoga Journal* is for readers at every level of familiarity with yoga. Articles range from interviews with New Age personalities such as Ram Dass to illustrated yoga *asanas* to self-care and nutrition.

Books

Michael Castleman. *Nature's Cures*. Emmaus, PA: Rodale, 1996. This book examines thirty-three natural self-care methods, from herbs, homeopathy, and vitamin supplements to music therapy, humor, and sleep. The reader can use a "cure finder" to pick the appropriate therapy for the particular concern.

Adriane Fugh-Berman, M.D. *Alternative Medicine: What Works*. Tucson, AZ: Odonian Press, 1996. Everything you wanted to know about alternative therapies, including which ones work. Fourteen therapies are examined, including many studies done on the therapies. The author feels that alternative therapies will ultimately become part of conventional medicine.

James S. Gordon, M.D. *Manifesto for a New Medicine: Your Guide to Healing Partnerships and the Wise Use of Alternative Therapies.* Reading, MA: Addison-Wesley, 1996. How to combine conventional medicine and complementary therapies.

Dee Ito. *Without Estrogen: Natural Remedies for Menopause and Beyond.* New York: Crown, 1994. This book shows how different alternative therapists approach treating the signs of menopause. If you thought there was only one way through menopause, this book will set you straight. It has an excellent section on how to choose a complementary practitioner.

Michael Lerner, Ph.D. *Choices in Healing: Integrating the Best of Conventional and Complementary Approaches.* Cambridge: MIT Press, 1994. This book covers choices in healing from serious illness, including mainstream and complementary therapies, pain control, and dying with dignity. Lerner founded Commonweal, the first cancer retreat center.

Carolyn Myss. *The Anatomy of Spirituality.* New York: Harmony Books, 1996. Carolyn Myss is a practitioner of energy medicine, a "medical intuitive," and a well-known speaker. In this book she addresses the seven body centers and discusses how you can access your own intuition and healing powers. Her many stories of healing make this quite an inspiring and intriguing book.

Dr. Gary Null. *The Woman's Encyclopedia of Natural Healing: The New Healing Techniques of 100 Leading Alternative Health Practitioners.* New York: Seven Stories Press, 1996. This book looks at causes, symptoms, tests, and treatments. One hundred practitioners were asked what approaches they found effective for treating different ailments, and the results are included in this book.

Angela Smyth. *The Complete Home Healer: Your Guide to Every Treatment Available for Over 300 of the Most Common Health Problems.* San Francisco: HarperSanFrancisco, 1994. Look up an ailment in this comprehensive A-to-Z home reference and find remedies for it from conventional medicine, traditional Chinese medicine, aromatherapy, herbalism, diet and exercise, and many more therapies.

Asara Tshai. *Principles of Radiant Health.* Oakland, CA: Touch of Life, 1996. This book for African American women addresses nutrition, exercise, and personal care, including skin care, external cleansing, and social and emotional issues from a natural health perspective. It also includes tips for finding a natural healer.

Andrew Weil, M.D. *Spontaneous Healing: How to Discover and Enhance Your Body's Natural Ability to Maintain and Heal Itself.* New York: Knopf, 1995. Dr. Weil uses stories of his patients to show that healing is possible through many channels. He also includes a very informative section on the properties and uses of various herbs and tonics. This book is inspiring and encouraging.

ACUPUNCTURE/TRADITIONAL CHINESE MEDICINE

Marie Cargill. *Acupuncture: Available Medical Alternative.* Westport, CT: Praeger, 1994. Learn about the history of acupuncture and its usefulness in the treatment of pain, the brain, the nervous system, the immune system, and mental health.

Dr. Hong-Yen Hsu and Douglas H. Easer. *Chinese Herbal Formulas for Women.* New Canaan, CT: Keats Publishing, 1982. This book addresses health concerns unique to women, such as endometriosis and menopause. It suggests Chinese herbal remedies designed to treat the underlying causes of chronic conditions rather than the symptoms.

F. M. Houston, D.C., D.D., Ph.D., *The Healing Benefits of Acupressure.* 2d ed. New Canaan, CT: Keats Publications, 1991. Learn about the art of acupuncture with this reader-friendly book. It has good illustrations and a glossary of terms.

Daniel P. Reid. *Traditional Chinese Medicine.* Boston: Shambhala, 1996. Chinese medicine aims to create harmony of mind, body, and spirit. To achieve this harmony it uses nutrition, exercise, herbs, acupuncture, massage, meditation and other restorative practices. This book looks at prevention, diagnosis, and treatment from this perspective and includes a discussion of chi and the history of Chinese medicine.

AROMATHERAPY

Susanne Fisher-Rizzi. *Complete Aromatherapy Handbook.* New York: Sterling Press, 1990. This book, translated from German, is easy to use and provides recipes as well as advice on the use of essential oils.

Jeanne Rose and Susan Earle. *The World of Aromatherapy.* Berkeley, CA: Frog Books, 1996. An anthology of aromatic history, ideas, concepts, and case histories by the National Association for Holistic Aromatherapy (NAHA).

Maggie Tissorand. *Aromatherapy for Women.* Rochester, VT: Healing Arts Press, 1996. Useful suggestions on using essential oils to support the immune system, reduce stress, enhance well-being, and improve sexual satisfaction. You can't ask for more.

AYURVEDA

Deepak Chopra, M.D. *Perfect Health: The Complete Mind/Body Guide.* New York: Harmony Books, 1991. Dr. Chopra, the foremost popularizer of Ayurveda in the United States, explains this system of medicine. Learn how to determine your body type and how to bring your body to balance.

Nancy Lonsdorf, M.D., Veronica Butler, M.D., and Melanie Brown, Ph.D. *A Woman's Best Medicine, Health, Happiness, and Long Life Through Ayur-Veda.* New York: Putnam, 1993. This book first helps you determine your body type and then explains how to bring balance into your life through mind–body approaches to wellness. Chapter 11 discusses menopause and offers some practical tips for aging.

HERBS

Amanda McQuade Crawford. *The Herbal Menopause Book: Herbs, Nutrition and Other Natural Therapies.* Freedom, CA: Crossing Press, 1996. This book gets right to the point: herbs for treating perimenopausal symptoms. It's easy to use and includes nutrition and mind–body approaches to better health.

Richard Makey, ed. *The New Age Herbalist.* New York: Macmillan, 1988. This book addresses ways to use herbs for healing, nutrition, body care, and relaxation. It contains beautiful botanical pictures.

Varro Tyler. *The Honest Herbal—A Sensible Guide to the Use of Herbs and Related Remedies.* 3d ed. Birmingham, NY: Haworth, 1993. How do you know how much to take of what? And what for? Read this book. It's a good source of information about herbs and plant remedies.

Susun Weed. *Wise Woman: Menopausal Years.* Woodstock, NY: Ash Tree Publishing, 1992. A useful book of botanicals to use when looking for ways to cope with the signs of menopause. The book also contains folk wisdom.

HOMEOPATHY

Dr. Christopher Hammond. *The Complete Family Guide to Homeopathy: Illustrated Encyclopedia of Safe and Effective Remedies.* New York: Penguin, 1995. This practical and well-illustrated guide details more than eighty homeopathic remedies. It has useful tables and is easy to understand.

MASSAGE/ACUPRESSURE/SHIATSU

Cathryn Bauer. *Acupressure for Women.* Freedom, CA: Crossing Press, 1987. This helpful book contains easy-to-use illustrations and instructions for acupressure for women. It looks at issues of concern to women and suggests acupressure treatments.

Lucinda Lidell. *The Book of Massage: The Complete Step-by-Step Guide to Eastern and Western Techniques.* New York: Simon and Schuster, 1984. This book on massage, reflexology, and Shiatsu stresses the need to have a pleasing environment and talks about the idea of the healing touch.

Ray Ridolfi and Susanne Franzen. *Shiatsu for Women.* San Francisco: Thorsons, 1996. Shiatsu is a Japanese massage therapy that is excellent for stress relief. This guide is very practical and focuses on women's health issues.

Diane Stein. *Essential Reiki, A Complete Guide to an Ancient Healing Art.* Freedom, CA: Crossing Press, 1996. To be a reiki healer, you need to have attunements from a teacher. But if you just want to learn about it, this book demystifies the ancient healing system and talks about the emotional sources of disease, chakras, and includes a special chapter on "Ki" exercises for women.

REFLEXOLOGY

Ann Gillander. *The Joy of Reflexology: Healing Techniques for Hands and Feet to Reduce Stress and Reclaim Health.* Boston: Little Brown, 1995. This book illustrates the body systems that are attended to in reflexology and explains the principles behind it. Color illustrations and ailment reference charts make this book easy to use.

Nicola Hall. *Reflexology for Women: Restore Harmony and Balance Through Precise Massaging Techniques.* San Franciso: HarperCollins, 1994. This book gives some history of reflexology and addresses conditions specific to women that respond to reflexology—for example, fibroids, endometriosis, and menopause difficulties. There is also a section on general conditions that respond to reflexology; illustrations are included.

Audio/Video

You can explore the world of complementary medicine on tape to your heart's content. In fact, there are so many tapes we gave up trying to list them. Instead, these catalogs are all good sources for audio- and videotapes on a wide range of therapies and paths. Other good catalogs include **Sounds True** (see Audio/Video, Chapter 5), **Living Arts** (see Audio/Video, Chapter 3), and **Layna Berman** (see Audio/Video, Chapter 4).

Conference Recording Service, 1308 Gilman St., Berkeley, CA 94706. Voice: (800) 647-1110. Fax: (510) 527-8404. Internet: newmed.com. The web site offers alternative medicine information, spiritual tapes, and conference recordings. You can also call for a catalog to receive a list of taped conferences, many on women's health and complementary medicine.

Meno Tapes, Menopause Center, 1108 Irwin St., San Rafael, CA 94901. Voice: (415) 459-5430. Meno Tapes is a list of primarily audiotapes that address natural remedies for menopause and places to get them. You can order the list for a small fee.

Sound Horizons, 250 W. 57th St., Suite 1517, New York, NY 10107. Voice: (800) 524-8355. Audiotapes on self-help, health, and relaxation. You'll find taped conferences and workshops along with some studio-produced tapes.

Tree Farm Communications, 23703 N.E. 4th St., Redmond, WA 98053. Voice: (800) 468-0464. Fax: (206) 868-2495. E-mail: 74117.720@compuserve.com. This company records conferences primarily on complementary medicine. It has an extensive catalog.

Wishing Well Distributing, P.O. Box 1008, Silver Lake, WI 53170. Voice: (800) 888-9355. Wishing Well has a large selection of New Age videos on many topics: acupressure, massage, Shiatsu, and more.

Online

The Internet is filled with resources to help you in your search for complementary therapies. Many of the organizations listed above have Internet addresses. You can search for the subject you're interested in using a search engine or start at one of the general sites listed below. Follow the many links in the general web sites.

MAILING LISTS

Subscribe to **The Holistic List,** a holistic health discussion group, at listserv@siucvmb.siu.edu. For **The Herblist, the Medicinal and Aromatic Plants Discussion List,** contact listserv@trearnpc.ege.edu.tr. **The Aromatherapy List** is run through listserv@idma.com. **The OrMed Mailing List,** an Eastern medicine mailing list, is run through listserv@bkhouse.cts.com.

News Groups

Discuss all aspects of complementary medicine at **misc.health.alternative**, or try a **sci.med** group. For herbs and natural foods, try **alt.folklore.herbs**, **bionet.plants**, **rec.gardens**, **rec.food.preserving**, or **sci.med.nutrition**. For aromatherapy, try **alt.aromatherapy**; for Ayurveda, try **alt.health.ayurveda**.

Web Sites

The Alternative Medicine Homepage, at www.pitt.edu/~cbw/altm.html, is a good place to start looking for Internet resources, news groups and mailing lists, commercial databases, and many links. **Natural Medicine, Complementary Health Care, and Alternative Medicine**, at www.amrta.org/~amrta, is a great place for alternative health care tips, lists of organizations, schools, training programs, and, of course, lots of links. **Dr. Bower's Alternative and Complementary Medicine Home Page**, galen.med.virginia.edu/~pjb3s/ComplementaryHomePage.html, is a great source for fact sheets on many complementary medicine topics and for information about ongoing research.

The **Doc Weil Database** at www.hotwired.com/drweil is the place to be if you've ever wanted to ask Dr. Andrew Weil a question about anything. It's a fun site, updated almost constantly, and quite addictive (in a positive way)! Check out the alphabetical database, where you can look up just about anything, from a specific herb, medication, or symptom ("from acne to zinc") to questions and answers to how to treat a cold, to how to find a complementary health practitioner in your area.

For specific areas, check out the following: **Acupuncture.com** at www.acupuncture.com; **The Homeopathy Homepage** at www.dungeon.com/~cam/homeo.html; **Medicinal Herb FAQ** at sunsite.unc.edu/herbmed/mediherb.html; **Natureopathic Medicine Network** at www.pandamedicine.com; **The Reiki Page** at www.crl.com/~davidh/reiki; and the **Chiropractic Page** at www.mbnet.mb.ca/~jwiens/chiro.html.

. . . .

What's Up, Doc?

Working with Your Western Health Practitioner

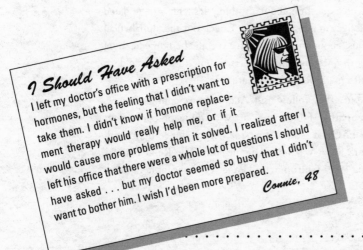

I Should Have Asked

I left my doctor's office with a prescription for hormones, but the feeling that I didn't want to take them. I didn't know if hormone replacement therapy would really help me, or if it would cause more problems than it solved. I realized after I left his office that there were a whole lot of questions I should have asked . . . but my doctor seemed so busy that I didn't want to bother him. I wish I'd been more prepared.

Connie, 48

. . . .

Menopause is not a disease. But no matter how healthy you are, midlife brings new health concerns related to aging and the decline in estrogen. Although you may never have given a thought to osteoporosis and heart disease before, in midlife they become a concern. The logical place to begin looking for answers to your questions on these health issues is with your health practitioner. And the best way to get answers that make sense is to find a doctor to whom you can talk freely and establish a good working relationship.

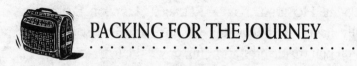

PACKING FOR THE JOURNEY

What Are the Health Concerns of Midlife?

Declining levels of estrogen mean more concern about heart disease, osteoporosis, and vaginal and genital health—whether or not you take hormone replacement therapy. The idea of "treating" perimenopausal symptoms with HRT presupposes that menopause is a "disease" that can be "cured." Clearly, this is not the case. However, conventional medicine can help women cope with some of the problems that crop up. For more on what Western medicine offers for coping with menopause, heart disease, and osteoporosis and to learn about breast cancer (a concern to women at almost any age), see the individual chapters on each subject.

How Can I Find a Doctor I Can Work With?

Many medical solutions are reached in tandem, doctor and patient working together. A doctor who knows you and respects you can be an important source of information and advice—no matter how much research you do, you can't know everything. When you and your doctor work as partners, you have a powerful team for good health. Here's how to start looking:

FIND ONE BEFORE YOU NEED ONE   If you don't already have a doctor, start looking now. When you're ill and feeling needy, it's much harder to be discriminating.

ASK FRIENDS TO RECOMMEND A DOCTOR   This is the easiest route to a good doctor. If your friends are happy, chances are you will be too.

CONTACT A COMMUNITY WOMEN'S HEALTH GROUP   Community groups are a good source of information. Many will have a list already prepared.

ASK ANOTHER PHYSICIAN WITH WHOM YOU HAVE HAD GOOD EXPERIENCES   Doctors know other doctors, and they know which ones are good. Ask a doctor who understands your needs, and you'll likely get some good referrals.

CONTACT A LOCAL HOSPITAL FOR A REFERRAL LIST OF DOCTORS
Hospitals usually have lists of doctors who are affiliated with them. Choose a hospital you trust, and start going down the list.

FIND A WOMEN'S HEALTH CENTER
Women's health centers are set up to respond to the special needs of women. Most are friendly places with staff who are willing and happy to talk with you. Look in the yellow pages or ask at a women's bookstore.

I Have to Go Where My Insurance Sends Me. How Can I Make Sure I'm Getting Good Treatment?

Most HMOs allow you to choose the doctor you're going to see, although you may have a limited number of choices. Some health plans provide short biographies of their physicians. If possible, speak to other patients, or ask nurses for recommendations. Then ask the HMO doctor the same questions that you would ask any other doctor. If you feel you're being herded through the system, put down your foot and insist on being treated as an individual. It's more work, but it's not impossible! Remember, under most managed care plans, your primary care physician will be a key player in your health care—making referrals and analyzing your health—so it's important to feel comfortable with your choice.

TRAVEL TIP

Looking for a Doctor? Go to the Source

One good way to find a doctor is to contact an organization specific to your needs. For example, the North American Menopause Society (NAMS) will send you a referral list of practitioners in your area who are members of this association, which offers annual conferences highlighting the latest menopause research and trends. You can also contact the American College of Obstetricians and Gynecologists. If you're looking for a physician who will prescribe natural hormones, call one of the compounding pharmacies listed in Resources for names of doctors in your area who use their products. See Resources for more information.

I'm Interested in Exploring Complementary Medicine, But I Don't Feel Comfortable Telling My Doctor

You can only find out if you ask, and you may be surprised at the answer. With the advent of the concepts of wellness and preventive medicine over the last twenty years or so, the lines between conventional medicine and complementary medicine are beginning to overlap. Some doctors are not interested, but many are open to a more integral approach. Some complementary techniques are being taught in medical schools today, so you may have luck with younger doctors. Insurance is catching

GUIDED TOUR:
Western Medicine

For the best health care, work in partnership with your doctor. Choose a doctor you can talk to, and do your best to ensure good communication. Prepare yourself with a knowledge of your family health history as well as your own medical history. If it's an important office visit, consider taking along a friend or relative.

WESTERN MEDICINE

Conventional Western medicine can help women cope with the health concerns of midlife, such as osteoporosis, heart disease, vaginal dryness or atrophy, and hot flashes. Consult a doctor if you are bleeding or in extreme pain or have some other acute symptom.

COMPLEMENTARY THERAPIES

More and more doctors are including aspects of complementary medicine in their treatment. Some insurance companies will cover acupuncture, chiropractic, and other alternative therapies. You may be able to find a health practitioner who is willing to work with such an integrated approach.

EXCERSISE

Medicine is increasingly recognizing the role of regular physical activity in helping us stay healthy and fight disease. For example, exercise, along with stress relief and a diet low in saturated fat, is recommended for heart patients as well as for people who want to prevent heart disease.

NUTRITION

What we eat has a great impact on our health. High-saturated-fat diets have been implicated in heart disease, breast cancer, and other illnesses, while a diet that includes monounsaturates such as olive oil seems to be beneficial for our health. You can find all the nutrients your body needs to stay healthy in a balanced diet that includes fruits, vegetables, nuts, grains, and lean protein.

Midlife Medical Tests

How many medical tests do you really need? If you have special health concerns, your doctor may suggest adding tests that aren't on this list. In general, these are the tests a healthy woman should have between ages forty and forty-nine:

- Mammogram: once a year
- Pap test and pelvic exam: once a year each
- Blood pressure check: once a year

And these are the tests she needs at age fifty and beyond:

- Mammogram: once a year
- Pap test and pelvic exam: once a year each
- Blood pressure check: once a year
- Colorectal cancer screening: get a baseline screening (frequency of subsequent testing may vary)
- Lipid profile: get a baseline screening (frequency of subsequent testing may vary)
- Bone density test: consider this if you think you may be at risk

How to Find an Open-Minded M.D.

- Ask your complementary practitioner for a referral to a physician.
- Contact the American Holistic Medical Association. Its members, from many disciplines, include M.D.s
- Contact the American Association of Naturopathic Physicians. Many naturopaths are also M.D.s.

up, too. For example, Washington and Connecticut have passed insurance equity laws, so health insurance policies in these states will cover some complementary treatments. If your doctor is not open to the avenues you want to explore, you may want to find another doctor. If you are having any kind of alternative treatments, keep your doctor informed.

How Can I Communicate Effectively with My Doctor?

A *Health*/Roper telephone poll asked 750 people, "What's the major source of problems in doctor-patient communication?" The two top answers were "Doctors don't explain things clearly" (34 percent) and "Patients aren't good at describing problems" (29 percent). Clearly, there's work to be done on both sides. Here are some hints.

DON'T MINIMIZE YOUR PROBLEM   Typically, even though you've suffered for a week, all the symptoms magically disappear when you go for an office visit. Nonetheless, it's important to tell your doctor exactly what brought you there as simply and straightforwardly as possible.

DON'T LEAVE ANYTHING OUT   Small, nagging symptoms may not seem important enough to bring to your doctor, but they may provide the clue your doctor needs to nail down your problem.

IF YOU DON'T UNDERSTAND SOMETHING, SAY SO   How many times have you gone home from a doctor's appointment and realized you don't know why you're supposed to take a prescribed medicine? You'll have better results sticking to the program your doctor gives you if you understand why you're doing it and what the benefits will be.

ASK QUESTIONS   Some doctors are chatty, some are silent. Doctors are people, too—they're all different. If you're not getting enough information to satisfy you, ask.

DON'T BE INTIMIDATED   If you're intimidated by your doctor, you may not get all the help you need. Doctors often move quickly from patient to patient. *You* are the one who knows what your needs are. If you feel you're not being taken seriously, or you feel you need tests that aren't being offered, say so (but be tactful!).

BE HONEST   It's easy to leave out information that's embarrassing—you stopped taking the pills your doctor prescribed because you forgot, you drink more than you think your doctor will approve of, you aren't really sticking to that exercise program. If you're not straight with your doctor, you won't get the kind of treatment you need.

IF ALL ELSE FAILS, FIND ANOTHER DOCTOR
If you've honestly tried to communicate with your doctor, but you continually feel confused, brushed off, short-changed, or intimidated, it's time to find another doctor!

How Can I Prepare for My Doctor's Appointment?

Doctors are often pushed for time. To get the most out of your appointment, it helps to plan ahead. Here are a few things you can do:

EXPECT THE BEST   When you go to see your doctor, go with the idea that she or he wants

POINT OF INTEREST
Avoid Medical Hexing!

Your doctor's attitude toward your healing may be crucial to your outcome. Here's what two doctors have to say:

Andrew Weil, M.D., in *Spontaneous Healing:* "Here are the complaints I hear most often: 'Doctors don't take time to listen to you or answer your questions.' 'They said there was nothing more they could do for me.' 'They told me it would only get worse.' 'They told me I would just have to live with it.' 'They said I'd be dead in six months.' The last four statements are particularly disturbing, because they reflect deep pessimism about the human potential for healing. At its most extreme, this attitude constitutes a kind of medical 'hexing' that I find unconscionable. Although it is easy to identify this hexing phenomenon in exotic cultures, we rarely perceive something very similar that goes on every day in our own culture, in hospitals, clinics, and doctor's offices."

Larry Dossey, M.D., in *Healing Words:* "Because it is generally agreed that a patient's attitudes are crucial to his or her response to a particular treatment, it is usually only the *patient's* beliefs that are considered when a particular therapy is entered. Is he or she cooperative? Will he or she give the medication a chance to work? Does he or she have a desire to get better? A will to live? Although it is essential to ask these questions, the beliefs of the patient are only one side of the coin. The physician's beliefs also shape the outcome of the therapy."

Tracking Down Your Family Health History

Although it can be successfully argued that living in ignorance can be bliss, ignorance of our family's health history can make us miss early signs of trouble that we might easily correct. According to Michael Crouch, a leading expert on inherited risks, "In the balance of things, learning more about your family history is about as close as you can get to controlling your destiny." Especially when you're facing a choice about your health, it can be crucial to know your family health history. Three areas are especially important for women at midlife:

1. Heart disease: If your father or brother had a heart attack before the age of fifty-five, or your mother or sister had a heart attack before age sixty-five, you may have an increased risk of heart disease.

2. Osteoporosis: If any family members had or have bone loss, you may be at increased risk for osteoporosis.

3. Breast cancer: Any history of breast cancer, on your father's side of the family as well as your mother's side, may put you at increased risk.

Risk factors that mean nothing to you may be red flags for your doctor. That's why the more detailed a history you can develop, the better chance you'll have of creating a realistic picture of your health risks and strengths and the better chance you'll have of being able to work with your doctor or other health professionals to make the best choices possible. You'll find a family medical history questionnaire in Part 2, Your Personal Companion. See Resources for some ideas on where to begin.

to help you and give you the best treatment possible.

MAKE A LIST   Write down your questions and concerns before you leave the house. That way you won't forget to ask that important question. Refer to your list during your appointment.

BRING AN ADVOCATE   If you tend to get nervous during a medical appointment, you might forget what was said by the time you get home. If this is an important appointment—to discuss surgery, serious medical treatment, or how to deal with menopausal symptoms—you may want to bring a trusted friend or your partner or spouse to the appointment with you. This person can help you pick up on ideas that may not be on your list. Later, your advocate can help you remember what was said.

BE ABLE TO EXPRESS YOUR REASON FOR THE VISIT   If you are going for a specific complaint, be as clear as possible about your symptoms—length of time you've had them, intensity, frequency, and so on. Let your provider know why you're there. If you want to explore options, say so.

PREPARE YOUR PERSONAL MEDICAL HISTORY   Be able to provide information about diseases or surgeries you have had in the past, medications you are currently taking, alternative treatments you may be involved in.

PUT TOGETHER YOUR FAMILY MEDICAL HISTORY   A family history of medical problems can alert your doctor to look for things that might otherwise escape notice. See "Tracking Down Your Family Health History" for pointers to family conditions that are particularly important for women at midlife.

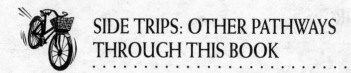

SIDE TRIPS: OTHER PATHWAYS THROUGH THIS BOOK

. . . .

CHAPTER 2: WHY IS THIS HAPPENING TO ME?   Menopause is not a disease, but midlife does have some new health concerns your doctor may be able to help you with. Look here for an overview of what to expect.

CHAPTER 7: THE HOLISTIC KIT AND CABOODLE   Western medicine is not the whole enchilada. Look here for an overview of approaches you may want to consider integrating into the way you care for your health.

CHAPTER 9: YES OR NO?   Your doctor is the first place to start when you're considering hormone replacement therapy. Look here to learn more about the pros and cons.

CHAPTER 10: THE WORLD DOWN UNDER   Your doctor may be able to help you cope with vaginal dryness, urinary incontinence, and uterine prolapse. Look here for more ways to cope.

CHAPTER 11: BONING UP   Loss of bone density is one of the major health concerns of women at midlife. Look here to learn what you can do to retard this loss.

CHAPTER 12: AND THE BEAT GOES ON   All women are at increased risk of heart disease after menopause. Look here to learn how you can protect your heart through lifestyle changes.

CHAPTER 13: WHAT ARE MY CHANCES?   Do you have to worry about breast cancer? Look here to learn more about this troubling disease.

CHAPTER 14: IS THIS REALLY NECESSARY? Look here to learn more about hysterectomy (one of the most-performed surgeries on women) and alternative treatments.

TRAVEL TIP

Think About Participating in a Clinical Trial

Yes, in some sense each woman is her own clinical trial. But this shouldn't prevent you from participating in an *official* clinical trial, if you so desire. Even if your participation does not benefit you directly, you will be contributing to the body of medical knowledge. Currently, clinical trials are being conducted in many areas, including tamoxifen therapy for women at high risk for breast cancer; on lipid-lowering drugs for people at high risk for coronary disease; on antihypertensive medication aimed at stopping kidney deterioration in African Americans with high blood pressure; and on hormone replacement therapy, dietary intervention, and/or calcium–vitamin D supplementation in postmenopausal women. Call (800) 54-CANCER to request the free booklet "What Are Clinical Trials All About?" See Resources for more information.

RESOURCES

Organizations and Services

In addition to the organizations in this section, take a look at the listings in Chapter 2, "Why Is This Happening to Me?," and the individual chapters on specific health problems.

American College of Obstetricians and Gynecologists (ACOG), Resource Center, 409 12th St. S.W., Washington, DC 20024-2188. Voice: (202) 638-5577. Fax: (202) 484-5107. Internet: www.acog.com. This national professional society publishes educational materials and video- and audio cassettes it has a public resource center of more than 10,000 books and 500 newsletters and medical journals. Write for "Reproductive Health," a free patient education pamphlet developed to help women make decisions about health care.

Boston Women's Health Collective, 240A Elm St., Somerville, MA 02144. Voice: (617) 625-0271. This group is responsible for the books *Our Bodies, Ourselves* and *The New Ourselves, Growing Older*. You can write or call to request information on women and aging. There is a small charge to cover costs.

Food and Drug Administration, 5600 Fishers Lane, Rockville, MD, 20857. Voice: (800) 532-4440. The FDA tests and approves drugs, among other things. Call the consumer's affairs number to ask questions about drugs and food supplements.

Institute for Natural Resources (INR), P.O. Box 4218, Berkeley, CA 94704-0218. Voice: (510) 450-1650. Fax: (510) 652-1859. E-mail: biocorp@aol.com. INR is a nonprofit scientific organization dedicated to research and education in the fields of science and medicine. INR provides continuing education for health providers, but interested laypeople can attend. The institute offers a number of women's health seminars all over the country. Send for information.

National Black Women's Health Project, 1211 Connecticut Ave., Washington, DC 20036. Voice: (202) 835-0117. The NBWHP acts as an advocate for African American women. The group has physician statements about African American women and selected health issues. Write or call to receive a packet of information.

National Health Information Center, P.O. Box 1133, Washington, DC 20013-1133. Voice: (800) 336-4797. E-mail: nhicinfo@health.org. Internet: nhic-nt.health.org. Speak with an information specialist who can put you in contact with the agency best able to respond to your needs. You can also request a list of 100 health-related hotlines.

National Institute of Aging, National Institutes of Health, Information Center, P.O. Box 8057, Gaithersburg, MD 20898-8057. Voice: (800) 222-2225. TDD: (800) 222-4225. Fax: (310) 589-3014. E-mail: niainfo@access.digex.net. Internet: www.nih.gov/nia. The NIA, the principal biomedical research agency of the United States government, is concerned with healthy aging. It has very good fact sheets and publications available on a number of different health topics, including osteoporosis, heart disease, menopause, and cancer. Request a publications catalog.

National Latina Health Organization, P.O. Box 7567, Oakland, CA 94601. Voice: (510) 534-1362. Call or write for information regarding conferences, forums, resources, and bilingual care.

National Women's Health Network, 514 10th St. N.W., Suite 400, Washington, DC 20004. Voice: (202) 347-1140. Fax: (202) 344-1168. Women's Health Clearinghouse: (202) 628-7814. Internet: www.womenconnect.com/or20550g.htm. This women's advocacy membership organization sponsors a wealth of resources, including the Women's Health Clearinghouse and the Women's Health Information Service Library. With membership you get a newsletter that updates you on all its activities. You do not need to be a member to purchase, for a low fee, their very informative packets of information. Use the network's "Doctor–Patient Checklist" as a continuing record of your health.

Native American Women's Health Education Resource Center, P.O. Box 572, Lake Andes, SD 57356-0572. Voice: (605) 487-7072. Fax: (605) 487-7964. E-mail: nativewoman@igc.org. This advocacy and educational organization also publishes a newsletter, *Wicozanni Wowapi*, covering health and environmental issues. Call about resources and educational materials for Native American women.

North American Menopause Society (NAMS), c/o Department of OB/GYN, University Hospitals of Cleveland, 11100 Euclid Ave., Cleveland, OH 44106. Voice: (216) 844-8748. Fax: (216) 844-8708. E-mail: nams@atk.et. Internet: www.menopause.org/all.html. The North American Menopause Society is a nonprofit professional organization of physicians, clinicians, scientists, and researchers. NAMS promotes the study and exchange of information about the climacteric in women. It also offers educational programs and maintains a list of menopause care providers. Send for a list of doctors in your area who specialize in treating women in midlife.

Office on Women's Health, U.S. Department of Health and Human Services, Humphrey Building, 200 Independence Ave. S.W., Washington, DC 20201, Room 712 E. Voice: (202) 690-7650. Fax: (202) 690-7172. The OWH is the coordinating office of the federal government for women's health issues. Its stated mission is "to improve the health of women across the life-span." It does this by educating women about healthful lifestyles, and working to provide more money for research into female health problems. Until now, women have been for the most part excluded from many health studies—research into heart problems, for example, was conducted only on men. Currently, OWH is putting together a women's health clearinghouse. Contact this very accessible agency to receive articles on the following topics: women and AIDS, menopause, women and domestic violence, women and heart disease, and more. The office also has information on and advocates for research and education regarding the concerns of women of color. Call for a complete list of articles.

Women's Health Initiative, National Institutes of Health, 7550 Wisconsin Ave., Room 6A09, Bethesda, MD 20892-9110. Voice: (800) 54-WOMEN or (301) 402-2900. Fax: (301) 480-5158. Internet: www.nih.gov/od/odp/whi. Write or call for a copy of the "Women's Health Initiative," which details the studies in progress and planned over the next fifteen years. The 800 number will refer you to your local center, from which you can request a list of clinical trial centers.

Women to Women, 1 Pleasant St., Yarmouth, ME 04096. Voice: (207) 846-6163. This women's medical clinic was founded by Dr. Christiane Northrup and three other practitioners. Dr. Northrup is a holistic physician and a member of the American Holistic Medical Association. She has produced audio- and videotapes, a newsletter, and the book *Women's Bodies, Women's Wisdom.* This group is committed to promoting health and balance and addressing the specific health concerns of women. The clinic offers a regular medical practice and also sponsors lectures and workshops and offers products, including tapes (see Audio/Video, below).

FAMILY HISTORY

If you're trying to track down your family health history, the following resources may be helpful. "To See Your Future, Look into Your Past," by Steven Finch, was printed in *Health* (October 1996): 93–101. This is an excellent article on the basics for anyone who wants to find out more about family health history.

Family History Library of the Church of Jesus Christ of Latter-Day Saints, 35 Northwest Temple, Salt Lake City, UT 84150. You do not have to be a Mormon to use this enormous (two billion names) genealogical resource. There are 1,800 Family Search Centers throughout the United States and Canada. Write for information or look in the yellow pages for your local center.

National Adoption Information Clearinghouse, 5640 Nicholson Lane, Suite 300, Rockville, MD 20852. Voice: (301) 231-6512. E-mail: naic@calib.com. Internet: www.calib.com/naic. If you're searching for your birth parents, this is a good place to start. The clearinghouse has a number of fact sheets, including "Searching for Birth Relatives." If you have Internet access, the web site has a lot of downloadable information.

National Genealogical Society, 4527 17th St. North, Arlington, VA 22207. Voice: (703) 525-0050. Internet: www.familytreemaker.com/00000141.html. This organization sponsors a library and publishes information designed to help you find your family health records. Its FamilyFinder Index contains approximately 115 million names.

RESEARCH REPORTS

The Health Resource Inc., 564 Locust St., Conway, AR 72032. Voice: (800) 949-0090. Fax: (501) 329-9489. E-mail: moreinfo@thehealthresource.com. Internet: www. thehealthresource.com. This medical information service will provide you with an individualized comprehensive research report on a specific medical condition. Reports contain information on both traditional and complementary therapies, current research, self-help, resource organizations, and specialist referral information.

Med Help International, Suite 130, Box 188, 6300 N. Wickham Road, Melbourne, FL 32940. Voice: (407) 253-9048. E-mail: staff@medhelp.netusa.net. Internet: medhlp.netusa.net. Med Help is the largest online medical information source for consumers. See Online for more information.

Planetree Health Resource Center, 2040 Webster St., San Francisco, CA 94115. Voice: (415) 923-3681. Fax: (415) 673-2629. Planetree is a health and medical library open without fee to the general public. The library contains a wide range of health information from conventional to alternative therapies. For a fee, Planetree can provide information packets on specific medical topics and diagnoses, or computer-searched bibliographies of the medical literature from databases of the National Library of Medicine and the National Cancer Institute. Call for prices and information about *The Planetree Health Catalog.*

Well-Connected, Nidus Information Services, 175 Fifth Ave., New York, NY 10010. Voice: (800) 334-WELL. Well-Connected publishes medical reports on a range of subjects. Eight-page reports are updated quarterly to reflect the latest research and information.

World Research Foundation, 20501 Ventura Blvd., Suite 100, Woodland Hills, CA 91364. Voice: (818) 999-5483. Fax: (818) 227-6484. Second address: 41 Bell Rock Plaza, Suite C, Sedona, AZ 86351. Voice: (520) 284-3300. Fax: (520) 284-3530. This organization offers computer and library searches on both traditional and complementary therapies for specific health problems. Also available are a catalog of books and tapes and a newsletter.

Hotlines

American Board of Medical Specialties: (800) 776-CERT. Call to check a physician's board-certification credentials.

FDA: (800) 532-4440. Call the FDA's consumer information line with questions about FDA-approved drugs or adverse reactions.

National Health Information Center: (800) 336-4797. Call for a list of 100 health-related hotlines.

National Institutes of Health, Women's Health Initiative: (800) 54-WOMEN. Call this hotline to be connected with the WHI center nearest you.

Office of Minority Health Resource Center: (800) 248-4344. Call for information on resources for people of color.

CLINICAL TRIALS:

African-American Study of Kidney Disease and Hypertension: (800) 277-2275.

Antihypertensive and Lipid-Lowering Treatment to Prevent Heart Attack Trial (ALLHAT): (800) 690-7870.

Breast Cancer Prevention Trial: (800) 4-CANCER.

Coordinating Center for Clinical Trials: (800) 690-7870.

Periodicals

Consumer Reports on Health, 101 Truman Ave., Yonkers, NY 10703-1057. Voice: (800) 234-2188. This six-page newsletter published by the nonprofit Consumers Union features articles on health and fitness issues. It also has information on current research as well as a nutrition update.

Harvard Women's Health Watch: Information for Enlightened Choices from Harvard Medical School, P.O. Box 420234, Palm Coast, FL 32142-0234. Voice: (800) 829-5921 This eight-page newsletter covers virtually every health topic of interest to women, including the environmental influences on breast cancer, the relationship between caffeine and women's health, eye surgery, and the curative ability of cranberry juice on urinary tract infections. It's always up to date, easy to understand, and highly informative.

Health, P.O. Box 56863, Boulder, CO 80322-6863. Voice: (800) 274-2522. This glossy magazine is available on newsstands as well as by subscription. Each issue is packed with interesting articles and news flashes about health topics of every sort, many aimed at women in midlife. It's intelligent and fun to read, and it has great graphics and layout.

Johns Hopkins Medical Letter: Health After 50, P.O. Box 420179, Palm Coast, FL 32142. This newsletter from Johns Hopkins University covers a wide range of health issues faced by men and women over fifty.

Network News, National Women's Health Network, 514 10th St. N.W., Suite 400, Washington, DC 20004. Voice: (202) 347-1140. Fax: (202) 344-1168. The National Women's Health Network's informative newsletter reports on current research, publications, and conferences regarding women's health issues. It also offers a feminist critique of health issues.

University of California Wellness Letter, P.O. Box 420148, Palm Coast, FL 32142. This publication covers a wide range of health issues and reports the latest findings in many areas. It's worth reading and informative.

Women's Health Access, 429 Gammon Place, P.O. Box 259690, Madison, WI 53725. Voice: (800) 558-7046. This bimonthly newsletter is offered by Women's Health America Group. It covers a wide range of women's health issues; it includes book reviews and offers products.

Women's Health Connection, P.O. Box 6338, Madison, WI 53716-0338. Voice: (800) 366-6632. This newsletter is published by the educational division of Women's International Pharmacy. It is issued six times a year and deals with PMS, menopause, and other hormone-related concerns.

Books

Diane L. Adam, M.D., ed. *Health Issues for Women of Color: Cultural Diversity Perspective.* Thousand Oaks, CA: Sage Publications, 1995. A collection of articles addressing the issues of health and diverse populations.

Tracy Chutorian Sempler. *All About Eve: The Complete Guide to Women's Health and Wellbeing.* New York: HarperCollins, 1995. This book can help you choose a doctor and sort through research. It also includes resources, signs and signals of illness, and preventive treatment.

Roselyn Payne Epps, ed., and American Medical Women's Association. *The Women's Complete Health Book.* New York: Delacorte Press, 1995. This big book gives state-of-the-art medical information for all stages of a woman's life. It's illustrated and includes diagnostic tests.

Paula B. Doress-Worters and Diana Laskin Siegal, with Boston Women's Health Collective. *The New Ourselves, Growing Older.* New York: Simon and Schuster, 1994. A wonderful and useful book to have as we age. This large book addresses many topics concerning women and aging, including women's health issues.

Directory of Women's Health Care Centers. To order: 4041 N. Central, No. 700, Phoenix, AZ 85012. More than 200 addresses and phone numbers of health care centers for women. $45.

Denise Foley, Eileen Nechas, and the Editors of Prevention Magazine. *Women's Encyclopedia of Health and Emotional Healing.* Emmaus, PA: Rodale, 1992. Advice from 150 female physicians, nurses, educators, and therapists on many issues of a woman's well-being, including aging and retirement. The book includes personal stories as well as practical advice.

Kary L. Moss, ed. *Man-Made Medicine, Women's Health, Public Policy, and Reform.* Durham, NC: Duke University Press, 1996. How the gender bias in the medical establishment affects women's health and the care they receive. Essays by doctors, activists, scholars, and lawyers all contribute to a new way of thinking about health care.

William Parker, M.D., with Rachel Parker. *Gynecologists' Second Opinion: The Questions and Answers You Need to Take Charge of Your Health.* New York: Penguin, 1996. This book addresses such topics as fibroids, hysterectomy, uterine prolapse, and cancer, to name a few, and has the latest information on drugs, tests, and surgery. The question-and-answer format helps readers find information and form questions for their doctor.

Gorun Sansioe, OB/Gyn. *Visual Diagnosis: Self-Tests on the Menopause and HRT.* Coral Springs, FL: Merit Publishing International, 1996. This book of diagnostic tests is structured around information, questions, and case histories, and is a clinician's book for diagnosis.

Eddie C. Sollie, M.D., OB/Gyn. *Straight Talk with Your Gynecologist: How to Get the Answers That Will Save Your Life.* Hillsboro, OR: Beyond Words Publishing, 1992. This book describes how to talk with your doctor and build a partnership. It also includes a good glossary of terms and explains types of tests and their interpretations.

Susan Swedo and Henrietta Leonard. *It's Not All in Your Head*. San Francisco: Harper-SanFrancisco, 1996. Are you sick, or are you imagining it? Personal tales of misdiagnosis and what to do if you think it's happened to you.

Linda Villarosa, ed. A National Women's Health Project Book. *Body and Soul: The Black Woman's Guide to Physical Health and Emotional Well-Being*. New York: HarperPerennial, 1994. This book is an inclusive look at health for African American women. There are sections on personal care, taking care of the body, menopause, love, and more.

Evelyn C. White, ed. *The Black Women's Health Book: Speaking for Ourselves*. Seattle: Seal Press, 1990. A collection of articles addressing African American women's health issues, lifestyles, and issues of diversity.

Audio/Video

You'll find a lot of good tapes on health and fitness as it relates to women. The catalogs below are all good sources. For tapes on complementary approaches to health, see Chapter 7, "The Holistic Kit and Caboodle."

Fanlight, 47 Halifax St., Boston, MA 02130. Voice: (800) 937-4113 or (617) 524-0980. Fax: (617) 524-8838. E-mail: Fanlight@TIAC.net. Internet: www.fanlight. com/index.htm. Fanlight distributes independently produced educational videos on health-related topics, including menopause, women's health, breast cancer, and caregiving. Call for a catalog, or access it online at the web site.

The Learning Lane, Total Marketing Services, 400 Morris Ave., Long Branch, NJ 07740. Credit card orders: (800) 469-7977. Fax orders: (800) 699-1744. Customer service: (800) 262-3822. Internet: www.learninglane.com/Learning/women.html. Learning Lane carries special-interest videos and CD-ROMs and has a number of women's health videos. Call for the catalog, or access it online.

The Planetree Health Catalog, Planetree Health Resource Center at California Pacific Medical Center, 2040 Webster St., San Francisco, CA 94115. Voice: (415) 923-3681. Books and tapes on aging, recovery, relaxation, women's health, and more.

The VideoFinders Collection, 425 E. Colorado St., B10, Glendale, CA 91205. Voice: (800) 799-1199. Fax: (818) 637-5276. A collection of more than 125,000 documentary and entertainment videos from public television, The Learning Channel, and other sources. If you've seen it on PBS, you'll find it here.

Women to Women, 1 Pleasant St., Yarmouth, ME 04096. Voice: (207) 846-6163. This women's medical clinic, founded by Dr. Christiane Northrup and three other practitioners, has a list of audiotapes by Dr. Northrup on a range of women's health issues.

VIDEOTAPES

Second Opinion. Carol Leonetti. Connecticut Public Television. 29 minutes. Available from Fanlight (see listing, above). An Emmy-nominated documentary about three women—one with breast cancer, one with heart disease, and one with AIDS—who fought the system to get the health care they needed. A resource for learning how to learn more about your own health care and what to do when you encounter resistance to getting that care.

Online

Online medical resources are seemingly unlimited. Every site has links to more sites, and more are being added every day. Look under women's health subdirectories in search engines such as Yahoo, check out the medical columns in magazines such as **Women's Wire** (www.women.com) and **PowerSurge** (members.aol.com/dearest). Here is a representation of what's available. To find your family health history, start by searching for the keyword *genealogy*. You'll find quite a number of resources.

MAILING LISTS

Mailing lists are available for a number of specific diseases and conditions. See other medical chapters in this book for listings, or search through comprehensive lists such as **Liszt**.

NEWS GROUPS

News groups are available for a number of specific diseases and conditions, many under the hierarchy **alt.support**. See other medical chapters in this book for listings, or access a complete list of Usenet news groups and find the one that interests you.

WEB SITES

You'll find a number of general medical sites. **Findings, the Woman's Healthcare Advocacy Service,** is at www.2cowherd.net/findings. Findings encourages women "to make thoughtful choices about their health by providing them with information and support." The service does this through web links, research on medical treatments and alternative medicine, support groups, and other resources. You'll find much information at the **Good Health Web** site at www.social.com/health—which has a database of 100 health organizations, discussions, a library of information, mailing lists, lists of newsgroups, FAQs, and more. A good place to visit. **Women's Health,** at www. feminist.com/health.htm, includes the category Womencare, for Women Over Forty, and many other links to women's health issues.

The **Health Information Resource Database** has toll-free health numbers, database searches, federal health information centers, publications, and more available at nhic-nt.health.org/Index.htm#Referrals.

If you've got questions, they've got answers. The Mayo Clinic makes cyberspace housecalls through the **Mayo Health O@sis** at www.mayo.ivi.com/ivi/mayo/

common/htm/index.htm. Ask questions and get answers on-line from dietitians, doctors, and nurses. You'll find **America's Housecall Network Women's Bulletin Board** at www.housecall.com/HyperNews/get/womenshealth.html. Post your questions here and get answers from other users, or read through the postings in the archives under a wide variety of health topics.

Med Help International, at medhlp.netusa.net, is the place to go online for research reports. This nonprofit organization provides qualified medical information on a wide variety of topics, and in nontechnical language that laypeople can understand. Some information is available free of charge, other information is available only to subscribers. A large file on women's health issues is available. There is a patient network where patients can be put in touch with other patients for information exchange and support; real-time health chat; and a public forum for specific questions, some answered directly by doctors or by patients with similar experience.

Online women's magazines like **Women's Wire,** at www.women.com, and **Power Surge,** at members.aol.com/dearest, have information about health the interviews with women's health professionals will keep you up to date on medical news. **Thrive: The Healthy Living Experience** is located at pathfinder.com/thrive. This user-friendly online health magazine covers a wide range of topics. It's easy to search through the online collection of medical abstracts and consumer publications. The site has fact sheets on symptoms, conditions, drugs, surgeries, resources; also included are summaries of magazine articles. A number of newsletters and magazines have web sites (see listings above). You'll even find the **New England Journal of the Medicine** at www.nejm.org.

The **U.S. Department of Health and Human Resources** site at www.os.dhhs.gov is your gateway to a huge resource of consumer information. The **Centers for Disease Control (CDC)** site at www.cdc.gov lets you access the CDC Prevention Guidelines discussion on environment and health, look at the section on women's health, or explore the CDC in cyberspace. The **American Medical Association** site at www.ama-assn.org has a lot of great links, including listings of regional, state, and county medical societies and organizations, U.S. government sites, scientific journals, and a database of more than 650,000 physicians. Another place to look for a doctor is the **Medseek** site, www.medseek.com, where you'll find more than 280,000 physician names. For information about clinical trials, go to **Clinical Trials Posting,** www.clinicaltrials.com.

If you have no idea where to start, try **Med Mark**'s site at medmark.bit.co.kr. Med Mark has bookmarks for more medical sites than you ever thought possible.

9

YES OR NO?

Hormone Replacement Therapy

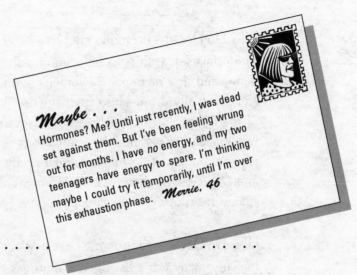

Maybe . . .

Hormones? Me? Until just recently, I was dead set against them. But I've been feeling wrung out for months. I have *no* energy, and my two teenagers have energy to spare. I'm thinking maybe I could try it temporarily, until I'm over this exhaustion phase. *Merrie, 46*

At some point, every woman approaching menopause confronts the question of whether or not to take hormone replacement therapy. Some women swear by HRT, some women prefer natural alternatives, some women do menopause cold turkey. In the end, the decision to use HRT is up to you. If you decide to take it and later feel it's not right for you, you can stop (but taper off slowly—consult your health practitioner about this). And if you decide it's not right for you now, that doesn't mean you can't decide to try it later.

What Is Hormone Replacement Therapy?

Hormone replacement therapy, or HRT, is primarily the administration of the female hormones estrogen and progesterone to treat the effects of fluctuating and declining ovarian hormone levels. In some cases, testosterone is also included in hormone therapy. Estrogen taken alone is called estrogen replacement therapy, or ERT. ERT, however, has been found to cause endometrial cancer and is no longer recommended for women who still have their uterus.

Why Do Doctors Prescribe HRT?

The primary reason is to help smooth the perimenopausal transition. Before and after menopause, women's hormone levels begin to fluctuate and eventually drop. This causes the best-known and least-loved signs of the change of life, such as hot flashes and vaginal dryness. Many women, and many health practitioners, choose to mediate the less pleasant effects of hormone fluctuation by readjusting the body's hormone levels with hormone replacement therapy. HRT also protects against heart disease and osteoporosis.

How Do Declining Hormone Levels Affect the Body?

In many, many ways. Estrogen and progesterone have a primary role in reproduction, but these powerful hormones are also involved in many other bodily functions. For example, estrogen receptor sites are located in the ovaries, heart, breast, skin, sex organs, bone, and brain; and estrogen is involved with regulating body temperature, vaginal secretions, the gastrointestinal tract, and bone health, to name just a few of its roles. With hormonal involvement in so many areas, it's no wonder a drop in estrogen levels can wreak such havoc!

What Are the Benefits and Risks of HRT?

The benefits of HRT are many: It may help alleviate some symptoms of menopause, including hot flashes and sweating, vaginal dryness, mood swings, exhaustion, and more. HRT also may retard osteoporosis,

GUIDED TOUR:
Hormone Replacement Therapy

Hormone replacement therapy offers women in midlife a number of benefits along with some risks. Not all women will want HRT, and not all women can take HRT. Review your family health history to determine your risks and think about the lifestyle choices you are willing (or not willing) to make. You can try HRT for a trial period—you don't have to make a lifetime commitment. It's important to work closely with your health practitioner to monitor your response to HRT. Many combinations of synthetic and natural estrogens and progesterone are available: Be sure you and your health practitioner are up to date on choices.

WESTERN MEDICINE

Before you make a decision on HRT, go to your doctor for a complete workup to determine what your needs really are. If you have a family history of heart disease or osteoporosis, HRT can help protect against these.

COMPLEMENTARY MEDICINE

Taking HRT does not exclude you from seeking balance in other ways, such as through acupuncture tune-ups or homeopathy. The combination of drug therapy and lifestyle change can work to your benefit.

EXERCISE

Even if you are taking HRT, you will still benefit from a program that includes weight-bearing exercise to build bone density and aerobic exercise to improve heart health.

MIND–BODY

Practices such as yoga, qi gong, t'ai chi, Alexander technique, Rosen work, the relaxation response, meditation, and biofeedback may relieve some of the same symptoms treated by HRT.

NUTRITION

Even if you are taking HRT, you still need to eat well. Be sure to include calcium to help build bone as well as foods that are low in saturated fats to help keep arteries clear. A number of foods, especially soy products, contain phytoestrogens that may help balance hormones.

Why Would I? Why Wouldn't I?

Why would I want to take HRT?

- To retard osteoporosis if you are at risk.
- To protect against cardiovascular (heart) disease if you are at risk.
- To protect against stroke if you are at risk.
- To improve memory and concentration.
- To help balance hormones if you have had a surgically induced menopause.
- To reduce or eliminate hot flashes and night sweats.
- To relieve vaginal soreness and dryness.
- To renew your energy and lift your mood.

Why wouldn't I want to take HRT?

- It may increase the risk of breast cancer.
- It costs money.
- It may cause symptoms of depression, anxiety, weight gain, and other unwanted side effects.
- It may cause irregular bleeding.
- Estrogen alone may increase the risk of uterine cancer.
- It may stimulate uterine fibroids (in rare cases).
- It may increase the risk of liver and gall-bladder disease (in rare cases).

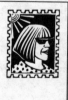

Much Better

HRT has made a huge difference in my sex life. Before, I was never sure if I would be wet or dry—and believe me, dry sex is not pleasant! *Marianne, 55*

protect against heart disease and stroke, and improve memory and concentration.

Risks and side effects may include weight gain, headaches, and resumption of menstrual flow. It may increase the risk of liver and gallbladder disease and breast cancer, and it may stimulate uterine fibroids.

Yes or No: Should I Take HRT?

Unfortunately, we can't give you a definitive answer to this question. First of all, because each woman's hormonal levels begin at a different point and decline at a different rate, each woman's experience will be unique. Second, each woman has different risk factors. For example, women with a family history of breast cancer are generally advised not to take HRT. Third, the pros and cons of HRT are still not as clear as we would like. As Dr. Sadja Greenwood points out, "New research is always coming out in this area. . . . What we think is true today may not be true tomorrow."

So, what should *you* do? Talk to other women about their experiences and keep up to date with the changing information. Talk to your doctor about your risks. To assess your needs, fill out the personal and family health history questionnaires in Part 2, "Your Personal Companion."

How Do I Take HRT?

Most women take HRT orally, in pill form. You can also take it transdermally (absorbed through the skin) with skin patches and creams. Although the creams are most widely used in Europe, you can have them specially formulated (see Resources for pharmacies that will do this).

Should I Use the Patch or the Pill?

This is something to work out with your health practitioner, depending on your health history and lifestyle. Both forms have pros and cons. For example, because the patch releases hormones directly into the bloodstream, levels tend to be steadier than with the pill. The pill is metabolized in the liver, where it helps out by raising levels of HDL (the good cholesterol). However, if you have liver problems, the patch is probably a better bet.

Can I Choose from More Than One Type of HRT?

You sure can. There are many options, especially if you include the natural hormone supplements also available. When it comes to taking HRT, every woman is her own clinical trial! Any regimen is something of an experiment. It's important to understand that there is no right way to take HRT: Each woman has different levels of her own hormones in her system at any one time, and we all metabolize hormones differently. So it's always a guess as to how much and what mix is optimal. Pay attention to how you feel, and work with your health practitioner to find the combination that works best for you.

The most commonly prescribed combination is Premarin and Provera—not because they are necessarily the best, but because they have been used in most of the research. Today, many other combinations are available. What's most important is finding the combination that's right for you. Some women who experience side effects with one combination experience no side effects with another. Make sure you and your doctor communicate and are willing to experiment if necessary.

How Long Will I Take HRT?

This depends on your reasons for starting hormone replacement therapy. If you are using HRT to get you past the discomfort of hot flashes

The Common Side Effects of HRT

These are the most common side effects of hormone replacement therapy. You may experience all, one or two, or none:

- You may gain a small amount of weight.
- You may retain fluids.
- You may experience nausea and headaches (about 10 percent of HRT users do).
- Your breasts may swell.
- You may have cramps.
- You may notice a vaginal discharge.
- You may notice mood swings.
- Your periods may start again.

and vaginal dryness, you'll take it during this transitional period. If you are using HRT to protect against heart disease and osteoporosis, you may take it for the rest of your life.

What Are Natural Hormones?

Natural estrogens and progesterone are manufactured from plants such as soybeans and have the same chemical structure as the natural hormones our bodies make. Many physicians are not aware of alternatives to synthetic hormones because they are not marketed by large pharmaceutical companies. If you or your doctor want more information, consult Resources for a list of pharmacies that sell natural hormones.

natural hormones Natural hormones are derived from plants. They are chemically equivalent to hormones that women produce in their own bodies.

How Do I Take Natural Estrogens?

Natural estrogens are generally available in pill form and as creams. You can get natural estrogen in a product such as Estrace, which is estradiol. You can also get a tri-estrogen product that combines estrone, estradiol, and estriol, which all occur naturally in our bodies. Even though they are "natural," you will need a doctor's prescription to take these hormones.

What Are Natural Progesterones?

Simply put, progesterones are naturally occurring hormones that play a role in reproduction. But when we're talking about natural progesterones and HRT, the definitions become more complex.

It's Hot in Here!

I'm a lawyer, and I have to see people all day. I couldn't bear to go to staff meetings or meet with clients—or God forbid, go to court!—because of the severity of my hot flashes. Somehow, I couldn't convince myself it was all right to take out my hanky, wipe my brow and upper lip, and say nonchalantly, "Oh, it's just a hot flash." Since I started taking HRT, I have no more hot flashes, and I'm comfortable again in the world of business suits. *Linda, 47*

PROGESTINS Progestins are synthetically made or derived from plant sources. Unlike natural progesterones, however, progestins do not provide the full range of biological activity. Many progestins are, in fact, chemically altered molecular forms of progesterone; the altered form is patentable by pharmaceutical companies.

NATURAL PROGESTERONE Natural progesterone is made from wild yams (*Discorea* roots—not the yams you buy in the grocery store) or soybeans, it is chemically equivalent to our own progesterones. Natural forms of progesterone are not patentable and therefore are less profitable. Natural progesterone is available in a nonprescription cream (a stronger formulation in cream and capsules is available by prescription), is an alternative to Provera, and seems to have fewer side effects. Lani Simpson, D.C., director of the East Bay PMS and Menopause Clinic in Oakland, California, says emphatically, "Natural progesterone is our choice to use instead of synthetic progestins, which have a wide range of side effects."

Why Am I Hearing So Much About Natural Progesterone Cream?

The guru of natural progesterone is John R. Lee, M.D., who has been a family practitioner in Mill Valley, California, for more than thirty years. He has opened the door to discussion of the role of progesterone in menopause. He says women can use natural progesterone cream, absorbed through the skin, to manage signs of declining hormones without side effects. His ideas are encouraging, but controversial, and the studies he cites are few and limited in numbers of participants. If you're interested in learning more about his theory, check out his book *What Your Doctor May Not Tell You About Menopause*.

How Do You Use Natural Progesterone Cream?

For treating symptoms of menopause, natural progesterone cream is rubbed into soft skin areas such as stomach, inner thighs, and buttocks, and absorbed through the skin (it is said to work better if you don't rub it into the same spot every time). The cream can take up to three

So many choices. Premarin and Provera are probably prescribed the most, but they are not the only choices when it comes to oral hormone replacement therapy. Here's a partial list of what's available:

- Oral estrogens include Premarin (made from the urine of pregnant mares), Estrace (a natural plant compound), Estratab, Menest (modified soy estrogens), Estraderm, Ogen, and Ortho-est (modified plant estrogen), tri-estrogens (estrone, estradiol, and estriol, modified plant estrogens).

- Oral progestins include Provera, Cycrin (medroxyprigesteribe acetate), Aygestin (norethindrone acetate).

- Oral progesterones include natural progesterone (made from wild yams or soybeans), Prometrium (micronized progesterone from a natural plant compound). Prometrium was used in the PEPI Trials and is awaiting FDA approval.

- Estrogen/progestin combinations include Prempro and Premphase.

- Estrogen/testosterone combinations include Estratest and Depo-Testodial.

TRAVEL TIP
A Little Dab'll Do Ya!

ProGest cream makes your skin look good and feel soft. But don't use it the same way you'd use a body cream. Remember: You're putting more progesterone into your system!

months to work its touted wonders and should not be used every day. This is newly charted territory: If you decide to try this treatment, be sure to monitor your reactions closely. If possible, work with a health practitioner.

How Much Progesterone Is in the Cream?

You can't always tell from reading the packaging how much is in the cream or how much is actually absorbed into your system. These creams are not regulated, so just because it's made from wild yam or calls itself a progesterone cream doesn't mean it has progesterone in it. Some call this the "yam scam." When it comes to natural progesterone creams, it's buyer beware: The amounts of progesterone in each vary wildly—from 0 percent on up.

Where Can I Buy Natural Progesterone Cream?

You can buy some brands of progesterone or wild yam cream in natural food stores or from health practitioners. An increasing number of pharmacies sell natural progesterone creams, capsules, and other natural hormones.

How Much Progesterone Is in My Body?

It's also important to be aware of your own progesterone levels—do you even need to use these creams? You may want to check your progesterone level before using one of these creams (and afterward, if you decide to use it). A saliva test is used to check your body's progesterone levels as well as other hormone levels. The saliva test is reported to be more reliable and less expensive than serum testing, and you can order it yourself. Remember, however, that hormone levels vary, even over the course of a day. You may want to consult your health practitioner to discuss the test beforehand or to help interpret the results. To find out more about the saliva test, check the progesterone content of a particular product, or receive a list of the progesterone content of a number of creams, contact Aeron Labs (see Resources).

Why Don't the Studies Always Agree?

When you're just trying to get the facts, it can be frustrating to run up against a wall of conflicting information. One problem is that we just don't know what "normal" means as it refers to perimenopausal, menopausal, and postmenopausal women—let alone anyone else! According to the National Institute on Aging's book *Menopause*, "Without knowing what normal is, scientists have difficulty judging the effect of a particular treatment."

"Another problem with past studies," continues the NIA, "is the 'healthy user effect.' In general, most physicians discourage women with a preexisting illness or long family history of breast cancer from taking HRT. This factor could skew study results to appear that non-users became ill or died more frequently simply because they failed to take estrogen. Only by randomly assigning participants to the treatment can this bias be overcome. Until more random trials are completed, the jury is still out on HRT." As Dr. Susan Love points out in *Dr. Susan Love's Hormone Book,* "There are no large prospective randomized controlled studies of postmenopausal women and hormones. . . . [We have only] circumstantial evidence . . . and it's flawed and subject to interpretation." Fortunately, thanks to

POINT OF INTEREST
The PEPI Trials

Since 1989, the National Institutes of Health have sponsored the Postmenopausal Estrogen/Progestin Intervention (PEPI) Trials. This study compares women who take estrogen alone with those who take it with progesterone or progestin. It also examines the effects of taking progestin both cyclically and continuously on cardiovascular risk factors, blood-clotting factors, metabolism, uterine changes, bone mass, and quality of life.

This study is ongoing. Early in 1995, the three-year results regarding heart disease were in:

- The study indicated that several hormonal therapies increased HDL levels—the "good" cholesterol associated with greater protection against heart disease—and improved two other risk factors.

- LDL, the "bad" cholesterol, was lowered, as was fibrinogen, which is involved in blood-clot formation.

- Women who took estrogen/natural progesterone and unopposed estrogen had the highest HDL levels; the increase for women on estrogen/progestin was not as great.

- The women on estrogen and natural progesterone also reported fewer side effects than those on estrogen and progestin (Provera).

- One-third of the women on unopposed estrogen developed endometrial hyperplasia, an overgrowth of cells indicating a potentially precancerous condition. These women were subsequently taken off the estrogen-unopposed treatments.

For a summary of the PEPI Trials in easy-to-understand language, contact the National Heart, Lung, and Blood Institute of the NIH Information Center. For a feminist critique of HRT that examines the claims of researchers and pharmaceutical companies, contact the National Women's Health Network. See Resources.

Some pharmacies, such as Women's International Pharmacy and Bajamar Women's Health Care Pharmacy, will send you free a thick packet of articles and information about their natural estrogens and progesterones and other formulations, including descriptions, studies, and resource lists. After you've read the information, call back to ask your questions. See Resources for more information.

1. Should all women take hormone replacement therapy? *No.*
2. Should any women take it? *Yes.*
3. Is it okay for some women and not for others? *Yes.*
4. Is it better to experience menopause naturally or with HRT? *It's up to you.*
5. Will I have to take HRT for the rest of my life? *It depends on why you're taking it.*
6. Will my period start again? *It might.*
7. Will it improve my energy level? *Probably.*
8. Will it help retard osteoporosis? *Yes.*
9. Will it help prevent heart disease? *It's likely.*
10. Will it cure my vaginal dryness? *Probably.*
11. Will it improve my mood? *It might.*
12. Will it stop my hot flashes? *Probably.*
13. Will it help protect against Alzheimer's? *It might.*
14. Will it improve my memory? *It might.*
15. Are natural estrogens and progesterone better than manufactured hormones? *The jury's still out.*

the PEPI Trials and the Women's Health Initiative, things are beginning to look better for the future of research into HRT.

What Are Some Other Ways to Cope with Hormonal Fluctuation?

Hormone replacement therapy is often the quickest solution to many concerns faced by midlife women, but it's certainly not the only solution. As soon becomes clear to every woman who plunges into the complicated world of hormones, there's no panacea. Even if you do decide to try HRT, you can still explore other lifestyle choices. We like this inclusive approach. Here are just a *few* of the many alternatives you'll find detailed elsewhere in this book.

EAT YOUR HORMONES American women are plagued by hot flashes during the menopausal years, while Japanese women rarely experience them. Why? A number of researchers suspect the answer is in the Japanese diet, which is high in soy foods and vegetables, many of which (soy especially) contain phytoestrogens, estrogen-like substances. Foods high in phytoestrogens include soybeans and their products (tofu, miso, tempeh, soy milk) and, to a lesser degree, cashews, peanuts, oats, corn, wheat, apples, and almonds.

LIFT WEIGHTS TO FIGHT OSTEOPOROSIS Resistance exercises, such as weightlifting, not only retard bone loss but can actually build new bone as well. No matter how old or out of shape you think you are, it's not too late to start lifting weights.

MEDITATE TO CALM ANXIETY Anxiety, depression, and worry are frequent complaints of women in midlife. Stress-reduction techniques, including meditation, deep breathing, the relaxation response, and biofeedback training, have all been shown to be very effective in smoothing out jangled nerves and clearing the head.

GET ACUPUNCTURE TREATMENTS TO BALANCE YOUR SYSTEM Women have used traditional Chinese medicine for thousands for years to help them through the rough spots of the midlife change. This knowledge has been around for a long time. Why not try it and see what it does for you?

FIGHT HEART DISEASE AND STROKE WITH EXERCISE AND DIET Two of the best things you can do for yourself are to get regular aerobic exercise and eat a balanced diet low in saturated fat and high in plant foods. You'll feel better, you may even lose weight if that's your goal, and you'll definitely be improving your odds for avoiding heart disease and stroke.

GET SUPPORT If you need a friend to walk with you on this sometimes rocky road, reach out. You'll find hands waiting to help you in peer support groups, on Internet chat groups, or in the office of a professional counselor or support organization.

> Any good natural regimen for healthy older women works to strengthen the entire immune system to help prevent the development of disease. But the approach is always multi-therapeutic and includes diet, exercise, body/mind techniques, and sometimes supplements—herbs, vitamins, minerals, and so forth. . . . Given the proper support, the body can often balance itself.
>
> DEE ITO, *Without Estrogen*

TRAVEL TIP
Become Part of a New Study

In 1992 the Women's Health Initiative began a study involving 70,000 postmenopausal women ages fifty to seventy-nine. This study focuses on long-term benefits and risks of HRT as it relates to cardiovascular disease, osteoporosis, and breast and uterine cancer. It will also determine the effects of calcium, dietary changes, and exercise on women in this age group. Results are a long way off, but efforts are now being made to include women in health research and to focus on diseases that are common to aging. This study will include a cross-section of the U.S. population, and many of the clinical centers will recruit primarily ethnically diverse populations—African Americans, Hispanics, Asian Americans, Pacific Islanders, and Native Americans. Women of all racial/ethnic groups are encouraged to participate in the study. For more information, contact the National Institutes of Health, Women's Health Initiative at (800) 54-WOMEN.

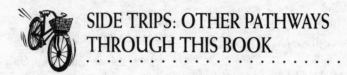

SIDE TRIPS: OTHER PATHWAYS THROUGH THIS BOOK

CHAPTER 3: KEEP ON MOVING   A good program of moderate exercise is not only important to overall good health but is also important in balancing your hormones. Look here for information and ideas to get started.

CHAPTER 4: ARE YOU WHAT YOU EAT?   Your diet can have a real effect on your general health and on how hormonal changes make you feel. Foods containing calcium can help with osteoporosis, and foods containing phytoestrogens provide substances similar to our own estrogen—and can help smooth out the rough edges of menopause. Look here for more on good nutrition for midlife women.

CHAPTER 7: THE HOLISTIC KIT AND CABOODLE   If you're interested in alternatives to HRT or want to live in balance with your body, check out the world of complementary therapies. Look here for tips on finding alternative health care and using it in conjunction with conventional medicine.

CHAPTER 8: WHAT'S UP, DOC?   If you're contemplating HRT, you'll need to find a doctor you can work with and make sure you're asking the right questions. Look here for the ins and outs of conventional medical treatment.

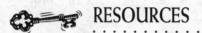

RESOURCES

Organizations and Services

Aeron Labs, 1933 Davis St., Suite 310, San Leandro, CA 94577. Voice: (800) 631-7900. Fax: (510) 729-0383. Do you really need progesterone cream? Call Aeron to find out about saliva testing to determine your current hormone levels. You or your physician can order the test kit to be mailed to you, and you can return your sample in the mail. The lab will send you the results, and you can talk with a doctor there and ask questions—the personnel are very helpful. The lab also provides a list of progesterone creams on the market and the progesterone content of each.

Food and Drug Administration, 5600 Fishers Lane, Rockville, MD 20857. Voice: (800) 532-4440. Call for information about FDA approval of prescription drugs. Prometrium, the natural progesterone used in the PEPI Trial, is pending FDA approval, and you can call here to find out its status.

National Heart, Lung, and Blood Institute, National Institutes of Health, Information Center, P.O. Box 30105, Bethesda, MD 20824-0105. Voice: (301) 251-1222. Call to request a copy of the PEPI Trial study and results.

National Institute of Alcohol Abuse and Alcoholism, Office of Scientific Affairs, P.O. Box 2345, Rockville, MD 20852. Voice: (800) 729-6686. Internet: www.niaaa. nih.gov. This agency has a quarterly publication, *Alcohol Alert.* Two issues are particularly important to women: "Alcohol and Women" and "Alcohol and Hormones," which describe how alcohol interferes with hormone actions and how this interference in turn alters blood sugar levels and so affects calcium metabolism and bone structure. It also discusses how hormones may influence alcohol-seeking behavior.

National Women's Health Network, 514 10th St. N.W., Suite 400, Washington, DC 20004. Voice: (202) 347-1140. Fax: (202) 344-1168. Women's Health Clearinghouse: (202) 628-7814. Internet: www.womenconnect.com/or20550g.htm. This women's advocacy group monitors federal policy on women's health issues and provides information and referrals on many topics, including current information on HRT research. The booklet "Taking Hormones and Women's Health: Choices, Risks, and Benefits" is available for a nominal fee. Also available are free quick-study brochures, "Heart and Bones" and "Hot Flashes and Hormones."

National Women's Health Resource Center, 2440 M St. N.W., #325, Washington, DC 20037. Voice: (202) 293-6045. This member-supported organization compiles information on women's health topics. The Center will do a customized search for members and nonmembers. It also prints a newsletter and provides reports and conference information. The report "The Menopause in Focus" is available for $20.

North American Menopause Association, c/o Department of OB/GYN, University Hospitals of Cleveland, 11100 Euclid Ave., Cleveland, OH 44106. Voice: (216) 844-8748. Fax: (216) 844-8708. E-mail: nams@atk.et. Internet: www.menopause. org/all.html. Contact NAMS about the latest information on HRT.

Women's Health America Group, 429 Gammon Place, P.O. Box 259690, Madison, WI 53725. Voice: (800) 558-7046. Fax: (888) 898-7412. Internet: www.womens health.com. This company was founded by a woman and has several divisions: Madison Pharmacy, which compounds natural hormones and has supplements especially for PMS and menopause, and Women's Health Access, which has information hotlines, the newsletter *Women's Health Access,* tapes, and books on menopause, PMS, and natural hormones. It also provides physician referral.

Natural Hormones

Bajamar Women's Health Care Pharmacy, 9609 Dielman Rock Island, St. Louis, MO 63132. Voice: (800) 255-8025. Fax: (314) 997-2948. E-mail: bmizes@mo.net. Internet: walden.mo.net/~bmizes/hormones.html. Bajamar compounds natural hormones and can refer you to a physician in your area who uses its services. Send for free information on hormone-related issues.

College Pharmacy, 833 N. Rejoin St., Colorado Springs, CO 80903. Voice: (800) 888-9358. Fax: (800) 556-5893. E-mail: collegep@rmi.net. Internet: college pharmacy.com. This pharmacy compounds natural hormones—transdermal, oral, and cream. They also offer prescription-only preservative-free injectable vitamins.

International Academy of Compounding Pharmacists, P.O. Box 1365, Sugar Land, TX 77487. Voice: (800) 927-4227. Internet: www.compassnet.com/~icap. Call for a referral to pharmacists in your area who compound natural hormones.

Madison Pharmacy Association, 429 Gammon Place, P.O. Box 259690, Madison, WI 53725. Voice: (800) 558-7046. This division of Women's Health America Group compounds natural hormones. It offers a range of services, and you can speak to a consultant about the wide variety of products. The pharmacy will also provide physician referral.

Research Reports

Want to order the latest research report on HRT? See the listings in Chapter 8, "What's Up, Doc?"

Hotlines

Food and Drug Administration: (800) 532-4440. Call with questions concerning FDA-approved drugs or side effects.

Women's Health Connection: (800) 366-6632. Call with questions about hormones and health. Sponsored by Women's International Pharmacy.

Women's Health America: (800) 222-4767. This line will put you in touch with a choice of access lines: PMS, Menopause, and Natural Hormones. Each line offers free printed material on the topic of choice and also a referral to a physician in your area. You can also order a free copy of *Women's Health Access Newsletter.*

National Institutes of Health, Women's Health Initiative: (800) 54-WOMEN for a recorded message and voice mail. Ask for information about the Women's Health Initiative and a list of clinical trial centers.

Products and Catalogs

Transitions for Health, 621 S.W. Alder, Suite 900, Portland, OR 97205. Voice: (800) 888-6814 or (800) 460-7853. Fax: (800) 944-0168. E-mail: etfh@progest.com. Internet: www.progest.com/index.html. This company makes and sells ProGest cream (the one used in Dr. Lee's study). It also offers herbal remedies, vitamins, homeopathic remedies, and a saliva test for measuring estrogen and progesterone levels. Call to receive a catalog. If you're online, you can submit questions to a doctor.

Vitamin Express, 1428 Irving St., San Francisco, CA 94122. Voice: (800) 500-0733. Internet: www.vitaminexpress.com. This is a neighborhood vitamin shop that does national and international shipping. It sells ProGest cream by mail at a competitive price.

Women's International Pharmacy, 5708 Monona Drive, Madison, WI 53716. Voice: (800) 279-5708. Fax: (800) 279-8011. Internet: www.wipws.com. Second address: 13925 Meeker Blvd., Suite 13, Sun City West, AZ 85375. Voice: (602) 214-7700. This pharmacy is particularly concerned with women's health issues. It sponsors women's health seminars and provide lists of books, organizations, and resources relevant to hormonal disorders. It will send a list of physicians in your area who prescribe natural hormones. Have your physician telephone or fax prescriptions.

Periodicals

All of the periodicals listed in Chapter 2, "Why Is This Happening to Me?," and Chapter 8, "What's Up, Doc?," include articles from time to time about the latest on HRT. For alternative therapies, see the newsletters listed in Chapter 7, "The Holistic Kit and Caboodle."

Books

Paula Brisco and Karla Morales. *The HRT Handbook: What Every Woman Should Know About Hormones.* Allentown, PA: People's Medical Society, 1996. A comprehensive guide to HRT: the various forms, effects, quantities, risks, and alternatives.

Sandra Coney. *The Menopause Industry: How the Medical Establishment Exploits Women.* Alameda, CA: Hunter House, 1994. The book to read if you are trying to make sense of research studies. Coney explains the different types of studies and what they mean, and explores the vested interest groups that constitute the menopause industry—hormone manufacturers, ad agencies, researchers, universities, national societies, and the medical establishment.

Gillian Ford. *Listening to Your Hormones.* Rocklin, CA: Prima Publishing, 1997. This book is especially for women with severe hormonal problems that affect their physical and emotional well-being. Ford experienced severely incapacitating hormonal problems and tells her story, along with those of other women. Also includes treatments.

Sadja Greenwood, M.D. *Menopause Naturally.* San Francisco: Volcano Press, 1996. The latest edition of this classic, very informative, and highly readable book on menopause and self-care offers even more complementary approaches. Also printed in a Spanish-language edition.

Dee Ito. *Without Estrogen: Natural Remedies for Menopause and Beyond.* New York: Crown, 1994. This book shows how a range of complementary practitioners treat the signs of menopause. It looks at a number of alternatives to HRT, including Chinese herbal medicine, acupuncture, chiropractic, aromatherapy, diet and nutrition, exercise, and many more.

John R. Lee, M.D. *What Your Doctor May Not Tell You About Menopause.* New York: Warner Books, 1996. If you're interested in natural progesterone, this is a more readable version of Lee's first book, *Natural Progesterone: The Multiple Roles of a Remarkable Hormone.* Lee talks about menopause and the role of progesterone and explains natural progesterones. He also discusses lifestyle and menopause.

Susan Love, M.D., with Karen Lindsey. *Dr. Susan Love's Hormone Book.* New York: Random House, 1997. This is an intelligent, thoughtful, and clearly written book full of information that can help you make a decision about whether or not HRT is right for you. Love explains all the issues, including how to understand the research. She covers menopause and all the medical topics, and her discussion of the alternatives to HRT is especially strong. A very good book.

Lila Nachtigall, M.D., and Joan Rattner Heilman. *Estrogen: A Complete Guide to Reversing the Effects of Menopause Using Hormone Replacement Therapy.* New York: HarperCollins, 1991. Dr. Nachtigall, who was involved in the first long-term study of estrogen replacement therapy, explores the use of HRT. A good book to read if you are considering using HRT.

Christiane Northrup, M.D. *Women's Bodies, Women's Wisdom: Creating Physical and Emotional Health and Healing.* New York: Bantam Books, 1994. Dr. Northrup is a holistic physician who combines Western medicine and mind–body approaches to health. She discusses natural and synthetic hormone replacement therapy and explains how to do a "trial run" of replacement therapy.

Linda Ojeda, *Menopause Without Medicine.* Alameda, CA: Hunter House, 1992. This book's emphasis is on nutritional supplementation, and it has a major nutrient guide. Also offers some herbal treatments for the signs of menopause.

Susan Perry and Katherine A. O'Hanlan, M.D. *Natural Menopause: The Complete Guide to a Woman's Most Misunderstood Passage.* Rev. ed. Reading, MA: Addison-Wesley, 1997. The newly revised edition of this classic reviews the latest studies on HRT. Perry and O'Hanlan thoroughly explore the decision-making process and closely examine the pros and cons.

Judith Reichman, M.D. *I'm Too Young to Get Old: Health Care for Women After Forty.* New York: Times Books, 1996. Dr. Reichman is straightforward, humorous, and informative, and doesn't hedge on her views. She has a lot to say about menopause and is heartily in favor of hormone replacement therapy. Read Chapter 7 of her book to get the lowdown.

Honora Lee Wolfe. *Second Spring: A Guide to Healthy Menopause Through Traditional Chinese Medicine.* Blue Poppy Press, 1990. A good book if you're interested in Chinese herbs or using a practitioner of Chinese medicine; it explains the theories of Chinese medicine and how they apply to menopause. Included are therapies for menopause as well as information on diet, exercise, and supplements.

Audio/Video

For catalogs of health and medical tapes, see the listings in Chapter 7, "The Holistic Kit and Caboodle," and Chapter 8, "What's Up, Doc?" You'll find other tapes on midlife and menopause in Chapter 2, "Why Is This Happening to Me?"

Online

See the Online Resources in Chapter 7, "The Holistic Kit and Caboodle," for alternatives to HRT. To keep current on the latest in HRT research, see the listings in Chapter 2, "Why Is This Happening to Me?," and in Chapter 8, "What's Up, Doc?"

10

THE WORLD DOWN UNDER
Vaginal Health, Incontinence, and Sex

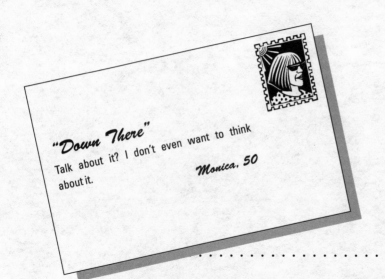

"Down There"
Talk about it? I don't even want to think about it.

Monica, 50

If Monica's thoughts ring a bell, you're in good company. When it comes to gynecological problems—to the parts of our body many of us grew up calling "down there"—a woman's life is just one thing after another. And in midlife, it seems, we're dealing with the seemingly disparate issues of vaginal changes, incontinence, and sex. The hormonal changes of midlife can cause loss of vaginal lubrication and thinning of vaginal walls; and the cumulative effects of childbearing and years of gravity may lead to urinary incontinence. Even women who are very comfortable with their sexuality may find these physical discomforts affecting their desire for sex, at least temporarily.

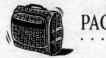

PACKING FOR THE JOURNEY

What Causes Vaginal Dryness and What Can I Do About It?

One effect of declining hormonal levels is less secretion of vaginal fluids. The vagina and vulva become dry, vaginal walls become thinner, we lose vaginal muscle tone, and we have an increased chance of vaginal and urinary tract infections. Fortunately, vaginal dryness is a problem you can do something about. For starters, stay away from hot tubs, bath oils, bubble bath, and deodorant soaps—these can cause irritation and even more dryness. You can minimize the rubbing, itching, and discomfort in a number of ways, including the following.

HORMONAL TREATMENTS   Because dryness is a result of dropping hormonal levels, replacing hormones is one solution. *Hormone replacement therapy* can prevent and even reverse vaginal dryness and thinning; women who begin hormone replacement early on may be able to avoid dryness altogether. Be sure to check your risk factors with your health practitioner. *Estrogen creams* can both moisturize and strengthen vaginal walls. (But don't use estrogen cream as a lubricant!) Topical estriol (a weaker form of estrogen) applied to the vagina is used in Europe with some success. *Natural progesterone cream* provides benefit to vaginal and urethral tissues after three to four months of use; topical prescription progesterone cream is also known to relieve vaginal dryness.

LUBRICANTS   *Non-estrogen water-soluble lubricants* such as Astroglide or K-Y Jelly can eliminate painful rubbing. (*Never* use petroleum jelly—it can block your own secretions.) Replens, a gel compound inserted into the vagina, imparts moisture to cell walls.

VITAMIN E   Vitamin E oil applied topically is helpful to some women in minimizing vaginal dryness. Vitamin E suppositories are also effective and healing.

BOTANICAL AND HOMEOPATHIC REMEDIES   For itching: Bathe the vagina in a warm chickweed infusion. For vaginal dryness: Try black cohosh root. You can also try topical applications of bryonia or calendula cream. For general perimenopausal symptoms including hot flashes and vaginal dryness, Dr. Susan Lark recommends a combination product called Formula I, which contains blue cohosh, false unicorn root, fennel, anise, and blessed thistle.

SEX   This remedy for vaginal dryness is free. According to the *Harvard Women's Health Watch*, "Sexual activity alone can preserve the vaginal epithelium presumably by increasing blood flow. . . . Sexual activity also helps maintain a more acidic original climate which offers substantial protection against infection."

Hold It
I can't even believe I'm talking about this. Truly. I cannot think of a more embarrassing problem for an adult than not being able to hold it when you have to.   *Barbara, 53*

What Is Urinary Incontinence?
Urinary incontinence is loss of bladder control—you pee when you don't want to. *Stress incontinence* means that you lose a few drops of urine when you sneeze, laugh, or cough. *Urge incontinence* means that you have the sudden, uncontrollable urge to urinate. *Overflow incontinence* occurs when the urethra is narrowed (by scar tissue or pressure from a prolapsed uterus). The pressure of a full bladder is too much for the sphincter muscle, and urine spills out. All of these can be a problem for women after menopause. In fact, it's estimated that 15 to 30 percent of all women are affected, and it may be more common than that. As one nurse practitioner put it, "This is the last women's health issue to come out of the closet."

What Causes Urinary Incontinence?
Urinary incontinence may have any of several causes. The pelvic-floor muscles, which support the bladder, may weaken. Thinning bladder walls caused by lower estrogen production, a prolapsed uterus pressing on the bladder, or simply a mild bladder infection may also contribute. Incontinence may also be a symptom of a more serious medical condition—consult a medical professional if you have this problem.

incontinence   The inability to hold urine in the bladder; uncontrolled leakage of urine.

GUIDED TOUR:
Vaginal Health, Incontinence, and Sex

Declining levels of hormones can harm vaginal health, causing dryness, pain, and itching; thinning vaginal walls; and weakening of the pelvic-floor muscles. It may also lead to urinary incontinence. Orgasmic potential does not necessarily change after midlife, but vaginal changes can make sex uncomfortable.

WESTERN MEDICINE

Vaginal dryness: Hormone replacement therapy, topical estrogen or progesterone cream, vitamin E oil or suppositories, non-estrogen water-soluble lubricants. *Urinary incontinence:* Hormone replacement therapy, surgery when appropriate, collagen injections, pelvic-floor muscle exercises. *Sex:* Testosterone replacement therapy may increase libido; vitamin E supplements.

COMPLEMENTARY MEDICINE

Vaginal dryness: Try bryonia or calendula cream, herbs (black cohosh root), naturopathy, or traditional Chinese medicine. *Urinary incontinence:* Homeopathic remedies (*Causticum, Pulsatilla*) and herbal remedies (buchu leaves, goldenlock tea) may help; acupressure may give relief. *Sex:* To help libido try herbal remedies (dong quai, sarsaparilla, red clover, damiana), supplements (evening primrose oil, zinc chelate), aromatherapy (clary sage and ylang ylang essential oils), biofeedback, and acupuncture or acupressure.

EXERCISE

For vaginal dryness: A regular exercise program and sexual activity may help stimulate lubrication. *For urinary incontinence:* Improve muscle tone with Kegels and pelvic-floor exercises; bladder control exercises can also help. *Sex:* Regular exercise can improve your physical condition, contributing to a more positive attitude toward sex; pelvic-floor exercises and Kegel exercises strengthen internal muscles and can make sex more pleasurable.

MIND–BODY

For vaginal dryness: Some yoga poses stimulate the endocrine system. *For urinary incontinence:* Use visualization, guided imagery, or biofeedback to enhance Kegel exercises or other treatments. *Sex:* Meditation, yoga, and other mind–body practices can help relieve tension.

NUTRITION

For vaginal dryness: Soy foods, alfalfa sprouts, and other foods containing phytoestrogens may help; avoid foods that irritate the bladder. *For urinary incontinence:* Avoid products with caffeine and other foods that irritate the bladder.

The best exercise to strengthen pelvic-floor muscles is the amazingly simple Kegel exercise, which you can do virtually anywhere—in your car at a stoplight, at your desk while you work, at the table while you read the paper. No one will ever know. And there may be an added bonus. In a letter to *Menopause News*, one fifty-five-year-old woman reported, "I've been doing Kegels for three years, and they have completely changed my sex life. I can't believe the orgasms I have now."

Here's how to do them: First, locate your pubovisceral (PV) muscle—it's the one you can tighten around a tampon. Tighten your pubovisceral muscle as if you were stopping your urine flow midstream, hold, and release. Do as many as you can in ten seconds, rest ten seconds, contract and hold for ten seconds (work up to this if you have to), and rest ten seconds. Repeat as many times as you can. Don't give up: It may take two to three months to see real results.

What Can I Do to Regain Bladder Control?

Take heart. Depending on the cause of your incontinence, you have a range of treatment choices. Behavioral techniques are often the most effective in promoting bladder control. Keep a journal of your activities and your losses to see if you can track down a cause. Do you wait too long before using the toilet? Do you seem to have a loss after eating certain foods? Once you've figured out a cause, here are some things you can try (see Resources for sources of information on behavioral techniques).

CHANGE YOUR STYLE   Try using the toilet more frequently. Work on emptying your bladder completely after every urination. Stay away from diuretics, including tea, coffee, and sodas with caffeine.

EXERCISE PLUS   You can strengthen your pelvic-floor muscles just as you can any other muscle. Exercise your pelvic-floor muscles by doing Kegel exercises (see the Point of Interest "The Mighty Kegel") or other pelvic-floor exercises. You may also consider speeding things up by using biofeedback to enhance the Kegels. Vaginal weights are another option to enhance Kegels. See Resources for sources.

BE KIND TO YOUR BLADDER   Something as simple as a low-grade bladder infection can cause incontinence. Try drinking a glass of bladder-friendly cranberry juice daily to keep bacterial growth at bay, and make sure you get your six to eight glasses of water a day. It may also be a good idea to stay away from foods and other substances that irritate the bladder, including tobacco, caffeine, alcohol, sugar, cold foods, acidic foods (citrus fruits and tomatoes), aspartame, and chocolate.

AVOID FORCEFUL SEX   Avoid forceful sexual activity when your bladder is irritated. Pressure on the bladder can cause more irritation.

MONITOR PRESCRIPTION DRUGS Some medications can contribute to incontinence. If incontinence is a problem and you are taking diuretics or sedatives, be sure to inform your doctor.

What Are the Medical Remedies for Incontinence?

When changing your behavior doesn't work, you may want to move on to the next step. Medical remedies include the following:

HORMONE REPLACEMENT THERAPY HRT can help correct incontinence caused by thinning of the vaginal wall. Dr. Christiane Northrup recommends "placing a small amount of estrogen cream directly on the part of the vaginal tissue that covers the outer third of the urethra." If this doesn't work for you, you may need more. Dr. Margaret Cuthbert suggests inserting an applicator full of estrogen cream three times a week for two weeks.

SURGERY Surgery will not correct urge incontinence, but hysterectomy or surgical repair of ligaments may be an option for stress incontinence caused by a prolapsed uterus pressing on the bladder. If this type of surgery is indicated, it can be successful, but the surgical failure rate is high. Get a second opinion.

COLLAGEN INJECTIONS Collagen injections into the urethra can control incontinence in some cases. Improvements are being made on this treatment.

Are There Any Complementary Remedies for Incontinence?

Homeopathic remedies include *Causticum* for stress incontinence and *Pulsatilla* for small involuntary losses of urine. Buchu leaves, which have mild antiseptic and antibacterial properties, may help with irritated bladders. Herbal remedies from traditional Chinese medicine may include golden lock tea, and acupressure massage may also be effective.

POINT OF INTEREST
Vaginal Mysteries

The vagina, point of entry into the world for most human beings, has a firm place in world mythology. The Indian goddess Kali, triple goddess of creation, preservation, and destruction, was also known as Kunda or Cunti, the root of words ranging from the sexual (cunnilingus) to the familial (kin and country). The *yoni,* the Tantric image of the vulva, represents the creative powers of the female and is the symbolic gateway to regeneration. Early symbols of the vulva and vagina in art and myth include triangles, spiraling circles, seeds and sprouts, and a bell shape with a dot to indicate the vaginal opening.

Feeling Sexier: Some Suggestions

Inhale: To encourage sensuality, try aromatherapy. Put a few drops of essential oil of clary sage or ylang ylang (or both) in your bathwater or in a diffuser, relax, and enjoy.

Relax: De-stress your life with biofeedback, a warm bath, candles, or a day at the spa. Go off for a few days with your partner to a romantic, exciting, or restful spot.

Get moving: Exercise stimulates blood flow, increases energy, and generally makes you more interested in everything.

Eat: According to Lissa de Angeles and Molly Siple in *Recipes for Change,* "Niacin, in fish, whole, grains, and sunflower seeds, has been shown to stimulate the formation of vaginal mucus."

Bend: A number of yoga exercises are recommended for directing energy to the female reproductive system and stimulating hormone production. They include forward bend poses such as Downward-Facing Dog (Adho Mukha Svanasana) and the wall hang.

Allow time for foreplay: Give yourself and your partner all the time you need for foreplay. Add variety to your routine, and have fun. Your partner will share the benefits!

Talk and listen: Talk to your partner about your changing needs. Let your partner know what you like and what you want. In return, listen to what your partner has to say. If you have relationship issues or unfinished business, talk about it. If necessary, consult a professional therapist or sex counselor.

Women's erotica: Enjoy women's erotic literature or videos, alone or with your partner. There's a great selection of erotica created by women for women. Virtually every woman can find a "turn on," regardless of sexual preference.

Always check with a qualified homeopath or herbal practitioner for the correct prescription and dosage.

Why Do Some Women in Midlife Report a Diminished Interest in Sex?

Although menopause does not affect a woman's orgasmic potential, a complex of emotional and physical factors may cause you to lose interest in sex temporarily. One major factor in sexual enjoyment is vaginal health. Although lower levels of estrogen do not seem to affect libido, lack of lubrication and thinning vaginal walls can make sexual intercourse painful. It's difficult to feel sexy when you're exhausted; the stress of coping with the midlife transition, as well discomfort with a changing body image, can also contribute. Yet another problem is aging partners who themselves may have less interest in sex. If you just don't feel like interacting, solo sex is a way to stay sexually active. It can be reassuring to discover that, yes, you are still responsive. And it is a real alternative if you are not in a relationship.

What's the Connection Between Testosterone and Sex?

Your testosterone levels generally affect your libido—your sex drive. As levels of estrogen and progesterone fall in menopause, levels of testosterone may also fall, and therefore libido is diminished: You're just not as interested in sex as you once were. Other symptoms of low testosterone levels include thinning pubic hair, diminished muscle mass, low energy, and memory loss. If lack of libido is a problem for you (and it's not for all women) or if you're concerned about any other symptoms, talk to your health care provider to find out more.

Is There Sex After Menopause?

Yes. In fact, according to *The New Ourselves, Growing Older,* "A study of people sixty to ninety-one years old revealed that 91 percent enjoyed sex for a variety of reasons: it reduces tension, makes women feel more feminine, helps people sleep, and provides a physical outlet for emotion. The people studied engaged in sexual relations an average of 1.4 times a week—about what they averaged when they were in their forties." Many women worry that in midlife their sexual feelings will disappear. But in this area, as with everything else, each woman's experience will be uniquely hers. Once they negotiate the rockier segments of the midlife passage, most women find that their sexual lives go on as before. Some women find that after menopause, they enjoy the new sexual freedom that comes from not having to worry about birth control. Others enjoy the release that comes from not having to think about sex all the time.

More Time Together

I heard stories of women losing interest in sex, and my doctor said I might experience vaginal dryness and painful sex. But my experience is that I enjoy sex more, I am more relaxed, and we have more time together. Once the children were gone we had to take time to renew our relationship and with it . . . a better sex life. *Dora, 53*

> When I was younger, there was a part of my brain back here that was always thinking about sex. . . . Going through menopause makes the difference. . . . All I can tell you is: it's wonderful. It doesn't mean you don't enjoy having sex when it happens, just that you don't *think* about it when it doesn't. . . . To young women I can only say, "Don't worry about it!"
>
> GLORIA STEINEM, *On Women Turning Fifty*

Can I Get Pregnant at My Age?

Remember those stories you've heard about unplanned middle-aged pregnancies? Thirty percent of women between fifty and fifty-four are theoretically fertile. If you haven't had a period for more than a year, it's unlikely you're still ovulating. But if you never know when your

Thinning vaginal walls provide an entryway for the HIV virus, and AIDS is a growing problem for women at midlife and beyond. Even if you can no longer get pregnant, be sure to practice safe sex.

period is coming or how long it will last, then you never know when you're ovulating. If you think that being in your forties means you can't get pregnant, think again. As Dr. Judith Reichman says, "Our fertility at age forty is about half that at twenty, and will continue to decline, yet that is not 'ground zero.' Neglecting contraception is as stupid in our forties as it was in the previous three decades."

From her body, Gaia made the land and the sea. She moved and her spine arched outward, forming the high mountains. In the mysterious hollows of her flesh she made valleys and caves where her voice still lingers. . . . Flowers grew upon her many breasts. From her body came all the life that would ever be. . . . She was always creating something from her mysterious being.

JAMAKE HIGHWATER, *Myth and Sexuality*

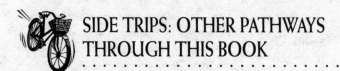

SIDE TRIPS: OTHER PATHWAYS THROUGH THIS BOOK

CHAPTER 3: KEEP ON MOVING   Movement and exercise programs to promote general health and well-being can also improve vaginal health. Look here to learn about what constitutes a good exercise program.

CHAPTER 4: ARE YOU WHAT YOU EAT?   Foods that contain phytoestrogens may help you balance your hormones. Look here to learn what they are.

CHAPTER 7: THE HOLISTIC KIT AND CABOODLE   Complementary therapies offer some help to vaginal dryness and urinary incontinence. Look here for an overview of what's out there.

CHAPTER 8: WHAT'S UP, DOC?   Your health practitioner may have solutions for your problems of vaginal dryness and urinary incontinence. Look here for some ideas on how you can work together.

CHAPTER 9: YES OR NO? Hormone replacement therapy can reverse or help prevent vaginal dryness, strengthen vaginal walls, and improve vaginal muscle tone. Look here to learn about the pros and cons.

CHAPTER 13: IS THIS REALLY NECESSARY? Hysterectomy may be the solution for severe uterine prolapse. Look here to learn more about this surgery.

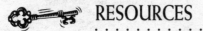 RESOURCES

Organizations and Services

URINARY INCONTINENCE

Incontinence Information Center, P.O. Box 9, Minneapolis, MN 55440. Voice: (800) 543-9632. Call to receive an information packet on this problem.

Krames Communications. Voice: (800) 333-3032. Internet: www.krames.com. This company publishes patient information in the form of illustrated, easy-to-understand, and very informative booklets. Call about ordering "Incontinence: Urinary Leakage" and "Urinary Tract Infections."

National Association for Continence, P.O. Box 8310, Spartanburg, SC 29305. Voice: (800) BLADDER. Fax: (864) 579-7902. E-mail: lverdell@globalvision.net. Internet: www.nafc.org. This organization, formerly called Help for Incontinent People, has information on services, treatments, and products for people with incontinence. Members receive a quarterly newsletter, *Quality Care*, and an informative catalog, *Resource Guide: Products and Services for Incontinence*.

National Kidney and Urologic Diseases Information Clearinghouse, 3 Information Way, Bethesda, MD 20892-3580. Voice: (301) 654-4415. Fax: (301) 907-8906. E-mail: nkudic@aerie.com. This publications clearinghouse has brochures and information packets on kidney and urologic diseases. Request a list.

Simon Foundation for Continence, P.O. Box 835, Wilmette, IL 60091. Voice: (800) 23-SIMON. Fax: (847) 864-9758. Call to request a free packet of information regarding incontinence and a sample of the foundation's absorbent product.

SEX

American Association of Sex Educators, Counselors, and Therapists, P.O. Box 238, Mt. Vernon, IA 52314. AASECT is devoted to the promotion of sexual health through the development and advancement of the fields of sexual therapy, counseling, and education. The association provides professional education and certification of sex educators, counselors, and therapists and encourages research related to sex education, counseling, and therapy. Send a stamped, self-addressed business-size envelope to receive a list of certified sex counselors and sex therapists in your state.

Sexuality Information and Education Council of the United States, 130 W. 42nd St., Suite 350, New York, NY 10036. Voice: (212) 819-9770. SIECUS serves as a clearinghouse for authoritative sex information for professionals of all disciplines. If you are in New York City, you have access to the SIECUS Information Service and Mary S. Calderone Library (noncirculating)—more than 6,000 books, eighty periodicals, and a number of pamphlets. Call to request a list of publications or a list of certified sex therapists in your state.

Products and Catalogs

Good Vibrations, 938 Howard St., Suite 101, San Francisco, CA 94103. Voice: (800) 289-8423. Internet: www.goodvibes.com/catalogs.html. Good Vibrations calls itself "a 'clean, well-lighted place' to shop for sex toys, books, and videos." The mail order *Catalog of Toys* and *The Sexuality Library* catalog of informational and erotic books and videos are intelligently designed and written. The catalogs arrive in an inconspicuous plain brown envelope, and your name and address are not sold or given to other businesses. Products include the Kegelcisor (tiny weights for exercising pelvic-floor muscles), lubricants, and safer sex supplies. With the easy conversational tone and staff tips ("I like to give Smoothies as first-time vibrator gifts—they're colorful, affordable and always appreciated"), this may be the most fun you've ever had reading a catalog!

Home Delivery Incontinence Supplies Co., Inc., 1215 Dielman Industrial Court, Olivette, MO 63132. Voice: (800) 538-1036. Fax: (314) 997-0047. Internet: www.hdisnet.com. Send for the catalog of incontinence products, including undergarments, absorbent protection, skin-care items, nutritional supplements, and more.

Periodicals

Quality Care. This very informative quarterly newsletter for members of the National Association for Continence (see listing in Organizations and Services, above) will keep you up to date on the latest medical advancements and products for people with incontinence. A letters column gives good insight into how people are dealing with this problem.

Sex Over Forty Newsletter, P.O. Box 1600, Chapel Hill, NC 27515. Voice: (919) 644-1616. Described as "a practical, authoritative newsletter directed to the sexual concerns of the mature adult," this eight-page monthly newsletter is directed toward both women and men. It publishes articles about many aspects of sexuality and answers questions from readers.

Books

VAGINAL HEALTH

Kathryn L. Bargio, Ph.D., K. Lynette Pearce, R.N., and Angelo J. Lucco, M.D. *Staying Dry: A Practical Guide for Bladder Control*. Baltimore: Johns Hopkins University Press, 1989. A how-to guide for controlling the bladder.

Paula B. Doress-Worters and Diana Laskin Siegal, with Boston Women's Health Collective. *The New Ourselves, Growing Older*. New York: Simon and Schuster, 1994). This book has an extensive and very informative chapter on urinary incontinence.

Judith Reichman, M.D. *I'm Too Young to Get Old: Health Care for Women After Forty*. New York: Times Books, 1996. Dr. Reichman's section on vaginal changes and urinary incontinence offers solid information along with ideas and suggestions for self-help. She also has an excellent chapter on "Contraception, Fertility, and Pregnancy After Forty."

SEX

Margo Anand. *The Art of Sexual Ecstasy: Cultivating Sexual Energy to Transform Your Life*. New York: Tarcher/Putnam, 1995. Anand, an internationally known expert and lecturer on Tantric sex, writes a gentle and sensual book about how to use erotic energy for personal and spiritual growth.

Lonnie Barbach, Ph.D. *For Each Other: Sharing Sexual Intimacy*. New York: Signet, 1984; and *For Yourself: The Fulfillment of Female Sexuality*. New York: Signet, 1976. These are the earlier works of therapist Barbach, author of *The Pause*. They've been around for a while, but they're still good books for women in and out of relationships.

Charlotte Hill and William Wallace. *Erotica II: An Illustrated Anthology of Sexual Art and Literature*. New York: Carroll and Graf, 1993. A blend of erotic art works, many from private collections, and literature, including forbidden literature from the West by authors such as Anais Nin and Emile Zola. A feast for the senses.

Sheila Kitzinger. *Women's Experience of Sex: The Facts and Feelings of Female Sexuality at Every Stage of Life*. New York: Penguin, 1988. This very nice book is warm and inclusive of all styles and ages. It has a good chapter on menopause and growing older.

Roselyn Payne, M.D., and Susan Cobb Stuart, M.D. *American Women's Medical Association Guide to Sexuality*. New York: Dell, 1995. This straight-ahead guide covers every aspect of women's sexuality, from medical concerns to reasons for lack of desire.

Marcy Sheiver, ed. *Herotica Four*. San Francisco: Down There Press, 1996. A collection of erotica by women that is pansexual, very diverse in approach, and addressed to all ages.

Saul Rosenthal. *Sex After Forty*. New York: Tarcher/Putnam, 1988. Rosenthal encourages sexual creativity and has many suggestions for a satisfying sex life despite medical conditions. He has a good chapter on hysterectomy and sexuality. This book is directed toward heterosexual couples.

Kensington Ladies' Erotica Society. *Ladies Own Erotica.* Berkeley, CA: Ten Speed Press, 1984. Kensington, an upscale "soccer-mom" suburb of San Francisco, is also home to a group of women who found their talent in writing women's erotic literature. Nonthreatening and good-humored fantasies.

Audio/Video

For catalogs of health and medical tapes, see the listings in Chapter 7, "The Holistic Kit and Caboodle," and Chapter 8, "What's Up, Doc?" You'll find other tapes on midlife and menopause in Chapter 2, "Why Is This Happening to Me?" The **Good Vibrations** catalog (see Products and Catalogs, above) is a good source for tapes on female sexuality.

Focus International, Inc., 1160 E. Jericho Turnpike, Suite 15, Huntington, NY 11743. Voice: (800) 843-0305. Internet: www.sex-health.com. A wide range of educational videotapes on sex and health. Call for a catalog, or access the catalog at the web site.

VIDEOS

Menopause and Beyond. 60 minutes. Available from Focus International, Inc. The sexual health issues that affect all women during menopause and the years that follow.

Menopause and Female Sexuality. Dr. Lonnie Barbach. 1992. Available from Focus International, Inc. Barbach, author of *The Pause* and other books, discusses the effect of menopause on women's sexual experience.

Sex After Fifty. Dr. Lonnie Barbach. 1991. 90 minutes. Available from Good Vibrations. Interviews with men and women over fifty shed light on the nature of sex in later life. Good Vibrations says, "An extraordinary educational tape with no sex depicted, but a world of wisdom to impart."

The Couples Guide to Great Sex Over 40. 2 videos. Available from Focus International, Inc. How maturity can enhance and reinvigorate sexual relationships.

Online

For vaginal health and urinary incontinence, check out the general health sites listed in Chapter 2, "Why Is This Happening to Me?," Chapter 7, "The Holistic Kit and Caboodle," and Chapter 8, "What's Up, Doc?"

MAILING LISTS

For support and suggestions with vaginal health issues, try the **MENOPAUS** (spelled without the final E) mailing list at LISTSERV@PSUHMC.HMC.PSU.EDU.

NEWS GROUPS

Try **alt.support.menopause** for issues of vaginal health.

WEB SITES

For vaginal health and urinary incontinence, check out the general health sites listed in Chapter 2, "Why Is This Happening to Me?," Chapter 7, "The Holistic Kit and Caboodle," and Chapter 8, "What's Up, Doc?" **Women's Wire** has a column called "Ask Sexpert," at www.women.com/body/qa.sex.html. There's no lack of Internet sites dealing with sex. Dr. Ruth's Sexnet, at www.drruth.com, is **Dr. Ruth Westheimer**'s web site. She features daily sex tips and answers e-mail questions about sex, and she has some links to other sites.

11

Boning Up
Osteoporosis

Osteoporosis, the condition in which bones become fragile and prone to fracture, is one of the major health concerns of women at midlife and beyond. When you hear that an older woman has fallen and broken her hip, osteoporosis is generally the culprit. Unfortunately, because the progress of osteoporosis is painless, your bones can be losing density for years and you never suspect it until you sustain a fracture, lose height, or develop a "dowager's hump." While it may not be possible to prevent bone loss completely, you can take steps to retard osteoporosis and even build bone density that has been lost.

osteoporosis Literally, "porous bone"; bone loss due to declining reproductive hormones, inadequate dietary calcium, and not enough physical stress on bones.

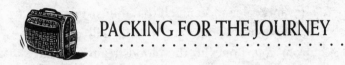

What Causes Osteoporosis?

Reduced hormone levels, inadequate dietary calcium, and a sedentary lifestyle all contribute to the development of osteoporosis, but doctors do not fully understand its cause. We do know that our bones are most dense in our mid-thirties. We begin losing bone density before menopause, and this loss increases around menopause and after. According to the National Osteoporosis Foundation, women can lose up to 20 percent of their total bone mass in the first five to seven years following menopause.

Am I at Risk for Osteoporosis?

Osteoporosis affects one out of four women today—and one out of three postmenopausal women. It's a real problem, but not all women will develop it. In general, African American women are far less likely to have osteoporosis than Caucasian women. (But if you are a thin, light-skinned African American woman, your chances of developing osteoporosis are higher.) Take a look at the list of risk factors in this chapter to see where you stand.

To reduce your risk of osteoporosis, you should:

1. Pay attention to your calcium intake.

2. Eat a balanced, low-sodium diet that includes a wide variety of fruits, vegetables, whole grains, and soy products.

3. Get plenty of exercise.

4. Discuss the benefits and risks of hormone replacement therapy with your doctor.

Why Is Calcium Important to Bone Health?

The body needs calcium for everything from muscle contraction to proper blood clotting.

TRAVEL TIP
Moo!

- Dairy products such as milk and yogurt are good sources of calcium, but they can also be sources of saturated fat. If you get calcium from dairy products, stick to nonfat.

- Yogurt with the active culture *Lactobacillus acidophilus* helps replenish friendly bacteria in your digestive tract, aiding health and digestion.

- Drinking one glass of milk a day may be enough to offset the calcium-draining effect of two cups of coffee. Next time, order a nonfat café latté.

- Just 1 tablespoon of nonfat dry milk has 85 milligrams of calcium. Add it to recipes for bread, muffins, pancakes, gravies, and anything else you can think of.

Evaluate Your Chances

Your risk of developing osteoporosis may be higher if:

- You are a fair-complexioned Caucasian or Asian.
- You are slender, petite, or small-boned.
- You have a family history of osteoporosis.
- You eat a diet high in meats and processed foods.
- You get very little exercise.
- You smoke.
- You drink alcohol daily.
- You are postmenopausal.
- You have had an early or surgically induced menopause.
- You have you been taking excessive thyroid medication or high doses of cortisone-like drugs for asthma, arthritis, or cancer.

Your risk of developing osteoporosis may be lower if:

- You are African American.
- You are overweight, tall, or large-boned.
- You eat a lacto-ovo vegetarian diet.
- You do not eat processed foods.
- You exercise vigorously three or more times a week.
- You are taking estrogen replacement therapy.

Don't Forget Vitamin D

A daily dose of vitamin D helps calcium absorption and stimulates bone formation. The recommended daily allowance is 200 IUs, which you can meet through supplements, good nutrition, dairy products fortified with vitamin D, or fifteen minutes of sunshine.

It wants calcium so much that if it isn't getting enough from your diet, it will pull calcium from your bones to the bloodstream to make the mineral available for the muscles and nerves. Taking a daily calcium supplement or eating adequate dietary calcium alone won't prevent bone loss, but it will help maintain the mineral balance your body needs for good bone health.

How Much Calcium Do I Need?

The National Institutes of Health recommend the following daily doses of calcium:

- Premenopausal women between the ages of twenty-five and fifty need 1,200 milligrams of calcium per day.
- Postmenopausal women under sixty-five who are taking hormone replacement therapy need 1,000 milligrams of calcium per day.
- Postmenopausal women under sixty-five who are not on hormone replacement therapy need 1,500 milligrams of calcium per day.

Can I Get the Calcium I Need Through Food?

The calcium your body absorbs best is dietary calcium—the calcium in food. You can eat the amount of calcium you need every day, but it means paying strict attention to what you are eating. Low-fat or nonfat dairy products, dark leafy greens, tofu, and canned salmon and sardines (it's the bones) are all good sources of natural calcium. Salad lovers will be especially happy to know that gourmet salad mixes con-

GUIDED TOUR: *Osteoporosis*

Osteoporosis is one of the major health concerns of women at midlife and beyond. Risk factors include menopause (women can lose up to 20 percent of their total bone mass in the first five to seven years following menopause), heredity, diet, and lack of exercise. A calcium-rich diet, weight-bearing exercise, and hormone replacement therapy can all help retard osteoporosis.

WESTERN MEDICINE

Hormone replacement therapy is often recommended for women at risk for osteoporosis; the use of natural progesterone for this purpose is still controversial. The nonhormonal drugs alendronate and calcitonin can help build bone. A bone-density test can help determine your current bone health if you suspect you are at risk.

COMPLEMENTARY THERAPIES

Herbal compounds high in calcium and other bone-building minerals are available in natural food stores. Traditional Chinese medicine may help osteoporosis in the early stages.

EXERCISE

Weight-bearing exercise (such as walking, stair climbing, strength training) can help build bone density at any age. A good exercise program will also promote balance that helps you avoid falls.

MIND–BODY

Chronic stress can leach calcium from bones. Mind–body practices such as biofeedback, meditation, and relaxation response can help reduce stress. Alexander technique, Rosen work, Pilates, qi gong, t'ai chi, and other movement programs can reduce stress and promote balance; some programs, including some yoga poses, can also build strength.

NUTRITION

Eat a balanced diet high in calcium-rich fruits, vegetables, and other foods and low in saturated fat, red meat, and sodium. Take calcium supplements and vitamin D to aid calcium absorption. Avoid or cut down on colas, nicotine, and caffeine.

taining arugula are a potent calcium source—just ¹/₂ cup of arugula (also known as rocket) has a whopping 309 milligrams of calcium, 30 percent of the recommended daily intake for premenopausal women. The traditional Japanese diet, which is low in meat protein but high in seaweed, soy products, and seafood, is another calcium bonanza. And while you're working so hard, be sure you're not eating foods that interfere with calcium absorption (see the Point of Interest "The Art of Calcium Supplements").

Which Calcium Supplement Is Best?

When it comes to supplements, the important thing is not the amount of calcium in the supplement but the amount of elemental calcium in the supplement that your body actually absorbs. This depends in part on the kind of supplement you take. The two most common forms of calcium are calcium carbonate and calcium citrate; calcium phosphate is also commonly used in supplements. *Calcium carbonate* has the highest amount of elemental calcium and is the least expensive, but often causes gas or constipation (take it on a full stomach). *Calcium citrate* tends to be more expensive, but is the one recommended by most health practitioners because it is the most easily tolerated. *Calcium phosphate* is easily absorbed, and can be taken with or without food. Avoid calcium supplements based on bone meal and dolomite, which may have impurities. If you tend to form kidney stones, consult your doctor: Calcium supplements may not be recommended for you.

What About Other Vitamins and Minerals?

A good bone health program also pays attention to adequate intake of minerals and vitamins that are crucial to calcium absorption and bone health. Chief among these is magnesium, which you'll find abundant in soybeans, spinach, turnip greens, dates, black-eyed peas, cornmeal, buckwheat, and cashews. You can

Some bottled waters can be a good source of calcium and magnesium, which is needed for calcium absorption. According to *The Good Water Guide* and *The Pocket Guide to Bottled Water,* San Pellegrino water contains more than 200 milligrams of calcium per liter, and Perrier has over 140 milligrams per liter. Do watch out for the sodium content of some brands. It can cause you to eliminate calcium in your urine. A santé!

How to Eat Your Calcium

Don't stop eating calcium-rich foods just because you take calcium supplements. Eating is the way our bodies are designed to get nutrients, and the calcium in foods is naturally better absorbed. You'll find calcium-rich foods everywhere.

Food	Calcium (milligrams)
FRUITS	
blackberries, 1 cup	46
figs, dried, 5	135
dates, dried, cut, or pitted, 1/2 cup	52
orange, 1 medium	58
apricots, dried, 1 cup	90
orange juice, calcium-fortified, 6 oz.	200
papaya, 1 medium	72
tamarind, raw, 1 cup	89
VEGETABLES	
arugula (rocket), 1/2 cup	309
bok choy, fresh, 1 cup	250
bean sprouts, 1 cup	100
carrot juice, 1/2 cup	83
broccoli, 1 cup	140
collards, 1 cup	300
turnip greens, 1 cup	200
okra, 1/2 cup, cooked	152
kale, 1/2 cup, cooked	134
mustard greens, 1/2 cup, cooked	184
spinach, 1/2 cup, cooked	98
SEAWEED	
agar-agar, 2 oz.	200
arame, 2 oz.	575
dulse, 3 1/2 oz.	213
hijiki, 2 oz.	700
kelp, 3 1/2 oz.	942
kombu, 2 oz.	400
nori, 3 1/2 oz.	188
wakame/alaria, 3 1/2 oz.	1,100
SEAFOOD	
sardines, canned, with bones, 3 oz.	258
salmon, canned, with bones, 3 oz.	212
clams, steamed, 3 oz.	78
lobster meat, 3 oz.	52
oysters, steamed, 3 oz.	76
mackerel, canned, 8 oz.	552

Food	Calcium (milligrams)
SOY	
tofu, firm, 1/2 cup	258
soybeans, green, boiled, 1 cup	175
soybeans, dry roasted, 1/2 cup	232
LEGUMES	
garbanzo beans, canned, 1 cup	150
navy, kidney, or great northern beans, cooked, 1 cup	120
white beans, cooked, 1 cup	161
NUTS AND SEEDS	
almonds, dried, 1/2 cup	170
Brazil nuts, 1/2 cup	130
sesame seeds, dry, 1/2 cup	85
sesame seed meal, 1/4 cup	270
sesame tahini, 1 tablespoon	64
sunflower seeds, 1 oz.	33
DAIRY PRODUCTS	
nonfat milk, 1 cup	302–316
nonfat milk powder, 1 tablespoon	85
yogurt, plain, nonfat, 1 cup	452
yogurt, fruit flavored low-fat, 1 cup	314
cottage cheese, low-fat, 1 cup	204
mozzarella, part skim, 1 oz.	145
feta cheese, 1 oz.	140
ricotta, 1 cup	669
GRAINS	
corn tortilla	60
corn flour (masa harina), 1/3 cup	77
soy flour, defatted, 1 cup	241
HERBS	
basil, dry, 1 teaspoon	30
fennel seed, 1 teaspoon	24
oregano, 1 teaspoon	24
poppy seed, 1 teaspoon	41
thyme, dry, 1 teaspoon	24
MISCELLANEOUS	
blackstrap molasses, 1 tablespoon	135

The Art of Calcium Supplements

Just swallowing your calcium supplement each day may not be enough. To make sure your body is absorbing as much calcium as possible, pay attention to the following guidelines:

- Spread the dosage out over an entire day rather than taking it all at once.

- Relax: High stress levels leach calcium from the bones.

- Eat foods that are high in calcium, especially fruits, vegetables, and grains.

- Avoid eating a diet high in saturated fats. But don't cut out fat altogether—small amounts of fat improve calcium absorption. (Try to limit your fat intake to between 20 percent and 30 percent of your total calories.)

- Avoid eating foods high in sodium—it robs your bones of calcium.

- Avoid or limit your intake of caffeine, alcohol, nicotine, and cola drinks, which interfere with calcium absorption.

- Avoid eating the following foods at the same time that you take your supplement (they interfere with calcium absorption):

Foods containing oxalic acid: spinach, rhubarb, Swiss chard, sorrel, parsley, beet greens, and unhulled sesame seeds.

Foods containing phytates: found in the outer layers of grain seed, such as wheat bran (sprouted-grain breads contain no phytates, but unprocessed bran does).

Foods high in phosphorus: red meat, cola drinks, and processed foods that have phosphorus additives.

also find combined calcium–magnesium supplements. Other important nutrients include zinc, copper, manganese, boron, silicon, and strontium, plus vitamins C, D, K, B_6, and beta-carotene. Yikes! You can eat your vitamins and minerals by getting a variety of fresh foods. Molasses and green leafy vegetables, for example, are high in both calcium and magnesium; sardines are high in calcium and vitamin D (needed for calcium absorption); papayas and broccoli are high in both calcium and vitamin C. You may also want to supplement. Check your natural food store for supplements that combine minerals and vitamins specific to good bone health.

Can Soy Products Help Retard Osteoporosis?

Could be. According to Mark and Virginia Messina in *The Simple Soybean and Your Health*, people who live in countries where protein intake is low and where most protein comes from plant foods maintain strong bones on low calcium intake. One reason may be that soy or soy protein causes less calcium to be lost in the urine than does animal protein. For more on the intriguing soybean, see Chapter 4, "Are You What You Eat?"

What About Exercise and Osteoporosis?

By all means, exercise. Not only is it good for your general health, but weight-bearing exercise (even walking) can actually help build up your bones and repair some of the damage as well. No matter when you begin, even if you don't start until after menopause, this kind of exercise can help.

You don't have to have expensive exercise equipment to reap these benefits. Weight-bearing activities that cost little or nothing include walking, jogging, hiking, aerobic dance, tennis, and climbing stairs. Free weights and weight machines can build bone mass and increase muscle and ligament strength, which can protect your bones. If you don't want to spend money on barbells or a gym, you can lift weights at home using equal-weight soup cans. Begin with the smallest size, and work your way up! As always, consult your health practitioner before starting any exercise program. For more information, see Chapter 3, "Keep on Moving."

Yoga exercises such as the Downward-Facing-Dog pose, in which the arms and upper body bear body weight, can also help increase bone strength. According to physical therapist and yoga instructor Judith Lasater, yoga also helps reduce stress, which is said to play a part in osteoporosis. "When you're more stressed out, your blood becomes slightly more acidic, which leaches calcium from the bones over time. When you're relaxed, your blood becomes more alkaline and doesn't leach out as much calcium." And Dr. Christiane Northrup observes that her patients who practice yoga "seem to show the least height loss. I believe that this is because yoga tends to keep the disc spaces between the vertebrae more supple and more open."

Should I Take a Bone-Density Test?

Probably not. A bone-density or bone-mass measurement is a test that uses small amounts of radiation to determine density or thickness

Bone-Density Testing

My mother had osteoporosis. I'm thin and blond, like her, although I'm way more athletic. But when I was forty-six, I decided to have a bone-density test—just to be comfortable. I was really shaken when I found out that my bone density was below average for someone my age. I am still not sure I want to use hormone replacement as a defense against osteoporosis, but the test was a wake-up call. I realize I cannot put off taking care of myself.   *Linea, 50*

EAT IT!
Cooking for Bone Health

If you take a look at the long list of calcium-rich foods in this chapter, you'll soon see that it's fairly easy to put together a meal that's good for your bones. Here are some simple ideas.

Italian Greens: Sauté the greens of your choice (chard, kale, mustard greens, bok choy, spinach) with chopped fresh garlic in a little olive oil. Add cubed tofu for even more calcium. Or steam Swiss chard and let it cool to room temperature. Drizzle on a little olive oil and lemon juice, and serve as a salad.

Middle Eastern Fruit Salad: Arrange dried figs, dates, and sliced fresh oranges on a bed of arugula. Make a sauce of nonfat or low-fat plain yogurt, with honey and ground cardamom to taste, and a dash of vanilla extract. Serve a dollop of sauce with the fruit salad.

Asian Sauté: Sauté minced fresh ginger (about a teaspoon), sliced bok choy, and tofu squares in a tablespoon of sesame seed oil. Add other vegetables (sliced mushrooms, carrots, and so on) according to your taste. Sprinkle with toasted sesame seeds with a little soy sauce or oyster-flavored sauce and serve over rice or noodles.

Deciding for Yourself:
The Calcium Chronicles

When it comes to making decisions in real life, it can be a tortuous path—at least for some people. I always feel the need to figure out everything for myself, so when my doctor told me that I should be taking 1,000 milligrams of calcium daily to prevent bone loss, it just wasn't possible for me to do the simple thing: Take the pills.

First, I went to the natural food store and stood in front of the seeming endless shelves of calcium. Oyster shell calcium (no, too many heavy metals end up in those oyster shells), calcium with vitamin D, calcium with potassium, calcium with fish liver oil. I picked up a couple of bottles and carried them around for a while. Should I take 1,200 milligrams? What if I already got sufficient calcium from my diet? Would I be overdosing? Even if I took 1,000 milligrams of calcium, would it all get absorbed? I was completely confused.

Then I realized why. I love food. I would rather eat my vitamins than swallow them in pill form. I was cheered to discover that women outside the United States need less calcium supplementation, by and large, because they eat diets lower in meat and so retain more of their dietary calcium. And I know that the body absorbs dietary calcium better than supplementary calcium. I like calcium-rich foods and there are plenty to choose from.

When I thought about it, it seemed to me that I was already doing pretty well. I eat a fairly balanced diet and get plenty of exercise, but I can add in more strength training. In the end, I decided to do what my doctor suggested: take 1,000 milligrams of calcium citrate a day. And I also decided to keep eating my calcium and start looking for a gym. But I left the supplements sitting on my counter for a week before I started taking them—just to keep up my image.

Naomi

of the bones in the hip, spine, and wrist. This test is expensive and rarely given. It's helpful if it can lead to a program of prevention or treatment; for example, if you are really on the fence about hormone replacement therapy, knowledge of your current bone density may help push you one way or the other. If you do need this test, the DXA (Dual-Energy X-Ray Absorptiometry) machine is said to be the most accurate. Ask your physician about this test, or contact the Foundation for Osteoporosis Research and Treatment (see Resources for more information). To find the bone-density testing center nearest you, call the National Osteoporosis Foundation Action Line: (800) 463-6700.

Can Hormone Replacement Therapy Help Retard Osteoporosis?

For many years the medical establishment has recommended hormone replacement therapy to prevent and treat osteoporosis. Although hormone therapy has been shown to slow down bone loss, it has not been shown to build bone that has already been lost. Results of studies are mixed, and no one knows for certain what the long-term effects of hormone therapy may be, natural or synthetic. If you are taking HRT to retard osteoporosis, you still need to get an adequate intake of calcium in your diet and do plenty of weight-bearing exercises. For more on hormone replacement therapy, see Chapter 9, "Yes or No?"

Can Natural Progesterone Help Osteoporosis?

John R. Lee, M.D., has popularized the use of natural progesterone in the United States. He says he has had success increasing bone density in menopausal osteoporotic patients with the use of a natural progesterone skin moisturizer. His claims that natural progesterone cream can increase bone density are controversial and not well substantiated. Doctors from the East Bay Menopause and PMS Center in Oakland have not seen the same results. In fact, on this regimen they have seen some bone loss. Clearly, more research needs to be done. Currently, these doctors are in the process of developing a research project that will be looking at natural progesterone and bone growth. For more on natural progesterone, see Chapter 9, "Yes or No?"

Are There Any Nonhormonal Bone Builders?

If you are at risk for osteoporosis but hormone replacement therapy is not an option, two nonhormonal drugs are now available. Alendronate (sold under the name Fosomax), a relatively new nonhormonal drug, shows real promise according to *Science News*. In a study of 994 postmenopausal women in sixteen countries, alendronate was shown to help maintain and even improve bone density and to cut the risk of vertebral fractures among women diagnosed with osteoporosis. The main side effect is esophageal irritation. A synthetic hormone, calcitonin (sold as a nasal spray under the name Miacalcin) is somewhat less effective than alendronate, but it does build bone. Check with your doctor to assess the risks and benefits of these drugs for you.

Are There Botanical Remedies for Osteoporosis?

A surprising number of herbs are high in calcium. Herbalist Susun Weed says, "Horsetail (*Equisetum arvense*) is my favorite herb for restoring bone density. Through its synergistic mineral actions, it helps the bone thicken and stabilize. A daily tea of dried, spring-picked herb helps reverse osteoporosis and speeds healing of fractures." In *The Herbal Menopause Book*, Amanda McQuade Crawford also suggests stinging nettle (*Urtica dioica*). Bone-All, a tablet containing calcium, horsetail, and a number of other bone-building compounds, is generally available in natural food stores.

Traditional Chinese medicine also treats problems associated with thinning bones. According to *The Complete Home Healer,* "Herbal treatment can help this condition if it is caught in the early stages. Practitioners of traditional Chinese medicine usually recommend *Angelica sinensis,* Chinese licorice, cibot rhizome, and eucomia bark." Consult an herbalist or Chinese medical practitioner before you embark on a treatment.

SIDE TRIPS:
OTHER PATHWAYS THROUGH THIS BOOK

CHAPTER 3: KEEP ON MOVING   Weight-bearing exercise helps promote bone growth. Look here for movement and exercise programs that build bone density and promote balance and good health.

CHAPTER 4: ARE YOU WHAT YOU EAT?   Your bones need calcium and other minerals to stay strong, and you can meet those needs through food and supplements. Look here for more on midlife nutritional needs.

CHAPTER 9: YES OR NO?   Hormone replacement therapy is one way to protect against bone loss, especially if you have a family history of osteoporosis. Look here to learn more on the pros and cons of HRT.

RESOURCES

Organizations and Services

Foundation for Osteoporosis Research and Education, 3120 Webster St., Oakland, CA 94609. Voice: (510) 832-BONE. Fax: (510) 208-7174. Internet: www. FORE.org. This nonprofit resource center and educational organization is a good place to begin your search. The foundation is involved in research and education, including several clinical studies. Write or call to request printed material and educational and research information. If you have Internet access, the web site has a lot of information.

Melpomene Institute, 1010 University Ave., St. Paul, MN 55104. Voice: (612) 642-1951. E-mail: melpomen@webspan.com. Internet: www.melpomene.org. This very helpful organization studies and promotes the role of exercise in all aspects of women's health. It has lots of solid information, including a packet on osteoporosis.

National Osteoporosis Foundation, 1150 17th St. N.W., Suite 500, Washington, DC 20036-4603. Voice: (202) 223-2226 or (800) 223-9994. Fax: (202) 223-2237. Internet: www.nof.org. This is a good resource for patients and health-care professionals seeking up-to-date information, support, and guidance on all aspects of osteoporosis, including studies and breaking news.

National Women's Health Network, 514 10th St. N.W., Suite 400, Washington, DC 20004. Voice: (202) 347-1140. Fax: (202) 347-1168. Internet: www.women connect.com/or20550g.htm. Send for a very informative packet on osteoporosis.

NATURAL HORMONE CREAMS/VITAMINS

Aeron Labs, 1933 Davis St., Suite 310, San Leandro, CA 94577. Voice: (800) 631-7900. Fax: (510) 729-0383. Do you really need progesterone cream? Call Aeron to find out about saliva testing to determine your current hormone levels. You or your physician can order the test kit to be mailed to you, and you can return your sample in the mail. The lab will send you the results, and you can talk with a doctor at the lab and ask questions—everyone there is very helpful. The lab also provides a list of progesterone creams on the market and the progesterone content of each.

Transitions for Health, 621 S.W. Alder, Suite 900, Portland, OR 97205. Voice: (800) 888-6814 or (800) 460-7853. Fax: (800) 944-0168. E-mail: etfh@progest.com. Internet: www.progest.com/index.html. This company makes and sells ProGest cream (the one used in Dr. Lee's study). It also offers herbal remedies, vitamins, homeopathic remedies, and a saliva test for measuring estrogen and progesterone levels. Call to receive a catalog. If you're online, you can submit questions to a doctor.

Vitamin Express, 1425 Irving St., San Francisco, CA 94122. Voice: (800) 500-0733 (mail order). Internet: vitaminexpress.com. This vitamin specialty shop sells ProGest cream by mail at a competitive price. Call to receive a newsletter. If you are on the Internet, the web site lists the products and prices.

Women's International Pharmacy, 5708 Monona Drive, Madison, WI 53716. Voice: (800) 279-5708. Fax: (800) 279-8011. Internet: www.wipws.com. Second address: 13925 Meeker Blvd., Suite 13, Sun City West, AZ 85375. Voice: (602) 214-7700. This pharmacy specializes in individual natural hormone treatment for women. Natural hormones are available by mail order—have your doctor fax or call in a prescription. The pharmacy will send information to you and your physician about its products, as well as copies of relevant studies, and pharmacists will answer any technical questions. The company can also provide you with a list of doctors in your area who have used their products. The pharmacists are very helpful.

RESEARCH REPORTS

See Chapter 8, "What's Up, Doc?," for a complete list of organizations that will do research reports on specific health issues such as osteoporosis.

Hotlines

Calcium Information Center: (800) 321-2681. Call for a recorded message explaining elemental calcium, to request a printed brochure on nutritional calcium and calcium's role in health, or to ask specific questions about calcium.

National Osteoporosis Foundation: (800) 223-9994. Call to request the brochure "Stand Up to Osteoporosis." Any specific questions you have will be routed to the National Foundation Office.

National Osteoporosis Foundation Action Line: (800) 464-6700. Call for bone-density testing sites in your area, information, and educational materials.

Women's Health Initiative: (800) 54-WOMEN. Call for the phone number of your local site for the Women's Health Initiative clinical trials on osteoporosis.

Periodicals

Virtually all of the newsletters and journals listed in Chapter 2, "Why Is This Happening to Me?," and Chapter 8, "What's Up, Doc?," cover breaking news about osteoporosis.

The Osteoporosis Report is devoted solely to news about osteoporosis. This quarterly publication is available by subscription from the National Osteoporosis Foundation, 2100 M St. N.W., Suite 602, Washington, DC 20037. Voice: (800) 223-9994.

Books

Sydney Lou Bonnick, M.D. *The Osteoporosis Handbook.* Dallas: Taylor Publishing, 1994. A medical approach to the prevention and treatment of osteoporosis.

Alan K. Gaby, M.D. *Preventing and Reversing Osteoporosis.* Rocklin, CA: Prima Publishing, 1994. Gaby, an expert on the natural treatment of bone loss, offers three concepts: the role of vitamins and minerals in addition to calcium, hormones other than estrogen, and the role of environmental pollutant contaminants.

Betty Kamen, Ph.D. *Hormone Replacement Therapy, Yes or No: How to Make an Informed Decision About Estrogen, Progesterone, and Other Strategies for Dealing with PMS, Menopause, and Osteoporosis.* Novato, CA: Nutrition Encounter, 1993. In this information-packed personal approach, Kamen admits to having formed fairly strong conclusions: She is an "advocate of using transdermally applied natural progesterone along with specific food supplements." She covers all the bases and explains how she reached her conclusions.

Ruth S. Jacobowitz. *150 Most Asked Questions About Osteoporosis: What Women Really Want to Know.* New York: Morrow/Hearst, 1993. The question-and-answer format really does answer women's most-asked questions in a way that's easy to understand.

John R. Lee, M.D. *What Your Doctor May Not Tell You About Menopause.* New York: Warner Books, 1996. If you're interested in natural progesterone, this is a more readable version of Lee's first book, *Natural Progesterone: The Multiple Roles of a Remarkable Hormone.* Lee talks about menopause and the role of progesterone and explains natural progesterones. He also discusses lifestyle and menopause.

Mark Messina, Ph.D., and Virginia Messina, R.D., with Ken Setchell, Ph.D. *The Simple Soybean and Your Health*. Garden City Park, NY: Avery Publishing, 1994. Explores the many nutritional advantages of soy foods and discusses their intriguing role in the possible prevention of a number of medical problems, including osteoporosis.

Audio/Video

See the catalogs listed in Chapter 8, "What's Up, Doc?," for more companies that carry general health tapes, and Chapter 7, "The Holistic Kit and Caboodle," for companies that carry tapes on complementary medicine. For tapes on hormone replacement, see Chapter 9, "Yes or No?" For exercise tapes, see Chapter 3, "Keep on Moving." For nutrition tapes, see Chapter 4, "Are You What You Eat?"

AUDIO

Every Woman's Guide to Osteoporosis. 1990. Available from P.O. Box 2, Wilmot, WI 53192. Voice: (800) 888-9355. Addresses the role of diet, exercise, and medical screening in the prevention of osteoporosis.

Online

Most of the resources in this chapter have web sites, and those web sites have links. **Power Surge,** located at members.aol.com/dearest, and **Women's Wire,** at www.women.com, cover midlife health issues on a regular basis. You'll also find news and help on osteoporosis in the medical sites and online magazines listed in Chapter 2, "Why Is This Happening to Me?," Chapter 7, "The Holistic Kit and Caboodle," and Chapter 8, "What's Up, Doc?"

MAILING LISTS

To discuss osteoporosis, try the **MENOPAUS** mailing list. To subscribe, contact LISTSERV@PSUHMC.HMC.PSU.EDU and note that MENOPAUS is spelled without the final "e."

NEWS GROUPS

Try **alt.support.menopause** if you're interested in sharing information about osteoporosis.

WEB SITES:

To go right to the source, try the **National Osteoporosis Foundation** site at www.nof.org, or the **Foundation for Osteoporosis Research and Treatment** site at www.FORE.org. Both include facts on risk factors, bone health, prevention, and treatment, as well as breaking news. For information about **Clinical Trials and Osteoporosis,** check out www.centerwatch.com/CAT111.HTM.

12

AND THE BEAT GOES ON

Heart Disease

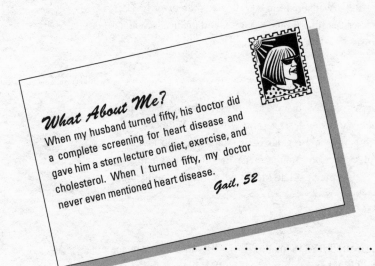

One of the biggest health concerns women begin to face in midlife may surprise you: It is heart disease. We've learned to think of this condition as a problem for middle-aged, overweight, overworked men, but heart attacks kill more American women than any other disease. In fact, heart disease is responsible for half of all deaths of women over age fifty. The American Heart Association puts it bluntly: "Clearly, heart disease is epidemic in women as well as in men. The main difference between the sexes is not *whether* women are likely to get heart disease, but *when.*" Fortunately, heart disease is one health problem that we can reverse and even prevent. It's never too early (or too late!) to begin to educate yourself about your risks and to begin to make healthful changes.

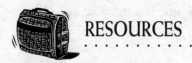

RESOURCES

What Is Heart Disease?

Heart disease is the term most people use to talk about cardiovascular disease, a group of diseases of the heart and blood vessels. The most common type of cardiovascular disease is coronary artery disease. In this condition, one or more of the coronary arteries that supply blood to the heart is blocked, and the blockage can lead to a heart attack. Stroke, rheumatic heart disease, and hypertension (high blood pressure) are all part of this group of diseases.

Why Is Heart Disease a Concern for Women in Midlife?

Estrogen gives women natural protection against heart disease for many years. The hormone's exact protective mechanism is not fully understood, but it appears to be related to the level of HDL (the good cholesterol) in the blood. As estrogen levels decline, we lose that protection. According to the American Heart Association, a woman's risk of heart attack ten years after menopause is almost the same as a man's. Women who have heart attacks are more likely to die than are men who have attacks, and heart surgery is also less successful for women than for men. Unfortunately, we know far less about women and heart disease than we do about men and heart disease. Most clinical trials have involved men, not women. Dosages of heart medication are based on studies of men, not women. The signs of heart disease in women may go unnoticed for many years, because the

POINT OF INTEREST
The Mystery of the Heart

Here at the end of the twentieth century, we have grown used to mechanical analogies: The brain is a computer; the heart is a pump. When you are thinking about taking care of your heart, it's healing to recall that the heart, the seat of love and compassion, has been central to the spiritual life of human beings in virtually all religions throughout recorded history. Jesus' divinity was "the moon dwelling in the heart," the Sacred Heart. In Eastern traditions, the fourth chakra is the Heart Chakra. In the words of Tantric therapist Margo Anand, "This is the turning point for the ascent of energy, because there are three chakras above and three below." In Jewish kabbalism this is *Tiferet* on the Tree of Life—beauty, where the Self resides. According to *The Woman's Encyclopedia of Myths and Secrets,* "So vital was the idea of the heartbeat in Oriental religions that the very center of the universe was placed 'within the heart' by Tantric Sages." For the ancient Egyptians, it was *Ab,* the heart-soul, that would be weighed in the balance after death. For the Greek philosopher Aristotle, the heart was the "unmoved mover" around which all else revolved. The alchemists considered the heart to be our inner sun; and in the Heart Practice Tibetan Buddhists visualize compassion as "tremendous rays of light [streaming] toward you . . . filling your heart up completely, transforming all your suffering into bliss."

symptoms are often silent and women are not routinely screened for heart disease.

Am I at Risk for Heart Disease?

With heart disease, as with everything else in life, each woman is unique and each woman's risks are different. All women share a higher risk for heart disease after menopause due to the loss of estrogen protection, but beyond this you will need to put your individual risk factors into the mix:

FAMILY HEALTH HISTORY   Do you know your family health history? You are more likely to develop heart disease if your mother or sister was diagnosed with it before age sixty-five or if your father or brother was diagnosed before age fifty-five. (For more on how to gather this information, see Chapter 8, "What's Up, Doc?" and the Family Health History in Part 2, Your Personal Companion.)

RACE   In general, African Americans are at greater risk for heart disease than white Americans, perhaps because of higher blood pressure and a higher average weight. Native American women seem to have a lower risk because they tend to have lower cholesterol levels.

HIGH BLOOD PRESSURE   High blood pressure (hypertension) is the continuous elevation of your blood pressure above 140/90. Unchecked, high blood pressure can lead to heart attack and stroke. More than half of all women over age fifty-five have high blood pressure, and it is a particular risk for African American women. According to Dr. Elizabeth Ross, "Two times as many women of color over the age of twenty have hypertension as white women." *You may be able to change this risk factor.*

CHOLESTEROL LEVELS   The concentration of fat and cholesterol in your blood (high LDL

GUIDED TOUR: *Heart Disease*

Heart disease is the number-one killer of women in the United States. It's a concern to every woman after menopause, when declining estrogen levels leave the heart more vulnerable. You may be able to prevent and even reverse heart disease through a threefold program of lifestyle changes: diet, exercise, and stress management.

WESTERN MEDICINE

See your doctor for a complete diagnostic screening for cardiovascular disease that includes checking blood pressure and blood levels of cholesterol and triglycerides. Hormone replacement therapy can protect against heart disease for women after menopause.

COMPLEMENTARY THERAPIES

Complementary medicine that seeks to balance the system and reduce stress is a good strategy for lifestyle change. Hawthorn berry and khella are two ancient herbs for heart problems.

EXERCISE

A program that includes regular aerobic exercise is particularly beneficial for the cardiovascular system. Try to fit exercise into your daily routine by climbing stairs, walking instead of driving, and so on.

MIND–BODY

Movement techniques such as yoga, t'ai chi, and qi gong, and mind–body practices such as meditation, biofeedback, and others that dissolve stress can help lower blood pressure and reduce strain on the cardiovascular system.

NUTRITION

A diet that is low in saturated fats and that includes plenty of fruits and vegetables, whole grains, antioxidants, omega-3 fatty acids, and light protein has been shown to lower blood lipids and promote cardiovascular health. Stop smoking, reduce alcohol consumption, and maintain a healthy body weight.

- Average cost of heart bypass procedures: Thousands of dollars and time lost from work, plus associated costs for doctor visits and drugs.

- Average cost of making changes in diet: You'll save money when you include more plant-based foods in your diet and eliminate some of the higher-priced meats.

- Average cost of making changes in your physical activity: Free.

- Average cost of quitting smoking: You'll save at least a dollar a day.

- Average cost of changing how you cope with stress: Free.

cholesterol levels and low HDL cholesterol levels) contributes to blocked arteries and is considered an indicator of whether or not you're headed for a heart attack. Women's cholesterol levels begin to rise at about age forty-five, as estrogen declines. *You may be able to change this risk factor.*

TRIGLYCERIDE LEVELS An elevated triglyceride level is another indicator for heart disease—even more for women than for men. Healthy levels range from 50 to 200 mg/dL, depending on age (they rise as we get older). When your doctor orders a diagnostic screen for heart disease, make sure triglycerides are included. *You may be able to change this risk factor.*

OBESITY If you are significantly overweight (20 percent or more above the average for your height), you are at risk for heart disease. Body shape is also an indicator: The "apple" person (who carries weight in her chest and stomach) is more at risk than the "pear" person (who carries weight in her hips). *You may be able to change this risk factor.*

DIABETES (HIGH BLOOD SUGAR) Diabetes makes women particularly vulnerable to heart disease and cancels the protection of estrogen. Diabetes can often be controlled by diet and exercise, so a program for diabetes will be just what you need to reduce your risk of heart disease. *You may be able to change this risk factor.*

Heart palpitations—bumps, pounding, jumps, flutters, racing—can be triggered by stress or too much caffeine. When they accompany hot flashes, they can be scary. Usually, they're nothing to worry about. If your palpitations are severe, painful, or leave you breathless, don't ignore them. Get them checked out by a physician right away. You might be having a heart arrhythmia that has more serious implications.

CIGARETTE SMOKING Smoking contributes to heart disease in a number of ways—by raising blood pressure, constricting arteries, and damaging coronary arteries and lungs. If you smoke, you've raised your risk of heart attack two to six times over that of nonsmokers. *You can change this risk factor.*

CIGARETTE SMOKING AND TAKING ORAL CONTRACEPTIVES Smoking stimulates blood clot formation, and oral contraceptives can do the same thing. Not surprisingly, this combination can be deadly. *You can change this risk factor.*

STRESS The stress response, a physical reaction to a perceived threat, can do real damage to our bodies and is particularly hard on the cardio-vascular system. *You may be able to change this risk factor.*

LACK OF PHYSICAL ACTIVITY Your heart needs exercise to stay healthy. If you're not active, you're more than twice as likely to develop heart disease. *You can change this risk factor.*

What Can I Do to Reduce My Risk Factors?

A lot! For starters, you can quit smoking, drink in moderation (for women in midlife this is one drink a day), and cut down on salt and sodium. You can actually prevent or reverse heart disease by making positive changes in how you eat, how much physical activity you get, and how you handle stress. Making changes in all three areas seems to work better than changing any one of them alone. Midlife is a time of changes you can't control, but it is also a tremendous opportunity to take charge of those parts of your life that you *can* control. We encourage you to embark on your journey with a healthy heart.

How Can I Make Positive Changes in My Diet?

If you feel that you're helping yourself by changing your diet rather than depriving yourself of things you love, you'll have a lot more success. Make changes slowly. Start by cutting down on the high-saturated-fat foods that clog your arteries and eating more plant-based foods that help keep your arteries clear and your blood pressure lower. For example, have a turkey burger or a lean quarter-pound hamburger instead of a half-pounder, and pile on the lettuce, tomatoes, and onions. Here's what you're aiming for:

EAT A LOW-FAT DIET

Most experts agree that a heart-healthy diet is low in artery-clogging fat and cholesterol and high in fiber (which helps remove cholesterol

TRAVEL TIP
Antioxidants Are Your Friends

Free radicals can do a lot of damage to the heart. Antioxidants like vitamin E, vitamin C, and beta-carotene are nutritional scavengers that eat up the free radicals and help achieve overall good health. If you take supplements, a daily dose of 400 International Units of vitamin E and 500 milligrams of vitamin C is currently considered preventive. You can also eat plenty of antioxidant-rich foods: yams, carrots, pumpkins, red and yellow squash, leafy green vegetables, citrus fruits, strawberries, bell peppers, chile peppers, potatoes, nuts, and seeds.

The human heart has long been thought of as the seat of our emotions, and our language reflects this feeling. If you doubt the negative effects of stress on your heart, ask yourself this: Have you ever had your heart broken? Felt heartsick? Had an aching heart (or an achey-breaky heart)? Has your heart dropped to your feet? Has your heart stood still? Relax. Enjoy. Listen to what the song says: Open up your heart and let the sun shine in!

from your blood). What they don't agree on is what they mean by "low." The American Heart Association recommends eating a diet no higher than 30 percent fat; Dr. Dean Ornish, who combines diet, exercise, and relaxation techniques to lower your risk for heart disease, recommends eating a diet no higher than 10 percent fat (a little higher if you don't have heart disease). Some research suggests that diets very low in fats may lower HDL cholesterol and lead to deficiencies in fat-soluble vitamins. Be sensible.

EAT LIGHT PROTEIN   Cutting out fatty meats doesn't mean cutting out protein. Fish, lean meats and poultry, tofu and other soy products, beans and legumes are all delicious and good for you, and they will give you energy.

EAT FOODS HIGH IN FOLIC ACID   According to a study of 5,000 men and women by Canada's health care agency, about 400 micrograms of folic acid per day seems to protect against heart disease. (Stay away from higher doses; too much can cause nerve damage.) You'll find this B vitamin plentiful in dark leafy greens and beans, and it's also being added to some packaged foods.

lipoproteins   Lipoproteins carry cholesterol in the blood. The "good" cholesterol, HDL (high-density lipoproteins), is believed to carry cholesterol out of the arteries to the liver where it is passed from the body. The "bad" cholesterol, LDL (low-density lipoproteins) tends to stay in the body and build up in the artery walls.

INCLUDE OMEGA-3 FATTY ACIDS   These are the good fats. You'll find them in cold-water fish like salmon, halibut, sardines, and mackerel, and in flaxseed oil as well.

EAT FOODS THAT LOVE YOUR HEART   Some foods are especially good for the heart. These include garlic, onion, celery, soy foods, whole grains and legumes, nuts and seeds, leafy greens, fresh fruits and vegetables, and foods high in vitamins E and C.

How Can I Make Positive Changes in My Physical Activity?

If you've been sedentary, any additional exercise will be a spectacular leap: Park your car a little farther away than usual, take the stairs instead of the elevator, rake your own leaves. A moderate and consistent program of exercise—particularly aerobic exercise—is great for your cardiovascular system. Exercise is also advised for most people who have had a heart attack (but check with your doctor before you embark on a program). Physical activity strengthens and improves the health of your heart and lungs in a number of ways, helps lower blood pressure, helps you lose weight (when combined with changes in diet), and makes you feel better. For more on exercise, see Chapter 3, "Keep on Moving."

What Can I Do to Relieve Stress?

The effects of stress can be deadly, but getting rid of stress can be bliss. Mind–body practices like meditation, biofeedback, relaxation response, yoga, and others can help you make an impressive turnaround when it comes to preventing or reversing heart disease. Dr. Dean Ornish is a pioneer in this area. For more on reducing stress, see Chapter 5, "Breathe Easy," and the section on mind–body practices in Chapter 3, "Keep on Moving."

Can Hormone Replacement Therapy Prevent Heart Disease?

For at least half of our lives, women's hearts are protected by estrogen. But after meno-pause this protection ends, and our risk of heart disease jumps. According to results of the PEPI (Postmenopausal Estrogen/Progestin Interventions) Trials, hormone replacement therapy (HRT) increased HDL levels (the "good" cholesterol), lowered LDL levels (the "bad" cholesterol), and lowered fibrinogen, a factor in forming blood clots. More research is currently being done under the Women's Health Initiative, a fourteen-year study, so the answers are not all in. If family health history or other factors put you at particular risk for heart disease, you may want to talk to your doctor about HRT and other preventive measures, such as

POINT OF INTEREST
Heart Tonics

Human beings have been treating heart disease for thousands of years—it's not new to the twentieth century. Seaweeds, popular in Japanese cuisine, help lower cholesterol and blood pressure. Hawthorn (*Crataegus monogyna*) berry and khella are two plant-based remedies that have stood the test of time. According to naturopathic doctor Michael T. Murray, N.D., "Hawthorn berry and flowering tops extracts are widely used by physicians in Europe for their cardiovascular activities," including reducing angina attacks and lowering blood pressure and serum cholesterol levels. Khella (*Ammi visnaga*), says Murray, is an ancient Mediterranean plant that "has been used in the treatment of angina and other heart ailments since the time of the pharaohs."

treating high blood pressure. See Chapter 9, "Yes or No?," for more information.

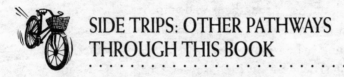

SIDE TRIPS: OTHER PATHWAYS THROUGH THIS BOOK

. . . .

CHAPTER 3: KEEP ON MOVING   Physical activity can help your heart get in shape and keep in shape. Look here to learn about the components of an exercise program you can stick to.

CHAPTER 4: ARE YOU WHAT YOU EAT?   Changes in how you eat can help you lose weight and maintain it and can take stress off your heart. Look here to learn more about the components of a good diet for midlife women.

CHAPTER 5: BREATHE EASY   Taking a load off your mind can take a load off your heart as well. Look here for some ideas on coping with stress.

CHAPTER 7: THE HOLISTIC KIT AND CABOODLE   Lifestyle changes can help you have a healthy heart, and most complementary medicines aim to strengthen the whole mind–body system. Look here to get an overview of what's out there.

CHAPTER 8: WHAT'S UP, DOC?   Is your physician paying attention to the health of your heart? Look here to learn more about working with your doctor for your good health.

CHAPTER 9: YES OR NO?   HRT may offer protection against heart disease. Look here for more on the pros and cons of hormone replacement therapy.

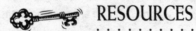

RESOURCES

. . . .

Organizations and Services

American Heart Association, National Center, 7272 Greenville Ave., Dallas, TX 75231-4596. Voice: (800) 242-8721. Internet: www.americanheart.org. The American Heart Association is the first place to begin when you're looking for information about women and heart disease. The organization has many publications, some for women only, such as "The Truth About Women and Heart Disease" and "What Every Woman Should Know About High Blood Pressure."

Coronary Club, The Cleveland Clinic Foundation, 9500 Euclid Ave., Cleveland, OH 44195. Voice: (216) 444-3690. This is a membership organization for people with heart disease. When you join, you get a newsletter with the latest research, treatment, and medications. This nonprofit group is dedicated to using education and understanding to improve the lives of those affected by heart disease.

Mended Hearts, c/o American Heart Association, 7272 Greenville Ave., Dallas, TX 75231. Voice: (214) 706-1442. Call for information about support groups for post–heart attack patients and their families.

Mind–Body Medical Institute, Mercy Hospital and Medical Center, Stevenson Expressway at King Drive, Chicago, IL 60616-2477. Mind–Body offers a cardiac risk-modification program that integrates Western medical practice with behavioral therapy and mind–body techniques in order to reduce blood pressure and cholesterol levels and control diabetes. Call to request a chapter registry listing 250 chapters across the United States.

National Heart, Lung and Blood Institute, National Institutes of Health, P.O. Box 30105, Bethesda, MD 20824-0105. Voice: (301) 251-1222. Internet: www.nhlbi.nih.gov/nhlbi/nhlbi.htm. This government agency has a wealth of educational information on heart disease and high blood pressure, including ways to improve your risk profile. You can also get information about the PEPI Trial, including the effects of HRT on the risk of heart disease.

National Women's Health Network, 514 10th St. N.W., Suite 400, Washington, DC 20004. Voice: (202) 347-1140. Fax: (202) 347-1168. This women's health advocacy and membership organization offers a very informative information packet (available to nonmembers) on heart disease.

National Center for Nutrition and Dietetics of The American Dietetic Association, 216 W. Jackson Blvd., Suite 800, Chicago, IL 60606. Voice: (312) 899-0040. Nutrition Hotline: (800) 366-1655. Customized nutrition information: (900) 225-5267. Internet: www.eatright.org. This association provides consumers with direct and immediate access to reliable food and nutrition information through the Nutrition Hotline, which has recorded food and nutrition messages and can locate registered dietitians in your area. Call the 900 number for customized nutrition information from a registered dietitian.

Dr. Dean Ornish, Preventive Medicine Research Institute, 900 Bridgeway, Suite C, Sausalito, CA 94965. Voice: (800) 775-PMRI. Call for information on residential programs that are aimed at reversing heart disease through low-fat diet, exercise, stress reduction, and psycho-social support. This program emphasizes "comprehensive lifestyle changes."

See Chapter 8, "What's Up, Doc?," for a complete list of organizations that will do research reports on specific health issues, including heart disease.

Hotlines

NHLBI Information Line: (800) 575-WELL. A recorded message about the prevention and control of high blood pressure and high blood cholesterol. Leave your name to receive more information about heart disease along with some heart-healthy recipes.

National Institutes of Health, Women's Health Initiative: (800) 54-WOMEN. A good source of information. Ask about clinical trials.

Periodicals

For general magazines and newsletters about health, see Chapter 7, "The Holistic Kit and Caboodle," and Chapter 8, "What's Up, Doc?" For periodicals about menopause and midlife, see Chapter 2, "Why Is This Happening To Me?" Most health periodicals have published articles on women and heart disease, and you can order back issues.

Cardiac Alert, George Washington University Medical Center, Phillips Publishing Inc., 7811 Montrose Road, Potomac, MD 20854. A newsletter devoted to heart news, education, and prevention.

Diet–Heart Newsletter, P.O. Box 2039, Venice, CA 90294. Published by health book author Robert Kowalski, author of *The 8-Week Cholesterol Cure.* Includes recipes and nutritional information and what's new at the grocery store in low-fat foods.

Harvard Heart Letter, Harvard Medical School Health Publication Group, P.O. Box 420234, Palm Court, FL 32143-0234. This newsletter is devoted to information and research about heart disease and how to have a healthy heart.

Heartline, The Cleveland Clinic Foundation, Coronary Club, Inc., 9500 Euclid Ave., E4-15, Cleveland, OH 44195-5058. (800) 478-4255. This is the Coronary Club's newsletter, written by surgeons, nutritionists, doctors, and scientists.

Books

American Heart Association. *The American Heart Association Cookbook,* 4th rev. ed. New York: David McKay, 1986. This is a good collection of low-fat recipes with an emphasis on getting a wide spectrum of nutrients. A favorite for many who have coped with having heart disease.

Morris Notelovety, M.D., Ph.D., and Diana Tonneson. *The Essential Heart Book for Women.* New York: St. Martin's Press, 1996. Written by a physician with twenty-five years of clinical research in women's health. This book includes special screening for women.

Dean Ornish, M.D. *Eat More, Weigh Less*. New York: Harper Perennial, 1987. Advice on how to cook low-fat meals from the well-known heart doctor. This book includes 250 healthy-heart recipes.

Dean Ornish, M.D. *Programs for Reversing Heart Disease—Stress, Diet, and Your Heart*. New York: Random House, 1990. This book gives you a lifetime program for your heart without drugs or surgery. It addresses stress management, deep relaxation, breathing, stretching, and more.

Helen Cassidy Page, John Speer-Spences, M.D., and Tara Coghlin Dickson, M.S. *The Stanford Life Plan for a Healthy Heart: Introduction to the Standard 25 Gram Plan*. San Francisco: Chronicle Books, 1996. This is a total plan of action, including exercise, relaxation, and eating low-fat foods. You'll find a section on women only, a self-assessment risk test, and even recipes.

Fredric J. Pashkow, M.D., and Charlotte Libov. *The Woman's Heart Book: The Complete Guide to Keeping Our Heart Healthy and What to Do If Things Go Wrong*. New York: Dutton, 1993. This book pays attention to how women can recover from heart disease and addresses the role of stress reduction and exercise for a healthy heart. The authors also offer a lot of medical information, including descriptions of diagnostic tests and possible operations.

Elizabeth Ross, M.D., and Judith Sachs. *Healing the Female Heart*. New York: Pocket Books, 1996. This book discusses medical knowledge of risk factors, tests used to diagnose heart disease, and treatments with holistic guidance—including nutritional supplements and diet that will help you give your heart the best care possible. Written by a woman cardiologist.

Audio/Video

See the catalogs listed in Chapter 8, "What's Up, Doc?," for more companies that carry general health tapes, and Chapter 7, "The Holistic Kit and Caboodle," for companies that carry tapes on complementary medicine. For tapes on exercise, see Chapter 3, "Keep on Moving." For tapes on nutrition, see Chapter 4, "Are You What You Eat?" For tapes on reducing stress, see Chapter 5, "Breathe Easy."

VIDEOTAPES

Heart to Heart: The Truth About Heart Disease. Dr. William Castelli. Available from Video-Finders Collection. Dr. Castelli, director of the Framingham Heart Study, discusses how heart disease affects both men and women. He speaks with compassion and some humor. This video is taped with a live audience.

Online

Don't forget to look at some of the general health sites listed in Chapter 7, "The Holistic Kit and Caboodle," and Chapter 8, "What's Up, Doc?"

MAILING LISTS

The discussion group for people with acquired or congenital heart disease is **percar**. For information, contact gerboni@unich.it.

WEB SITES

The **American Heart Association** site at www.amhrt.org will tell you just about everything you ever wanted to know. Its A-Z guide to heart attack and stroke covers an amazing range of topics, from aspirin and heart attack to women and heart disease. It's a very helpful site. The **Heart Information Network** at www.heartinfo.org is another comprehensive site with a great FAQ, a directory of lipid clinics, and personal stories.

13

WHAT ARE MY CHANCES?
Breast Cancer

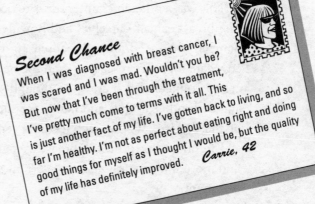

Second Chance

When I was diagnosed with breast cancer, I was scared and I was mad. Wouldn't you be? But now that I've been through the treatment, I've pretty much come to terms with it all. This is just another fact of my life. I've gotten back to living, and so far I'm healthy. I'm not as perfect about eating right and doing good things for myself as I thought I would be, but the quality of my life has definitely improved.   *Carrie, 42*

Our breasts are a topic very close to our hearts—literally and figuratively. At one time or another breasts have been the subject of awe, of worship, of love, of lust, of nourishment. They are symbols of life and regeneration, even as the source of the stars in the Milky Way, yet their image is used to sell everything from magazines to power tools. We spend a good part of our lives complaining that they're too big, too small, too hard, too soft, too pointy, too saggy. Yet we treasure them and, if possible, we want to keep them. When something threatens them, as breast cancer does, we worry.

In 1964 a woman in the United States had a one-in-twenty chance of developing breast cancer in her lifetime. Today, by the time she reaches age eighty-five, her chances are one in eight. At age forty, the odds sound somewhat better—one in twenty-three—but they increase as you get older. Breast cancer is now the leading cause of death for women between forty and forty-five.

These are scary statistics. Is it really as bad as it sounds? Not necessarily—statistics are confusing. Some researchers think breast cancer may only seem to be increasing. In an *Atlantic Monthly* article, Dr. David Plotkin states, "Some of the increase is more apparent than real. Because women today are less likely to die in childbirth or die of infectious disease, they live long enough to develop diseases of middle and old age, breast cancer among them." He cites other factors as well: the increase of women in that age group and early diagnosis due to mammography. Some good news: The National Cancer Institute reports that, overall, the breast cancer rate dropped 5 percent between 1989 and 1993.

This was a difficult chapter to write because we both felt fears of getting breast cancer ourselves and how devastating it might be. We recognized the need for all people to talk about breast cancer and advocate for more research—and the need for women with breast cancer to connect and share their thoughts and feelings with each other and with other friends and family for support and more understanding of the disease. We have collected a lengthy assortment of resources and information regarding breast cancer. Use it as a starting place to find more information and stay current with changes in detection and treatment.

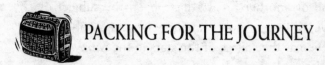

PACKING FOR THE JOURNEY

What Is Breast Cancer?

Breast cancer is an uncontrolled growth of abnormal cells that can result in a number of types of tumors. The most common type is ductal cancer, which begins in the lining of the ducts, small tubes that terminate in the areola. When breast cancer spreads outside the breast (this is called metastatic breast cancer), cancer cells are often found in the lymph nodes under the arm.

GUIDED TOUR: *Breast Cancer*

The incidence of breast cancer may or may not be increasing, but we are increasingly aware of it. Although causes and cures are uncertain at this time, certain lifestyle changes may decrease your risks of getting this disease.

WESTERN MEDICINE

Breast self-exam and mammograms (yearly for women over fifty) can help you detect breast cancer early. Treatment is individual, according to each case. It may include lumpectomy, mastectomy, radiation therapy, chemotherapy, and hormone therapy.

COMPLEMENTARY THERAPIES

Systems such as traditional Chinese medicine, Ayurveda, yoga, and others are useful for balancing the system and for stress reduction; they may improve outcomes when used in conjunction with conventional therapies.

EXERCISE

There is a correlation between aerobic exercise and lowered breast cancer rates in women under forty; research is underway for postmenopausal women.

MIND–BODY

Meditation, visualization, and other techniques are a part of the program at many cancer wellness centers and may help patients do better during treatment and recovery.

NUTRITION

A diet low in saturated fats and high in fiber, cruciferous vegetables, and soybeans shows promise in reducing risk of breast cancer.

SUPPORT

Breast cancer patients who participate in support groups have a higher survival rate; support is also available for partners of women with breast cancer. Cancer retreat centers offer emotional and spiritual support for cancer patients and their family and friends. Internet news groups are another kind of support network for women with breast cancer and their families and partners.

What Is My Risk of Getting Breast Cancer?

These are the general risks associated with 30 percent of breast cancer cases:

- A family history of the disease (your risk is higher if your mother was affected before sixty)
- Menstruation at an early age (before twelve)
- Menopause starting later in life (after fifty-five)
- No children or few children
- First child after thirty
- A high-fat diet
- Obesity, especially if you are predisposed to carry your weight in your tummy
- Some research points to the risk of prolonged use of estrogen replacement therapy after menopause, but the jury is still out on this

What Causes Breast Cancer?

As with many cancers, no one really knows what causes breast cancer. We know the risk factors, but we also know that not every woman who has these risk factors will develop breast cancer. Breast cancer research can be confusing. Different studies come up with opposite results or with different results for different age groups. For example, a recent study found no correlation between low-dose birth control pills and breast cancer for women who are still ovulating, but the results are still inconclusive regarding continued hormone replacement therapy (HRT) for postmenopausal women. Researchers are exploring a number of possible causes, including lifestyle choices (such as a high-fat diet and lack of exercise) and HRT (the jury's still out on that one). Another recent study indicated a correlation between high bone density and increased risk of breast cancer. Other re-

POINT OF INTEREST

Know the Symptoms of Breast Cancer

Early breast cancer does not cause pain, and in many cases there are no symptoms at all. As the cancer grows, it can cause visible changes. See your physician if you notice these or any other changes in your breasts:

- A lump in the breast
- A thickening in or near the breast
- A change in shape or size of the breast
- A discharge from the nipple
- A change in color or feel of the skin of the breast, areola, or nipple, such as dimpling, puckering, or scaliness

searchers are exploring the influence of alcohol consumption on breast cancer rates. Genetic factors and environmental factors are two other important areas of study.

GENETIC FACTORS Scientists believe that a small percentage of women (5 to 10 percent) have an inherited tendency toward breast cancer. Some of these women carry the recently discovered BRCA gene, which causes them to have the highest known risk of any women; other genes may also play a part. Other genetic predispositions to breast cancer are the subjects of ongoing research. It's important to assess breast cancer history as well as ovarian and prostate cancer history on *both* sides of the family—in some cases, your father's family health history is as important as your mother's. If your doctor doesn't ask for this information, bring it up.

ENVIRONMENTAL FACTORS One controversial area of research concerns xenoestrogens (literally, foreign estrogens). These by-products of our industrial civilization include pesticides such as DDT, emissions from burning of fossil fuels, petroleum by-products, and polychlorinated biphenyls (PCBs). Xenoestrogens mimic natural estrogens and attach themselves to our natural estrogen receptor sites. They're strong, have a lengthy half-life, and stay in the body a long time. As a result, our bodies overload on estrogen, which some researchers think could cause breast cancer.

What Are the Chances of Surviving Breast Cancer?

According to the Arizona Cancer Center at the University of Arizona, "More than 90 percent of women whose breast cancer is found

You can gain a measure of control in your treatment if you are as well-informed as possible about your illness. In "What You Need to Know About Breast Cancer," the National Cancer Institute suggests asking your doctor the following questions:

1. What kind of breast cancer do I have? Is it invasive?

2. What stage is my breast cancer?

3. What did the hormone receptor test show? What other lab tests were done on the tumor tissue, and what did they show?

4. How will this information help the doctor decide what type of treatment or further tests to recommend?

and treated early with no spreading beyond the breast will survive." Early detection can be a lifesaver. Socioeconomic factors seem to make race an ingredient in survival. For example, although there are thought to be fewer cases of breast cancer among Hispanic women, they tend to be diagnosed at later stages. And survival rates are also lower for Native American women than for white women. African American women are more than twice as likely as white women to die of breast cancer, in large part because their disease more often reaches an advanced stage before it is diagnosed. According to an article in the *New York Times*, "Black women should see themselves as being at risk for breast cancer, and they should do all that's in their power to reduce their chances of being killed by breast cancer."

How Can I Distinguish a Breast Lump from Lumpy Breasts?

Whether or not you have had lumpy breasts before, in midlife you may find benign lumps; this condition is called fibrocystic breast disease. If you've been performing regular breast exams, you're familiar with how your breasts usually feel. But even if you think it's a benign breast lump, suddenly encountering one can be scary. Play it safe and get it checked out by your doctor. Remember: Eight out of ten breast lumps are *not* cancer.

Here are some things you can do to discourage lumpy breasts:

- Eat a low-fat diet.

- Exercise to bring blood circulation to your breasts (and everywhere else).

- Cut down on caffeine or eliminate it altogether.

- Make sure you're getting enough selenium (it's in whole wheat, brown rice, low-fat dairy products, lean meats, fish, other seafood).

- Take vitamin E supplements.

- Take evening primrose oil supplements.

Is There Any Way to Prevent Breast Cancer?

Although the cause, cure, and prevention of breast cancer remains unknown, health care practitioners, scientists, and breast cancer activists have recommended some steps that may reduce your risk of getting breast cancer.

BREAST SELF-EXAMINATION   It's hard *not* to find information about breast self-exams. They're illustrated in many books, in videos, and in brochures available at screening centers and medical offices. Nonetheless, many women manage to avoid examining their breasts regularly. If you do a breast self-exam faithfully, once a month, you may catch a tumor before it has a chance to do you harm.

FOLLOW AN ANTICANCER DIET   The American Cancer Society recommends eating cruciferous vegetables, like broccoli and cabbage, and foods high in beta-carotene, like carrots and yams. High fiber intake is associated with lower risk of breast cancer, as is a low intake of saturated fat. Soy products also appear to have anticarcinogenic effects.

EXERCISE   Three to four hours of aerobic exercise a week may reduce the risk of breast cancer in premenopausal women, and research is being done to study the effects of exercise in reducing the risk of breast cancer in postmenopausal women. Just do it—it can't hurt!

REDUCE YOUR INTAKE OF ALCOHOL   Alcohol has been shown to elevate estrogen levels, which can increase cell multiplication and therefore the risk of cancer. If you're taking hormone replacement therapy and drinking beer, wine, or liquor, check with your doctor.

MAMMOGRAMS   Discuss your need for a mammogram with your physician. Currently, the American Cancer Society advises women aged forty and over who have no personal risk

Love 'Em/Hate 'Em

It's time for my annual mammogram—I'm over fifty, and I have to endure this torture annually. It brings up very ambivalent feelings about my breasts. On the one hand, they make me feel feminine and attractive. On the other hand, they represent the possibility that I could have a life-threatening disease. Even though I know I should do the breast self-exam every month, sometimes I don't, because I just don't want to deal with what could happen. I don't remember having these feelings ten years ago.   *Tina, 51*

**Questions to Ask Your Doctor
Before Treatment Begins**

In "What You Need to Know About Breast Cancer," the National Cancer Institute suggests asking these questions:

1. What are my treatment choices? Which do you recommend for me? Why?

2. What benefits can I expect from each kind of treatment?

3. What are the risks and possible side effects of each treatment?

4. Would a clinical trial be appropriate for me?

or family history of breast cancer to have mammograms every year.

What Foods May Help Prevent Breast Cancer?

Some foods, particularly fruits and vegetables, seem to have anticancer properties. *Soy foods* may help to reduce the risk of breast cancer. Soybeans are rich in anticarcinogens, such as isoflavones. One of these, genistein, is a weak estrogen look-alike that can plug into estrogen receptor sites and prevent estrogen overload. Genistein may also prevent small blood vessels from forming around the cancer cells, cutting off oxygen and nutrients. Some *crucifers,* such as broccoli and cabbage, contain a treasure trove of cancer-fighting substances. Some boost the production of enzymes that defuse carcinogens and flush them out of the body. Others, called indoles, affect the metabolism of estrogen, prompting the body to make benign forms of the hormone that don't promote breast cancer.

What Is the Treatment for Breast Cancer?

No single type of treatment fits every woman. Age, menopausal status (cancers seem to be faster-growing in premenopausal women), type of breast cancer, the stage, additional laboratory test results (especially those that indicate if the tumor is estrogen-receptive or not), and its degree of invasiveness all help determine the treatment. Treatment for breast cancer doesn't have to start right away. According to *Understanding Breast Cancer,* women have at least six weeks to learn about and choose their treatment options.

LUMPECTOMY   Removal of just the breast lump and a margin of normal tissue around it.

PARTIAL MASTECTOMY   Removal of the tumor and some normal breast tissue around it and the lining over the chest muscles below the tumor.

TOTAL MASTECTOMY   Removal of the entire breast.

RADICAL MASTECTOMY Removal of the entire breast, nearby lymph nodes, and underlying chest muscles. This was the standard for years, but it is less common now.

RADIATION THERAPY The use of high-energy rays to damage cancer cells and stop them from growing. This can be done by external radiation or by radioactive materials placed directly in the breast.

CHEMOTHERAPY The use of drugs to kill cancer cells. It's given either orally or by injection. This is a systemic therapy because the drugs travel throughout the body.

HORMONE THERAPY A treatment to keep the cancer cells from getting the hormones they need to grow. There are two treatment choices: taking a drug, such as tamoxifen, or removing the ovaries, which make hormones.

What Does Complementary Medicine Offer for Breast Cancer?

Harvard Women's Health Watch recommends that complementary therapies—such as massage therapy, acupuncture and traditional Chinese medicine, yoga, meditation, and many other techniques—be used as supplements to conventional treatments, not as substitutes. If you do need to endure the rigors of Western treatment, these can nurture you, soothe you, relieve stress and symptoms, and help you remember that you are a whole human being, not just a "cancer patient."

Can I Combine Complementary and Conventional Treatments?

More and more, doctors are taking an integral approach to cancer treatment. For example, in *Spontaneous Healing*, Dr. Andrew Weil suggests taking astragulus root (a popular herb in traditional Chinese medicine) to strengthen the

TRAVEL TIP
Support for Partners of
Women with Breast Cancer

Partners of women dealing with breast cancer often get lost in the shuffle. Y-ME remedies this with a hotline specifically for partners of women with breast cancer. Callers will be matched with trained peer counselors and with someone whose partner is a survivor. Also available from Y-ME is the brochure, *When the Woman You Love Has Breast Cancer*. See Resources.

POINT OF INTEREST
Tamoxifen

Tamoxifen is often prescribed for women with breast cancer. It's a systemic therapy, with side effects that include irregular periods, aggravated hot flashes, and an increase in uterine cancer. Nonetheless, according to Scandinavian studies and the NCI, the benefit of taking tamoxifen outweighs the risk of getting endometrial cancer because the recurrence rate drops by one-third. Research is continuing in this area, so stay informed!

Survivors in Search of a Voice

If you have access to the Internet, you can view this lovely and moving collection of artwork, photographs, and essays by 100 artists who are also breast cancer survivors. Canadians Barbra Amesbury and Joan Chalmers put this project together in 1995, to "give voice to the thousands of women suffering with this disease." Look for it at aorta.library.mun.ca/bc.

immune system during conventional treatment. According to *Center News*, the newsletter of the Women's Cancer Resource Center, Keith Block, M.D., makes an individualized treatment plan for each patient. He urges his patients to take charge of their treatment and pursue alternatives such as attitudinal changes, nutrition (a diet of 15 percent to 18 percent fat, mostly grains, fruits, and vegetables), supplements (omega-3 fatty acids, antioxidants), exercise and massage, and biofeedback and meditation. He uses surgery, radiation, and chemotherapy only if the patient "chooses to do so if non-invasive therapies fail." Block's advice to women with breast cancer shines like a light in the wilderness: "Maintain hope, a life-affirming attitude. Your attitude can beneficially impact your immune system. What you eat and how you think communicates with your cells."

I Don't Want to Go Through Breast Cancer Treatment Alone. How Can I Find Support?

Being diagnosed with breast cancer can be particularly frightening because it touches women on so many levels: fear of dying, fear of losing our femininity, fear of losing our partners. This is a time when we really need support. In fact, studies done at Stanford University indicate that breast cancer patients who were in support groups while undergoing therapy actually lived longer than those who received medical treatment alone. To find an ongoing group, check with your hospital or local women's center. See Resources for more.

> At first [after my breasts were removed] it was difficult to look in the mirror at myself because I looked like a little girl who had never developed. Someone once said, "You don't even have the raisins on a breadboard." After nine years I've learned to live with it. I still have a hard time going to public swimming pools and dressing in front of other people. I am conscious of the fact that I don't have breasts and maybe, as a caretaker, I'm more concerned about upsetting the other person than about myself.
>
> BARBARA EDDY, from *On Women Turning Fifty*

What Are Cancer Retreat Centers?

A growing number of cancer patients find support in retreats and centers specially dedicated to people who are living with cancer. These centers, which promote spiritual as well as physical healing, offer a variety of services: professional and peer support and counseling, information about treatment choices, deep relaxation techniques, massage, complementary therapies, and more. Many encourage the involvement of friends and family. See Resources for more information.

SIDE TRIPS: OTHER PATHWAYS THROUGH THIS BOOK

CHAPTER 3: KEEP ON MOVING   Regular aerobic exercise is associated with lowered risk of breast cancer. Look here to learn more about your exercise choices.

CHAPTER 4: ARE YOU WHAT YOU EAT?   A good diet may be instrumental in lowering your risk of breast cancer and fortifying your body to withstand treatment. Look here for more information.

CHAPTER 5: BREATHE EASY   Stress reduction can help you support your immune system. Look here for ideas on how to relax.

CHAPTER 7: THE HOLISTIC KIT AND CABOODLE   More and more conventional medical practitioners are adopting an integral approach to treatment. Look here for an overview of the world of complementary medicine.

CHAPTER 8: WHAT'S UP, DOC?   If you are diagnosed with breast cancer, you will be spending a lot of time with health practitioners. Look here for suggestions on how to work with your doctor.

CHAPTER 16: GETTING HELP   Emotional support is a necessary part of any cancer treatment. Look here for ideas on how to get the help you need.

CHAPTER 17: THE INNER JOURNEY   Confronting life-and-death issues often brings us face to face with our spiritual nature. Look here for discussion of dimensions beyond the physical.

RESURCES

RESOURCES

Organizations and Services

American Cancer Society, 1599 Clifton Road N.E., Atlanta, GA 30329-4251. Voice: (800) ACS-2345. Internet: www.cancer.org. Provides information and educational programs such as Reach to Recovery, an assistance program for women with breast cancer, and Look Good Feel Better, which helps those going through cancer treatment improve their appearance. Voice: (800) 395-LOOK

ENCORE *plus*, YWCA of the U.S.A., Office of Women's Health Initiatives, 624 9th St. N.W., 3rd Floor, Washington, DC 20001. Voice: (202) 628-3636. Fax: (202) 783-7123. E-mail: hn2205@handsnet.org. ENCORE *plus* provides breast and cervical cancer early detection education and screening services to medically underserved women—particularly those over the age of fifty, those who are minorities, and those with limited income. In addition, support and exercise programs are offered to all postdiagnostic women. Call the YWCA of the U.S.A or your local YWCA for more information.

Foundation for Alternative Cancer Therapies, Old Chelsea Station, P.O. Box 1242, New York, NY 10113. Voice: (212) 741-2790. This is a referral agency and educational group with information on alternative treatment options for cancer patients. It has a newsletter, *Cancer Forum.*

The Komen Alliance, Susan G. Komen Foundation, Occidental Tower, 5005 LBJ Freeway, Suite 370, Dallas, TX 75244. Voice: (972) 233-0351. Fax: (972) 385-5005. This is a comprehensive program for research, education, diagnosis, and treatment of breast disease. The alliance provides information on screening, BSE, treatment and support, including the booklet "Caring for Your Breasts."

Krames Communications. Voice: (800) 333-3032. Internet: www.krames.com. This company publishes patient information in the form of illustrated, easy-to-understand, and very informative booklets. An extensive list of publications about breast health, including breast lumps and mammography, is available. Call for titles.

The Mautner Project, 1707 L St. N.W., Suite 1060, Washington, DC 20036. Voice: (202) 332-5536. This group provides support to lesbian cancer patients and their partners and caregivers. It also provides educational information at no cost.

National Alliance of Breast Cancer Organizations (NABCO), 9 E. 37th St., 10th Floor, New York, NY 10016. Voice: (800) 719-9154 or (212) 719-0154. Fax: (212) 689-1213. E-mail: NABCOinfo@aol.com. Internet: www.nabco.org. This breast cancer information network of more than 370 organizations provides information on detection, treatment, and care to hundreds of thousands of American women. Ask about resource lists, the newsletter, and other information.

National Black Women's Health Project, 1211 Connecticut Ave. N.W., Suite 310, Washington, DC 20036. Voice: (202) 835-0117. Fax (202) 833-8790. E-mail:

nbwhpdc@aol.com. This organization offers public information, education, and policy regarding African American women's health issues, including printed material about breast cancer.

National Breast Cancer Coalition, 1707 L St. N.W., Suite 1060, Washington, DC 20036. Voice: (202) 296-7477. Fax: (202) 265-6854. Internet: www.natlbcc.org. Founded in 1991, this organization describes itself as a "grassroots effort in the fight against breast cancer." With 350 member organizations nationwide and thousands of members, the coalition has helped bring about changes in funding for breast cancer research and more. Contact the group for information.

National Cancer Institute Cancer Information Service, 9000 Rockville Pike, Bethesda, MD 20892. Voice: (800) 422-6237. Fax: (301) 402-5874. This service will provide free, up-to-date written material on current research questions and answer sheets on tamoxifen and genetic studies. Request "What You Need to Know About Breast Cancer," Publication No. 93-1556. You can also ask to talk to a cancer specialist.

National Women's Health Network, 514 10th St. N.W., Washington, DC 20004. Voice: (202) 347-1140. Information clearinghouse: (202) 628-7814. This network offers publications on a wide variety of women's health topics, including breast cancer.

Strang Cancer Prevention Center, 428 E. 72nd St., New York, NY 10021. Voice: (212) 794-4900. National High-Risk Registry: (800) 521-9356. This is a free national resource for breast cancer risk counseling and research into breast cancer risk. Strang operates a National High-Risk Registry for breast and ovarian cancer and also publishes a newsletter.

University of California at Los Angeles, The Revlon–UCLA Breast Center, 200 Medical Plaza, Surgery Suite 530, Los Angeles, CA 90095. Voice: (800) 825-2144. This research and teaching medical center is a place to go for risk evaluation, breast cancer diagnosis, or a second opinion as well as treatment. It draws people from all over the world.

Y-ME National Breast Cancer Organization, 212 W. Van Buren St., Chicago, IL 60607-3908. Voice: (800) 221-2141. Latina hotline: (800) 986-9505. Fax: (312) 294-8597. E-mail: michyme@aol.com. Internet: www.yme.org. Y-ME is a gold mine. This not-for-profit organization provides information, hotline counseling, educational programs, self-help meetings, and a resource library. The hotline is staffed with trained peer counselors who are survivors of breast cancer. The group publishes informative booklets for single women with breast cancer and for partners of women with breast cancer. Membership includes a bimonthly newsletter, *Y-ME Hotline*, with up-to-date information and resources.

CANCER RETREAT/SUPPORT CENTERS

These educational centers (they are not treatment programs) support an integral approach to healing that combines physical, emotional, and spiritual techniques.

Commonweal Cancer Help Program, P.O. Box 316, Bolinas, CA 94924. Voice: (415) 868-0970. Fax: (415) 868-2230. This is the program on which all the others are based. Begun a decade ago by Michael Lerner, author of *Choices in Healing*, Commonweal was featured in the PBS documentary "Wounded Healers." Ongoing programs allow cancer patients and their family and friends to explore physical, emotional, and spiritual healing. Vegetarian diet, massage, art, poetry, and dreams are explored, as are choices in conventional and complementary therapy. This popular center usually has a waiting list.

Okamana Kaho'ola, P.O. Box 1236, Kamuela, HI 96743. Voice: (808) 885-0995 or (808) 885-7547. Fax: (808) 885-4998. Modeled on the Commonweal program, this seven-day residential retreat includes yoga, support groups, Ayurveda, vegetarian diet, Chinese medicine, and more. This is an educational program, not a treatment program. Located on the Kona coast of the big island of Hawaii.

Smith Farm Cancer Help Program, 1501 32nd St. N.W., Washington, DC 20007. Voice: (202) 338-2330. Fax: (202) 338-2333. Smith Farm offers weeklong retreats in Potomac, Maryland. Sessions are closely based on the Cancer Help Program at Commonweal.

Wellspring Cancer Help Program, P.O. Box 317, Lyme, NH 03768. Voice: (603) 795-2144. Wellspring's five-day residential retreats are modeled directly on the Commonweal program. It also offers women-only retreats. Call or write to request the free newsletter, which gives dates, information, and the latest news.

The Wellness Community, 2716 Ocean Park Blvd., Santa Monica, CA 90405-5207. Voice: (310) 314-2555. The Wellness Community provides free psycho-social support as an adjunct to conventional medical treatment for people and families fighting cancer. The Community has sixteen treatment facilities nationwide, aimed at enhancing the quality of life and the possibility of recovery. The program is free; the organization also sponsors lectures and offers participant groups and networking breast cancer groups.

RESEARCH REPORTS

Keep up to date on breast cancer research by sending for the latest research reports. See the listings in Chapter 8, "What's Up, Doc?," for resources.

Hotlines

American Cancer Society, Cancer Response System: (800) ACS-2345. Call with questions about breast cancer.

American Hair Loss Council: (800) 274-8717.

Breast Cancer Prevention Trial: (800) 4-CANCER to find out about this clinical trial.

Chemocare: (800) 55-CHEMO. This national agency pairs cancer patients with a volunteer who had a similar diagnosis. The volunteer writes or visits to offer emotional support. This is a free service and confidential.

FDA (Food and Drug Administration) Breast Implant Information Line: (800) 532-4440. Call with questions about breast implants.

Komen Alliance: (800) IM-AWARE. Call with questions about breast cancer or to request free literature.

National Cancer Institute, Cancer Information Service: (800) 4-CANCER. CIS information specialists have extensive training in providing up-to-date and understandable information about cancer and cancer research and will provide information about cancer-related services and resources in your area. English and Spanish.

National High-Risk Registry: (800) 521-9356. Call if you have a family history of breast cancer.

Nolvadex (Tamoxifen) Patient Assistance Program: (800) 424-3727. Call for information about tamoxifen.

Reconstruction Counseling: (800) EIN-STEIN (only available in the Pennsylvania area) or (215) 456-7383. A support program staffed by trained volunteers who have had post-mastectomy reconstruction. Part of the Einstein Medical Center's Breast Cancer Program in Philadelphia.

Y-ME 24-Hour Hotline: (800) 221-2141. Staff and volunteers who have had breast cancer provide information, support, and access to thousands of resources. Male volunteers are also available for male partners.

Y-ME Latina Hotline: (800) 986-9505. Special hotline for Spanish-speaking callers.

Products and Catalogs

Feminine Image. Voice: (800) 730-1123. This catalog features a wide variety of clothing designed especially for women who have undergone a mastectomy.

TLC, Hanover, PA 17333-0080. Voice: (800) 850-9445. TLC has a collection of difficult-to-find products, such as scarves and hats to hide hair loss as well as bras that disguise breast surgery. The catalog has articles about surgery, sex after cancer, and support; it also offers tips on how to feel better about yourself.

Periodicals

Look at the listings in Chapter 7, "The Holistic Kit and Caboodle," and Chapter 8, "What's Up, Doc?," for publications that address complementary and traditional medical approaches.

The Newsletter of the Strang Cancer Genetics Program, Strang Cancer Prevention Center, 428 E. 72 St., New York, NY 10021. (212) 794-4900. This free newsletter has up-to-the-minute news about breast cancer and genetics, useful information, and lots of support.

NABCO News, National Alliance of Breast Cancer Organizations, 9 E. 37th St., 10th Floor, New York, NY 10016. Voice: (800) 719-9154 or (212) 719-0154. Fax: (212) 689-1213. E-mail: NABCOinfo@aol.com. Internet: www.nabco.org. This quarterly newsletter for NABCO members publishes material concerning the latest developments in medicine, science, services, and policy, including risk factors, early detection, and treatment options.

Y-ME Hotline, Y-ME National Breast Cancer Organization, 212 W. Van Buren St., Chicago, IL 60607-3908. Voice: (800) 221-2141. This bimonthly newsletter for Y-ME members keeps readers up to date with articles by experts in the field of breast cancer. If you have Internet access, you can check out back issues at the Y-ME web site.

Books

American Cancer Society. *Questions and Answers About Pain Control: A Guide for People with Cancer and Their Families (45180-PS)*. This publication, developed by Yale Comprehensive Cancer Center and National Cancer Institute, discusses pain control using both medical and nonmedical means. The emphasis is on explanation, self-help, and patient participation. To purchase, call (800) ACS-2345.

Sharon Batt. *Patient No More: The Politics of Breast Cancer*. Milford, CT: L.P.C./InBook, 1994. A look at the reality of breast cancer and how it is replaced by unrealistically optimistic assessments of various treatments. The book also addresses how little understanding and treatment of breast cancer have changed over the years. An exposé as well as an invitation for women to get more involved in the politics of breast cancer.

Harold H. Benjamin, Ph.D. *The Wellness Community: A Guide to Fighting for Recovery from Cancer*. New York: Putnam Books, 1987. This book explores strategies cancer patients can use to strengthen the immune system, including visualization, nutrition, exercise, and enhanced personal relationships.

Elizabeth Berg. *Talk Before Sleep*. A novel about women who face the crisis of breast cancer and how that redefines the meaning of friendship and unconditional love.

Breast Cancer Action Group and Women's Caucus for Art. *Healing Legacies*. P.O. Box 5605, Burlington, VT 95402. Voice: (802) 863-3507. Fax: (802) 863-3140. This is a collection of art and writing for and by women with breast cancer. National exhibitions are curated from a slide registry. The collection is open and ongoing.

Nancy Bruning. *Coping with Chemotherapy*. A matter-of-fact, objective, and comprehensive overview of medical, physical, and emotional aspects of chemotherapy treatment. Contains a list of standard drugs and their side effects and a glossary of terms.

Linda Dackman. *Affirmations, Meditations, and Encouragements for Women Living with Breast Cancer*. San Francisco: HarperSanFrancisco, 1992. Quotes and recollections offer insight into what women with breast cancer feel but don't always reveal.

Lisa De Angelis and Molly Siple. *Recipes for Change*. New York: Penguin, 1996. This recipe book addresses the nutritional needs of midlife women and includes a section on breast cancer.

Ronnie Kaye. *Spinning Straw into Gold: Your Emotional Recovery from Breast Cancer.* New York: Simon and Schuster, 1991. This book offers personal tools to deal with the impact of breast cancer.

Michael Lerner, Ph.D. *Choices in Healing: Integrating the Best of Conventional and Complementary Approaches.* Cambridge: MIT Press, 1994. This book covers choices in healing from serious illness, including mainstream and complementary therapies, pain control, and dying with dignity. Lerner founded Commonweal, the first cancer retreat center.

Susan M. Love, M.D., with Karen Lindsey. *Dr. Susan Love's Breast Book.* Rev. ed. Reading, MA: Addison-Wesley, 1995. A very important book! Comprehensive information on the breast, its health and disease states. Lots of resources, including a state-by-state list of breast clinics and physicians.

Jon J. Michnovicz, M.D., Ph.D. *How to Reduce Your Risk of Breast Cancer.* New York: Warner Books, 1996. This book looks at prevention through nutrition, with a good section on phytochemicals. Includes recipes.

Ralph Moss, Ph.D. *Cancer Therapy: The Independent Consumer Guide to Non-Toxic Treatment and Prevention.* New York: Equinox Press, 1992. Discusses nontoxic or less toxic modes of cancer prevention and treatment. Documentation of the effectiveness, safety, and disadvantages of the methods.

Marilyn Yalom. *A History of the Breast.* New York: Knopf, 1997. Yalom, a scholar, explores changing ideas about women's breasts in all their glory: sacred, erotic, commercialized, domestic, political, medicalized, and more. Illustrated with paintings, photos, and even advertising, this book is fun to read as well as enlightening.

Books and Pamphlets from Agencies

National Association of Breast Cancer Organizations (NABCO). *Breast Cancer Resource List.* A list of resources for breast cancer services, including books, treatment choices, research, organizations, and more. To purchase the latest edition, contact NABCO, 9 East 37th St., 10th Floor, New York, NY 90016. Voice: (212) 889-0606. Fax: (212) 689-1213.

National Cancer Institute. *After Breast Cancer: A Guide to Follow-up Care.* Phone: (800) 4-CANCER. For the woman who has completed treatment. Explains the importance of continuing BSE, regular physical exams, possible signs of recurrence, and managing the physical and emotional side effects of having had breast cancer.

National Cancer Institute. *Clinical Practice Guidelines, Cancer Pain Guidelines.* Voice: (800) 422-6237. This is a critical synthesis of research and knowledge in the field designed to help any clinician work with cancer patients.

National Women's Health Network. *Breast Cancer: Environmental Causes.* Contact the National Women's Health Network, 14 10th St. N.W., Suite 400, Washington, DC 20004. Voice: (202) 628-7814. This impressive compilation of articles and resources is a good place to start for anyone who wants to know more about this issue.

U.S. Government Printing Office. *Unconventional Cancer Treatments.* Both a summary and full report of a four-year study of unconventional cancer treatments by the

Congressional Office of Technology Assessment. Examines many of the better-known and most controversial therapies and diet regimens. Contact the U.S. Government Printing Office, Washington, DC, 20402-9325. Voice: (202) 783-3238.

Y-ME. *For Single Women with Breast Cancer.* A forty-page booklet offering practical guidance and support for coping with breast cancer based on testimonies and advice from single women who have experienced breast cancer. Contact Y-ME, Box SB, 212 W. Van Buren, 4th Floor, Chicago, IL 60607.

Audio/Video

See the catalogs listed in Chapter 8, "What's Up, Doc?," for more companies that carry general health tapes, and Chapter 7, "The Holistic Kit and Caboodle," for companies that carry tapes on complementary medicine.

AUDIO

Creating Breast Health. Christiane Northrup, M.D. Available from Sounds True (see Audio/Video, Chapter 7). This audiocassette includes facts and skills you need to reclaim control of your breast health. It touches on healthful eating, family history, and self-exams.

VIDEOTAPES

A Sense of Balance: Breast Reconstruction. John B. Goodale. 30 minutes. Available from Fanlight (see Audio/Video, Chapter 8). An overview of what's involved in breast reconstruction and alternatives to breast implants. It includes a study guide.

Beyond the Loss of the Breast. Sherry Thomas-Zon. 25 minutes. Available from Fanlight (see Audio/Video, Chapter 8). This video looks at the value of poetry and art as self-expression for women with breast cancer. Two women living with breast cancer, and the filmmaker, whose mother died of the disease, speak about their experiences and share their poems and creations.

The Breast Center Video. Available from The Learning Lane (see Audio/Video, Chapter 8). Breast cancer does not necessarily mean death or even the loss of a breast. This video dispels the many myths about breast cancer and contains up-to-date information on low-dose mammography, step-by-step self-examination, nutrition, treatment options, and reconstruction.

Women's Health Series—Breast Cancer: Replacing Fear with Facts. 37 minutes. Available from The Learning Lane (see Audio/Video, Chapter 8). The risks of breast cancer and the proper method of breast self-examination.

Online

The number of breast cancer resources on the Internet is staggering. The easiest way to find new sites is to access the home page of one of the major organizations listed here and look for recommended links. You can also find links in some search engines under the subdirectory *health* or *women's health;* **PowerSurge** (members.aol.com/dearest) and **Women's Wire** (www.women.org) keep up to date with the latest news.

NEWS GROUPS

Breast cancer postings are welcome at **alt.support.cancer** and **sci.med.diseases. cancer,** both ongoing discussions about all kinds of cancer. Many people write with questions regarding their own breast cancer or treatment for a friend or loved one, or to discuss the latest buzz on treatment and alternate therapies.

MAILING LISTS

Medinfo calls itself "the central location of all the cancer discussion list archives." To get on the **Breast Cancer Listserv,** access the Medinfo web site at www.medinfo. org/lists/cancer/bc-about/html.

WEB SITES

Most of the major breast cancer organizations have excellent web sites (see Organizations, above, for locations). If you have access to the Internet, you can get most information immediately instead of waiting for your mail to be delivered. Sites worth a visit include the **Breast Cancer Information Clearinghouse** at nysernet.org/breast/default.html, **National Alliance of Breast Cancer Organizations, National Breast Cancer Coalition,** and **Y-ME.** The National Cancer Institute's **CancerNet** site, at wwwicic.nci.nih. gov, has all sorts of information and will tell you how to receive a PDQ statement on breast cancer via e-mail.

Breast Care Online, at breast-care.louisville.edu/breast-care, includes excellent breast cancer information and links, but with a new twist: The people who put together this site are also attempting to make it user-responsive by constantly collating and updating women's online questions and concerns. This site tries hard to make users feel like individuals rather than patients.

Edu Care Inc.'s Breast Health and Breast Cancer Network, at www.cancerhelp. com, is a very warm site that answers a wide range of questions asked by patients and their partners. Resources include a woman's guide to breast health services, breast cancer support groups, and networking opportunities.

For comprehensive links to anything from medical journals to alternative treatments, check out **Oncolink,** cancer.med.upenn.edu, a major cancer site from the University of Pennsylvania with many breast cancer resources. **Medinfo** at www.medinfo. org, has a searchable breast-cancer list archive of online support groups and more.

14

IS THIS REALLY NECESSARY?

Hysterectomy

Hysterectomy is one of the surgeries most often performed on women in the United States—and one of the most controversial. Opinion on hysterectomy swings back and forth, like a pendulum. In our mothers' day, when fewer people saw the need to have a uterus after the childbearing years were over, hysterectomies were performed almost routinely, many unnecessarily, and for all sorts of reasons. Today's women have learned to speak up and are not as willing to go quietly to the surgeon's table: We want to keep our body parts, whenever possible!

Our general wariness of the need for hysterectomy is not unfounded. The *Harvard Women's Health Watch* says, "There is evidence that an estimated 15 percent of hysterectomies are performed for conditions for which removing the uterus has no clear benefit and another 25 percent for reasons that are considered questionable." Nonetheless, for many women, hysterectomy is the right choice. It may save your life or vastly improve the quality of your life. When you're making a decision about hysterectomy, consider your own situation and your own feelings. Make a decision based on your own health and emotional needs, not on political correctness or the opinions of those closest to you. Learn as much as you can, work closely with your doctor, and *always* consider getting a second opinion.

 ## PACKING FOR THE JOURNEY

What Is a Hysterectomy?

Did she have a hysterectomy, or didn't she? Only her doctor knows for sure! In common usage, hysterectomy may mean removal of the uterus, the uterus and ovaries, the uterus above the cervix . . . you can see where this is going. Much of the confusion about hysterectomy stems from the fact that in common usage, a number of surgeries are often lumped together under the same term. In all cases, hysterectomy implies surgery: Something will be removed. If your doctor suggests a hysterectomy, make sure you know what kind of surgery you're in for. See the definitions on the next page to clear up any doubt.

> Hysteria was given its present meaning by Renaissance doctors who explained women's diseases with a theory that the womb sometimes became detached from its place and wandered about inside the body, causing uncontrolled behavior.
> —BARBARA G. WALKER, *The Women's Encyclopedia of Myths and Secrets*

When Should a Hysterectomy Be Considered?

In the case of certain cancers, hysterectomy can save your life. When your life is not threatened, but you've reached the limits of your tolerance for pain and discomfort (from excessive menstrual bleeding, rapidly growing fibroids, endometriosis, and genital prolapse, for example), your doctor may also recommend hysterectomy. Get a second opinion, and be sure you have explored all of the alternatives before you commit to surgery.

How Is a Hysterectomy Performed?

How your hysterectomy is performed will depend on a number of factors that your doctor will have to determine. Some hysterectomies can be performed vaginally, requiring no abdominal incision, but most do involve an abdominal incision. Some hysterectomies are done with a combined abdominal/vaginal approach. All are major surgeries that require a recovery period—shorter in the case of the vaginal technique, longer for the abdominal surgery.

What Are the Possible Side Effects?

If you do need a hysterectomy, it's important to understand the possible side effects of the surgery beforehand. Knowing ahead of time what may happen can make it easier to deal with side effects if and when they occur. It's also important to be emotionally *ready* to have a hysterectomy. Some women attribute symptoms such as bone and joint pain, insomnia, memory loss, and loss of libido to hysterectomy, but it is more likely that these are at least in part a response to distress surrounding the issue of surgery.

subtotal hysterectomy Surgical removal of the uterus only, above the cervix.

total hysterectomy Removal of the cervix and uterus only.

total hysterectomy with a bilateral salpingo-oophorectomy Removal of uterus, cervix, both ovaries, and fallopian tubes.

subtotal hysterectomy with a bilateral salpingo-oophorectomy Removal of the uterus above the cervix, both ovaries, and fallopian tubes.

SURGICAL RISK The risks and complications of hysterectomy are those of other surgeries, including infection, bleeding, blood clots, and side effects from anesthesia.

SEXUAL PLEASURE Some women who have had both uterus and cervix removed, and who have obtained pleasure in the past from uterine contractions or pressure against the cervix, report missing these sensations.

GUIDED TOUR: *Hysterectomy*

Hysterectomy may be your only choice if your life is threatened by cancer or if pain and bleeding from other causes has destroyed your quality of life. With less serious uterine problems, there are a number of alternatives to try first. In the case of fibroids and endometriosis, the decline of estrogen after menopause will probably make the problem disappear.

WESTERN MEDICINE

For uterine prolapse: Alternatives to hysterectomy include pessary, electric stimulation of the pelvic floor, surgery to strengthen uterine ligaments. *For fibroids:* Alternatives to hysterectomy include hormone treatment, myomectomy. *For endometriosis:* Alternatives to hysterectomy include hormone treatment, pelviscopic surgery.

COMPLEMENTARY THERAPIES

For fibroids and endometriosis: Acupuncture, acupressure, homeopathy, and botanical remedies may be effective in controlling symptoms.

EXERCISE

For uterine prolapse: Kegel exercises done regularly can help strengthen the pelvic floor. Sometimes fibroid or endometriosis pain is the overriding reason for hysterectomy. A regular program of exercise may help you alleviate chronic pain, preventing the need for surgery.

MIND–BODY

For fibroids and endometriosis: Massage, t'ai chi, visualization, reiki, and other techniques may be effective in controlling symptoms.

Yoga, qi gong, t'ai chi, Rosen work, and other techniques, combined with meditation, can be effective in calming the system and helping you cope with pain that is not life-threatening.

- In 1991, 546,000 hysterectomies and 458,000 oophorectomies were performed on women in the United States.

- The most common reasons for hysterectomy: fibroids, endometriosis, excessive bleeding, uterine prolapse, pelvic inflammatory disease, complications of childbirth, cancer.

- Average age at which women have a hysterectomy: 42.7.

- According to the *Harvard Women's Health Watch,* "It is one of the most common surgical procedures performed on women; as many as one-third of us may have a hysterectomy before we reach sixty-five."

HEALING After surgery, your body will need time to heal itself. You may feel tired and in pain for longer than you want to. Complete recuperation can take anywhere from a few weeks to a number of months.

HORMONE REPLACEMENT Removal of your ovaries means that you will experience an immediate withdrawal of reproductive hormones. You will most likely be started on hormone replacement therapy immediately, to avoid experienc-ing hot flashes, vaginal dryness, and other effects.

How Can I Be Sure I Need a Hysterectomy?

As with all recommendations for surgery, don't be afraid to get a second or even third opinion. Discuss the alternatives with your physician. The more emotionally ready you are for surgery, the better chance you have of a speedy recovery.

What Are the Alternatives to Hysterectomy?

Alternatives depend on the presenting problem—the most common non-life-threatening reasons for hysterectomy are uterine prolapse, pain and bleeding due to fibroids, and endometriosis. Depending on the severity of the problem, you may have a number of options. See the individual discussion of each of these issues for specific suggestions.

Buying Time

When I was perimenopausal, I was troubled with excessive bleeding due to fibroids. I decided I would enlist all my will-power and determination to make some changes. I gradually eliminated sugar, alcohol, dairy, and animal protein. I began to eat a macrobiotic diet of lots of cooked vegetables and grains. I felt great, my fibroids decreased, and the bleeding lessened. When I went through menopause, my fibroids continued to shrink and I was symptom-free.

Mary, 55

What Is Uterine Prolapse?

Uterine prolapse is an uncomfortable condition where the pelvic muscles become less able to support the uterus. The uterus drops and may press against the bladder and other organs (causing urinary incontinence); in some cases the uterus or bladder can actually come through into the vagina.

The usual causes are stretching of ligaments due to childbearing, age, and decline in estrogen.

What Are the Treatment Options for Uterine Prolapse, Other Than Hysterectomy?

Clearly, a hysterectomy to remove the uterus will clear up the problem immediately. But there are other solutions, depending on the degree of prolapse.

SURGERY   Surgery may be able to tighten up the ligaments that hold the uterus in place. Unfortunately, this type of surgery is not always effective in the long term.

PHYSICAL DEVICES   You may be helped by using a pessary, a ring (similar to a large diaphragm) that is inserted into the vagina to support the uterus. Electric stimulation can aid in strengthening pelvic floor muscles to support the uterus in mild to moderate cases of prolapse.

EXERCISE   Consistent practice of Kegel exercises can help strengthen pelvic floor muscles to support the uterus in mild to moderate cases of prolapse. For instructions, see Chapter 10, "The World Down Under."

What Are Fibroids?

Fibroids are benign growths of muscles and fibrous tissues in the uterus. They tend to grow in the presence of estrogen. Fibroids are troublesome if they grow large and press on the bladder, causing urinary discomfort. They may also cause pain and abnormal bleeding. Excessive bleeding can lead to anemia.

What Are the Treatment Options for Fibroids, Other Than Hysterectomy?

When it comes to fibroids, you may have a number of alternatives.

DRUG TREATMENT   A class of estrogen-lowering drugs, called GnRH agonists, is sometimes used to shrink fibroids before surgery to make them easier to remove. When

TRAVEL TIP
Call HERS for Help

If you are considering the alternatives to hysterectomy, you may want to call HERS (Hysterectomy Education Resources and Services) for a telephone counseling session to explore your choices. See Resources for more information.

the problem is excessive bleeding, doctors will prescribe either synthetic progestin or natural progesterone capsules (these are less likely to cause depression and other unpleasant side effects). Recently, low-dose birth control pills have become an option for nonsmoking women between the ages of forty and fifty who have no other contraindications. This treatment can make a significant difference in controlling uterine bleeding and may make it possible to avoid a hysterectomy that would have been inevitable just a few years ago.

SURGERY   If your fibroids are few enough and small enough, you can elect to have a myomectomy, in which the fibroids are removed from the uterus. Doctors and patients both like this surgery because it preserves fertility and allows a woman to preserve her uterus for whatever reason. Side effects are comparable to those of hysterectomy, although a myomectomy may involve more blood loss during surgery.

STRESS REDUCTION   Stress can stimulate the adrenal glands to produce hormones, which have an effect on fibroids. Reducing the amount of stress in your life, and learning to cope with what's left, can really help.

COMPLEMENTARY MEDICINE   Acupuncture, massage, t'ai chi, or qi gong may help by increasing the circulation and energy flow through the pelvic area. Some women have had success in decreasing bleeding by using homeopathic remedies. Botanicals include vitex (chaste tree) to shrink small fibroids and cotton root bark (*Gossypium*) to stop excessive bleeding due to fibroids.

VISUALIZATION   Visualize your fibroids shrinking and eventually disappearing. Here's a suggestion from *The Complete Home Healer:* "Lie or sit in a relaxed position in a quiet atmosphere. Let your attention go to the area of the fibroids. Focus your attention on them and experience how they feel. Try to create an image of the fibroids . . . keep focusing on that image, allowing it to change and evolve. Then try to form an image of something that could be done to make the fibroids reduce in size. Finally, visualize what the womb looks like without the fibroids."

FORM A SUPPORT NETWORK Talking to other women who are trying to live with fibroids can give you great emotional support. See Chapter 16, "Getting Help," for ideas on peer support. If you have Internet access, check out women's mailing lists and news groups.

WAIT IT OUT If your fibroids are not causing you pain or excessive bleeding, you can probably just ignore them. Fibroids shrink naturally after menopause, when estrogen levels decline. If your fibroids are not too troublesome, this is the easiest solution.

What Is Endometriosis?

Endometriosis is a strange, often painful, and little-understood condition in which the endometrial lining that grows inside the uterus somehow migrates outside and attaches itself to pelvic organs, the pelvic wall, and other sites, causing pain and bleeding. The only sure way to diagnose endometriosis is to look inside the abdomen through laparoscopy or laparotomy.

What Are the Treatment Choices for Endometriosis, Other Than Hysterectomy?

Endometriosis can seem hopeless, but you do have treatment choices, depending on the severity of the problem. Some women have had success with pelviscopic surgery, which removes the endometrial implants but leaves the uterus intact. Because endometriosis is estrogen-sensitive, it can be treated with birth control pills. Many of the alternative treatments suggested for fibroids also apply to endometriosis. According to Christiane Northrup, M.D., massage can be effective in reducing the pain of endometriosis. Finally, as with fibroids, you can wait it out. Endometriosis will diminish when estrogen levels drop after menopause.

TRAVEL TIP
Be Nice to Your Abdomen

Apply a warm castor oil pack to your abdomen to start heat and energy moving through the area. You can make a castor oil pack yourself: It consists of wool flannel saturated with castor oil, a plastic bag, and a hot water bottle or other nonelectric heat source. You can also order one ready-made from a catalog. See Resources.

What Is Surgical Menopause?

Surgical menopause is cessation of ovulation that occurs before a woman's natural menopause as a result of the removal of the uterus, both tubes, and ovaries. Unlike natural menopause, in which your body may have years to gradually adjust to falling hormone levels, surgery jolts your body into menopause and can cause extreme symptoms such as heavy hot flashes and night sweats, mood swings, and difficulty sleeping. Generally, women are started on hormone therapy immediately after surgery to try to prevent these problems before they begin.

Can Surgical Menopause Occur If Only My Uterus Is Removed?

It's not impossible. Some women do experience a bout of postsurgical menopausal signs (hot flashes and the rest) when only the uterus is removed. One reason may be that surgery has interfered with the blood supply to the ovaries, interrupting their usual functioning. These symptoms continue until the ovaries have readjusted. In some cases, women who have had chemotherapy or radiation treatment for cancer will also experience premature menopause.

SIDE TRIPS: OTHER PATHWAYS
THROUGH THIS BOOK

CHAPTER 3: KEEP ON MOVING   Some problems that can lead to hysterectomy can be moderated by exercise. Look here for more on exercise to promote health.

CHAPTER 5: BREATHE EASY   Stress is associated with growth of fibroids and endometriosis. Look here to learn more about how you can cope with stress.

CHAPTER 7: THE HOLISTIC KIT AND CABOODLE   If you are considering alternatives to hysterectomy, you may want to explore the world of complementary therapies. Look here for an overview of what's out there.

CHAPTER 8: WHAT'S UP, DOC?   When your health problems are serious enough for you to be considering hysterectomy, you'll want to make sure you have a good working relationship with your physician. Look here for pointers on finding a doctor you can work with.

CHAPTER 10: THE WORLD DOWN UNDER   The problems that can necessitate a hysterectomy can be part of the changes in hormonal levels that also influence vaginal health. Look here to learn more about what can happen and what you can do about it. And don't forget to do your Kegels!

 RESOURCES
. . . .

Organizations and Services

American Association of Sex Educators, Counselors, and Therapists, P.O. Box 238, Mt. Vernon, IA 52314. Send a stamped, self-addressed envelope for a referral to a certified sex therapist in your area. From that list you can select a sex therapist or counselor experienced in dealing with problems and feelings that arise after a hysterectomy.

American College of Obstetricians and Gynecologists, Resource Center, 409 12th St. S.W., Washington, DC 20024. Voice: (204) 638-5577. Fax: (202) 484-5107. Internet: www.acog.com. Send a self-addressed, stamped, business-size envelope to receive the free booklet, "Understanding Hysterectomy." This organization also offers patient and physician education, information packets, and educational audiocassettes on issues of women's reproductive health. Request a list of gynecologists in your area who specialize in surgery and cancer.

DES Action, 1615 Broadway, Suite 510, Oakland, CA 94612. Voice: (800) DES-9288. Fax: (510) 465-4815. E-mail: desact@well.com. If you are the daughter of a women who took the drug DES during pregnancy, you may be subject to a range of disorders. Call or write for information to help you understand your options.

Endometriosis Association, 8585 N. 76th Place, Milwaukee, WI 53223. Voice: (800) 992-3636. Fax: (414) 355-6065. This self-help membership organization of women with endometriosis provides educational support and research. Staff members will consult with you and can refer you to an endometriosis support group in your area. With membership you get a newsletter with up-to-date information. This is a good source for tapes, videos, booklets, and more. You do not have to be a member to receive low-cost informational packets.

Endometriosis Treatment Program, St. Charles Medical Center, 2500 N.E. Neff Road, Bend, OR 97701. Voice: (800) 446-2177. This treatment program is based on the laparoscopy/laparotomy for endometriosis developed by Dr. Redwin. Send for a packet of information about the facility and treatment. Instructions for how to obtain an evaluation are also included. Also available is a newsletter, St. Charles Medical's *Endometriosis Newsletter.*

Hysterectomy Education Resources and Services Foundation (HERS), 422 Bryn Mawr Ave., Bala Cynwyd, PA 19004. Voice: (610) 667-7757. Fax: (610) 667-7757. HERS is serious about finding alternatives to hysterectomy. The Foundation offers telephone consultations and information about getting second opinions, legal referrals, and the alternatives to and consequences of hysterectomy. You can be referred to other women who have dealt with making a decision about a hysterectomy; telephone counseling is also available. The organization has a library of publications and videos.

Krames Communications. Voice: (800) 333-3032. Internet: www.krames.com. This company publishes patient information in the form of illustrated, easy-to-understand, and very informative booklets. Call for information about ordering "A Guide to Managing Endometriosis," "Uterine Fibroids," "Abnormal Uterine Bleeding," and "Hysterectomy."

Masters and Johnson Institute, 1 Campbell Plaza, Suite 4B, St. Louis, MO 63139. Voice: (314) 781-1112. Fax: (314) 781-2859. The institute can refer you to sex therapists in your area.

National Institute of Child, Health, and Human Development, NIH-NICHD-PIC, 9000 Rockville Pike, Bldg. 31, Room 2A32, Bethesda, MD 20892. Voice: (301) 496-5133. You can request information on such women's health concerns as fibroids, endometriosis, and hysterectomy.

National Women's Health Network, 514 10th St. N.W., Suite 400, Washington, DC 20004. Voice: (202) 347-1140. Fax: (202) 344-168. Call or write for more information on this group's wealth of resources, including the Women's Health Clearinghouse and the Women's Health Information Service Library. You do not need to be a member to purchase, for a low fee, the very informative packets of information on endometriosis and fibroids.

National Women's Health Resource Center, Columbia Hospital for Women, 2425 L Street N.W., Washington, DC 20037. Voice: (202) 293-6045. Internet: www. womenshealth.com/NWHRC.html. This membership organization offers low-cost educational packets to members and nonmembers about recent research and new developments in women's health care. You can get a research packet on such concerns as hysterectomy, fibroids, and endometriosis.

RESEARCH REPORTS

Keep up to date on hysterectomy research by sending for the latest research reports. See the listings in Chapter 8, "What's Up, Doc?," for resources.

Products and Catalogs

Home Health Products, 949 Seahawk Circle, Virginia Beach, VA 23452. Voice: (800) 468-7313. Catalog: (800) 284-9123. Call for information about castor oil and wool flannel to make castor oil packs and for a catalog of other natural health and beauty aids.

Women to Women, 1 Pleasant St., Yarmouth, ME 04096. Voice: (207) 846-6163. Dr. Christiane Northrup's organization. Call or write for information about the supplements, books, tapes, and other products offered.

Periodicals

Look at the listings in Chapter 2, "Why Is This Happening to Me?," for periodicals dealing with midlife and menopause. Refer to Chapter 7, "The Holistic Kit and Caboodle," and Chapter 8, "What's Up, Doc?," for newsletters dealing with a variety of complementary and traditional medical approaches.

Books

Mary Lou Ballweg and the Endometriosis Association. *The Endometriosis Sourcebook.* Chicago: Contemporary Books, 1995. A book that addresses many issues that arise when a woman has endometriosis. It examines a wide range of options, from medical treatments, to surgery, to transcendental meditation.

Winnifred B. Cutler. *Hysterectomy Before and After.* New York: Perennial Library, 1990. Cutler, an international authority, explains all aspects of women's health choices and provides the reader with the facts she needs to make informed choices. She also discusses dietary considerations and recovery for women who undergo surgery.

Herbert A. Goldfarb, M.D., and Judith Greif, M.S. *The No-Hysterectomy Option.* New York: John Wiley, 1990. This book explores the many alternatives to hysterectomies.

Adelaide Haas and Susan Puretz. *The Woman's Guide to Hysterectomy.* Berkeley, CA: Celestial Arts Publishing, 1995. After undergoing surgery, both authors found themselves frustrated by the lack of information on hysterectomies and decided to write a comprehensive guide. This book is written with compassion and the reassurance of women who have taken charge of their health choices.

Vicki Hufnagel, M.D. *No More Hysterectomies.* New York: Penguin, 1989. An easy-to-read, well-illustrated guide that discusses options and alternative treatments. Provides excellent resource lists in all related subjects.

Gale Malesky and Charles B. Inlander. *Take This Book to the Gynecologist with You.* Reading, MA: Addison-Wesley, 1991. This book examines hysterectomies, ovary removal, and hormone therapy. It has a good section on medical terms and is helpful in preparing women to speak and work with doctors.

Ivan K. Strausz. *You Don't Need a Hysterectomy: New and Effective Ways of Avoiding Major Surgery.* Reading MA: Addison-Wesley, 1993. A look at women's options and health issues related to making a decision not to undergo surgery. This book is comprehensive in discussing the medical concerns and provides excellent resource lists for additional reading.

Stanley West, M.D., and Paula Dranov. *The Hysterectomy Hoax.* New York: Doubleday, 1994. Thinking about having a hysterectomy? Read this book first. Also describes why up to 90 percent of all hysterectomies are unnecessary and has information to help you decide. You'll find a good section on questions to ask your surgeon and information on alternatives.

Audio/Video

Hysterectomy Education Resources and Services Foundation (HERS), listed in Organizations and Services, above, has a list of tapes available. See the catalogs listed in Chapter 8, "What's Up, Doc?," for more companies that carry general health tapes, and Chapter 7, "The Holistic Kit and Caboodle," for companies that carry tapes on complementary medicine. You may also be interested in the tapes listed in Chapter 2, "Why Is This Happening to Me?"

VIDEOTAPES

Endometriosis. Available from The Learning Lane (see Audio/Video, Chapter 8). The signs and symptoms of endometriosis and an explanation of laparoscopy.

Fibroids. Available from The Learning Lane (see Audio/Video, Chapter 8). How fibroids are detected, how they grow, and potential problems.

Endometriosis at Time of Diagnosis. A Time Life Medical Video. Call to find out if a pharmacy in your area has this video available for rent.

Trial of 12 Women with Uterine Fibroids, by Linda Showler. Available from Tree Farm Communications (see Audio/Video, Chapter 7).

Online

For information on fibroids, endometriosis, uterine prolapse, and hysterectomy, check out the general medical sites listed in Chapter 7, "The Holistic Kit and Caboodle," and Chapter 8, "What's Up, Doc?"

NEWS GROUPS

For support and discussion of endometriosis, try **alt.support.endometriosis**.

MAILING LISTS

For discussion of hysterectomy (before and after), try the **Sans Uteri** mailing list. For subscription information, access the web site at www.2cowherd.net/findings/

sans-uteri.html. The **WITSENDO** mailing list is for endometriosis sufferers. (WIT-SENDO stands for "We're Interested in Treatment and Support for Endometriosis.") For subscription information, contact listserv@listserv.dartmouth.edu.

WEB SITES

Endometriosis Links, at www.frii.com/~geomanda/endo, is the place to go for everything about endometriosis, including links to organizations and even full-color pictures of endometriosis implants.

15

EVERYBODY NEEDS ME NOW

Caregiving

Today, one of every five working Americans is caring for an aging relative. This sudden and unavoidable need to provide care for aging parents, relatives, partners, or friends can come as a great shock. Just when you think you'll have more time to spend exploring your own interests and reaching for long-put-aside dreams, you may find yourself having to put your energy into caring for someone else. For women who started families in their thirties or early forties and are also actively raising children, the care burden is doubled. If you find yourself in this situation, you are a member of what has been aptly and uncomfortably called "the sandwich generation."

Women are the traditional caregivers, and midlife may well bring this issue home to you. If you are not caring for someone now, you might want to take this opportunity to look ahead and become familiar with the territory.

caregiver A person caring for a close relative or another person who is chronically ill or dying, either in the home, in a care facility, or from a distance.

PACKING FOR THE JOURNEY

What Is Caregiving?

When a person you love is chronically ill or dying, he or she may need a wide range of services, from financial support to physical care, from assistance with daily activities to help in making life decisions. You may care for your friend or relative in your home or be in charge of finding care outside the home. But no matter what is required to meet physical needs, he or she will always need your empathy and emotional support—and the reassurance that, despite any incapacity, you know your loved one as the person he or she has always been.

When the lives of our loved ones turn out so miserably different from what we had hoped, it can be hard to see any good in it. Life is a mystery, and the question of why someone we love has to suffer is one we can't really answer. Our only options in such a situation lie in how we choose to act. We may not be able to change as many things as we'd like, but we can try to respond in a way that allows compassion, respect, and forgiveness—in regard to the ailing person and to ourselves. If we provide as well as we can and make sure we deal with our own stress and conflicting emotions, we may be able to experience the deep satisfaction that comes from knowing we have given to someone else the loving support and recognition that we ourselves would hope to have in the same situation.

Is Caregiving Stressful?

Caregiving is not for the faint of heart! Often, in midlife, we are giving care to a person who does not get better. It is always hard to see people you love suffer; and it is especially difficult when your parents, on whom you have depended for comfort and support—and who used to seem invincible—become unable to care adequately for themselves. Slowly, you begin to experience role reversal. In addition, seeing your parents age so dramatically can bring you face to face with your own mortality and fears about what may lie ahead.

If you're caring for a friend or relative in your home, the stress of the situation is always with you. But even if you are looking after someone's welfare from a distance, you are putting out a serious amount of emotional energy. This is an especially important time to make sure you get the breaks you need, and it's an excellent chance to begin to think about how you want to live out the latter years of your life.

Why Is This Responsibility Falling on Me?

Women, like it or not, have traditionally been the caregivers, whether for the very young or the very old. In earlier times, when extended families were the norm, women had many others to help shoulder the burden. Today, when most of us live more isolated lives, we seem to feel we must take on this role ourselves—even when we know we have other options. If you choose to take on caregiving, one key to success is figuring out when you can assist an ailing loved one and when you truly cannot. This is not being selfish: Meeting your own needs actually allows you to help others more effectively. Caregiving because you feel you have to or because you just can't say no—or taking on all the responsibility yourself—is not a successful solution for anyone.

How Can I Avoid Caregiver Burnout?

TAKE CARE OF YOURSELF Make sure you're meeting your own physical and emotional needs.

GUIDED TOUR: *Caregiving*

There are many resources that can help you with caregiving—from groups providing information about aging and diseases of the elderly to groups that will advise you on getting the help you need with home care and nursing care to groups that will offer emotional support and much more. Don't neglect yourself in this time of stress. Burnout and depression are a real possibility.

WESTERN MEDICINE

Hospitals and clinics have medical and social work resources to help you with your needs. It may be up to you to make sure the person you are caring for is getting regular medical treatment.

EXERCISE

Caregiving can take a physical toll on the caregiver. Diffuse your tension and improve your mood with regular exercise.

MIND–BODY

Practices such as yoga, t'ai chi, and Rosen work as well as meditation, relaxation response, and similar techniques can give you some personal time, tension relief, and perhaps even a broader perspective during times of continued stress.

NUTRITION

Eat foods that will support you through this period. Avoid stimulants and non-nutritive foods like sugar and fat-laden fast foods.

SUPPORT

Many support groups exist for caregivers, and they are a good way to share with others who understand what you're going through. A counselor or therapist can help you get over the really rough spots.

Are You Suffering from Caregiver Burnout?

If you're not careful, caregiving can consume your life. Caregiver burnout, a recognized condition, is the gradual wearing down of one's physical and emotional resources, and it can eventually lead to depression. Ironically, we often don't realize the toll that even a small amount of caregiving can take. The symptoms of burnout are much like the symptoms of stress (see Chapter 5, "Breathe Easy"). Watch for the warnings. For example, you may find yourself giving up friends and activities you have long enjoyed, experiencing vague or not-so-vague aches and pains, changing your sleeping and eating patterns, or being more easily angered.

If you have these signs, you may need to pull back, take a break, and get some assistance or support. You can't do it all yourself. Sometimes it's hard to let go and delegate responsibilities, especially when a loved one is involved. But recognizing limits is a strength. Strides have been made in resources and services for physically and mentally impaired elders. A good place to start looking for help is with your local county or state office of aging, your local senior center, Eldercare, and AARP. Check Resources for information.

KNOW YOU ARE NOT ALONE You do not have to do this by yourself. Take advantage of the many resources available to you. Community services offer adult day care, senior centers, transportation, home-delivered meals, and home health aides.

KNOW YOUR LIMITS AND RESPECT THEM It's not necessary to work to the point of exhaustion in order to care for someone effectively—in fact, it's impossible. If you sense that you are nearing emotional or physical burnout, ask your doctor or a mental health professional for help.

GET OTHERS TO HELP Enlist the aid of other family members, develop a shared caregivers' network, or hire a care manager.

JOIN A SUPPORT GROUP FOR CAREGIVERS No one knows what you're going through as much as others who are going through the same thing. A support group is not only a place to honestly deal with your feelings, it's also a place to exchange information, ideas, and resources.

TAKE TIME OUT You need a break. Make sure you get a change of scene, even if it's only for a day.

ACKNOWLEDGE WHAT YOU'VE ACCOMPLISHED You're doing a great job on a difficult task. Give yourself the credit you deserve.

CONSIDER A CHANGE OF CARE If the caregiving job has grown to be more than you can handle, your relative may need to move from your care to an assisted-living residence, a board and care home, a skilled nursing facility, or a hospice.

What Are My Care Options?

You have a number of options, depending on the person's need for care.

SENIOR RESIDENCES OR COMMUNITIES This option allows independent living for older adults in low-upkeep houses, duplexes, or apartments in secure communities. It includes many social and recreational opportunities, and limited medical services.

HOME CARE IN YOUR LOVED ONE'S HOME Most people want to remain at home as long as possible. You may need to help your loved one find a home health aide. Check into adult day-care services (many have home pick-up and drop-off).

HOME CARE IN YOUR OWN HOME Even if you are providing most of the care, you may still want to hire a home health aide for additional help. You can also use adult day-care services.

ASSISTED-LIVING RESIDENCE Residents live in apartments with a small kitchen in which they can cook meals, or they can eat prepared meals in a common area with other residents. This is a good option for people with a measure of independence but who may need graduated levels of care. It also offers many social opportunities.

BOARD AND CARE A small number of residents live in a home that provides meals and assistance with daily living and doctor's visits, but has limited on-site medical services.

SKILLED NURSING FACILITY A small or large residential facility that provides twenty-four-hour care for the elderly, including medical care.

Setting Limits
My uncle has Parkinson's and ended up in a skilled nursing facility. Half the time he's hallucinating from the drugs and doesn't know me; sometimes I get a glimmer of who he used to be. I was visiting him really often and it was tough. I realized I had to visit with him from a place of joy and compassion, not obligation and fear. If I couldn't be that way, then I didn't need to go that day. Once I made that decision to go consciously, I almost never missed a visit. It all worked.
Remy, 38

HOSPICE   Hospice services—interdisciplinary medical, emotional, and spiritual support for a terminally ill person and his or her family—may be provided in a separate facility or in your own home. The aim is to enable the person to die with comfort and dignity, surrounded by family and friends.

How Can I Find a Care Facility?

Finding a care facility may seem a daunting task at first, but help is available. Many of the organizations listed in Resources have local referral services. In addition, Eldercare suggests talking to people closer to home: Hospital discharge planners or social workers, your family physician, religious organizations, state nursing home associations, and close friends or relatives. Find out if any of these sources have personal experience with facilities, and then arrange to check the facility for yourself. Many of the organizations listed in Resources provide information and suggestions on how to choose the right facility for your needs.

How Am I Going to Pay for All This?

Caregiving can be draining emotionally, physically, and financially. Short of winning the lottery, there is no easy solution. If possible, talk to your loved ones ahead of time to find out about their financial situation and their wishes for care as they age. If you can plan ahead, take your time to get the facts, talk with a legal professional, and review options together. It can also help to talk with others who have already faced these decisions. Some of your options may include spending savings, liquidating investments and real property, getting a reverse mortgage (the lending institution buys your house and gives you a monthly payment while you reside there), long-term care insurance (bought ahead of need), Medigap insurance (covers copayments and medicine), Medicare (for age sixty-five and older), and other state, federal, and privately funded programs. See Resources for information.

I'm Not in This Situation Now, But I May Be. What Can I Do to Be Prepared?

Preparing ahead of time for the eventuality of caring for a friend or relative can save you a lot of stress down the line. Realistically, you may also want this information for yourself some day. In terms of estate planning and ensuring that you will be cared for as you wish if you become incapacitated, it's always advisable to get professional advice from a knowledgeable and experienced attorney who specializes in estate planning and elder law. To get some background information, contact AARP, which has materials for sale prepared by Legal Counsel for the Elderly, Inc., called "Planning for Incapacity: A Self-Help Guide" (see Resources). Here are some areas to explore—remember, laws vary from state to state:

LIVING WILL/DURABLE POWER OF ATTORNEY FOR HEALTH CARE   Spell out your wishes about whether or not you want lifesaving measures in the case of terminal illness. This document lets you appoint an agent to speak on your behalf if such decisions become necessary.

SOPHISTICATED DURABLE POWER OF ATTORNEY   Authorize someone to act for you in case of temporary or permanent incapacity. This includes making financial transactions on your behalf.

REPRESENTATIVE PAYEE   A government agency, generally the Social Security Administration, appoints a "payee" to manage your benefits if you are unable to manage them yourself.

Long-Distance Care: Geriatric Care Managers Can Help

It's a big country, and many of us live hundreds or even thousands of miles away from our families. If this is you, you're not alone: It's estimated that one-third of the people caring for elderly relatives today are trying to do it from a long distance, which only adds additional stress and guilt. Trying to assess the needs of your loved ones and their financial ability to pay for increased care is difficult to do from afar. Nonetheless, quality caregiving doesn't mean you have to move back home or spend all your free time attending to the needs of your loved ones. Geriatric care or case managers are well-qualified professionals who specialize in assessing the needs of the elderly, pulling together available fragmented services, monitoring, and intervening in crisis situations. Price of this service varies: A geriatric care manager can be an employee of an agency or can be hired privately. Some managed-care health plans also provide geriatric case managers when necessary. To locate a geriatric care or case manger in your area, call the National Association of Private Geriatric Care Managers. (See Resources for this and other agencies that will provide references to geriatric care or case managers.)

MULTIPLE-PARTY ACCOUNT You can have a bank account that gives withdrawal authority to more than one person, which allows money to be accessed in case of emergency, incapacity, or death of one of the signers.

WILL OR TRUST State how you want your assets to be dealt with upon your death, regardless of the size of the estate. A trust addresses how to manage or disburse assets both before and after death and is an important tool for dealing with estate taxes.

LEARN ABOUT TAXES Your home or real property—or other investments—may have greatly increased in value over the years. Sale of these assets may mean large capital gains. Get professional help to understand your tax options.

LEARN ABOUT CARE OPTIONS AHEAD OF TIME Do the research now. How much will long-term care cost? Are savings and income adequate to cover it? Is there insurance that will pay for this? What kinds of resources are available nearby?

IS HOME CARE AN OPTION? Some long-term-care insurance pays home-care benefits, and you may be eligible for assistance through county or privately funded agencies. Medicare sometimes pays for services delivered at home. Insurance coverage for nursing-home care varies, and many restrictions apply. Check the policy carefully.

> If we really want to live, we must have the courage to recognize that life is ultimately very short, and everything we do counts.
>
> ELISABETH KÜBLER-ROSS, *Death: The Final Stage of Growth*

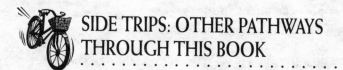 # SIDE TRIPS: OTHER PATHWAYS THROUGH THIS BOOK

CHAPTER 3: KEEP ON MOVING Exercise is a great stress reliever. Look here for ideas on how to get moving and keep moving.

CHAPTER 5: BREATHE EASY You can't adequately care for others if you are not caring for yourself at the same time. Look here for suggestions on how to deal with stress.

CHAPTER 16: GETTING HELP   Caregiving can be draining emotionally as well as physically. Look here for ideas on finding counseling or support.

CHAPTER 17: THE INNER JOURNEY   Caregiving can be a conscious practice of compassion. Look in this chapter to find resources for finding spiritual support and meaning for a fragmented time.

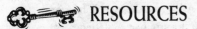 # RESOURCES

Organizations and Services

American Association of Retired Persons (AARP), 601 E St. N.W., Washington, DC 20049. Voice (202) 434-2277. Hotline: (800) 424-3410. E-mail: member@aarp. org. Internet: www.aarp.org. AARP is an organization for people fifty years or older. Membership brings you many benefits, including a number of ideas for caregivers. The AARP brochure "Manage Your Money" explains reverse mortgages, money management, where to store important documents—and what they are! "Planning for Incapacity: A Self-Help Guide," available for every state, will give you key information regarding legal requirements for such things as health directives, living wills, and power of attorney. "The Caregiver Rescue Kit" has a number of items to get you started.

The Alzheimer's Association, 919 N. Michigan Ave., Suite 1000, Chicago, IL 60611-1676. Voice: (800) 272-3900. Fax: (312) 335-1110. Internet: www.alz.org. E-mail: info@alz.org. This group offers local support groups, help lines, pamphlets on research developments, caregiver training, and referrals for assistance in your area.

The American Association of Homes and Services for the Aging, Department 5119, Washington, DC 20061-5119. Voice: (800) 508-9442. Fax: (301) 206-9789. Call for publications related to choosing a nursing home or assisted-living facility, a directory of continuing-care retirement communities, and information on long-term-care insurance. There are fees for these services; the organization also publishes free brochures on issues concerning aging.

American Self-Help Clearinghouse, North West Covenant Medical Center, 25 Pocono Road, Denville, NJ 07834. Voice: (201) 625-7101. Fax: (201) 625-8848. E-mail: ashc@bc.cybernex.net. Internet: www.cmhc.com/selfhelp. This clearinghouse has a national database of support groups. Ask for a referral to agencies that will help you find caregiving support groups in your area. The organization also has information on how to set up your own support group.

American Seniors Housing Association, 1850 M St. N.W., Suite 540, Washington, DC 20036. Voice: (202) 659-3381. Fax: (202) 775-0112. Contact this association for information on housing options.

Association of Jewish Family and Children's Agencies, P.O. Box 248, Kendall Park, NJ 08824-0248. Voice: (800) 634-7346. Fax: (908) 821-0493. E-mail: ajfca@ aol.com. If you're trying to provide care from a long distance, the AJFCA offers an elder support network that will put you in touch with the Jewish Family Service nearest your elderly loved one. A professional will do an assessment, coordinate services, and keep you informed. There is a fee for these services.

Children of Aging Parents (CAPS), 1609 Woodbourne Road, Suite 302A, Levittown, PA 19057. Voice: (800) 227-7294. Fax: (215) 945-8720. Internet: www.experts. com. CAPS offers information, referral, and support for caregivers as well as for professionals and agencies dealing with the elderly. Ask about the manual for starting a support group. Membership will also bring you the group's newsletter.

Choice in Dying, 200 Varick St., Suite 1001, New York, NY 10014-4810. Voice: (800) 989-9455. Fax: (212) 366-5337. Internet: www.choices.org. Choice in Dying is a not-for-profit organization offering advice on living wills, power-of-attorney transfer, and other issues related to end-of-life decision making. Online counseling services are also available.

Council of Better Business Bureaus, Publications Department, 4200 Wilson Blvd., Suite 800, Arlington, VA 22203. Voice: (703) 276-0100. Ask about the informative brochures on housing and care.

American Heart Association Stroke Network, 7272 Greenville Ave., Dallas, TX 75231. Voice: (800) 553-6321. E-mail: strokeaha@amhrt.org. Internet: www. amhrt.org. This network provides information and online support to stroke victims and families. It has a list of nationwide support groups.

Eden Alternative, RR1, Box 31134, Sherburne, NY 13460. Voice: (607) 674-5232. Fax: (607) 674-6723. Dr. William Thomas's organization is aimed at improving the quality of life in nursing homes by "enlivening" the environment with plants, animals, and people of all ages. Call for a directory of organizations with the same philosophy.

The Family Caregiver Alliance, 425 Bush St., Suite 500, San Francisco, CA 94108. Voice: (800) 445-8106. Fax: (415) 434-3508. E-mail: gen-info@caregiver.org. This group can provide information on long-term health care resources, research, and advocacy on health care issues for the elderly.

Legal Services for the Elderly, 130 W. 42nd St., 17th Floor, New York, NY 20046-7803. Voice: (212) 391-0120. Fax: (212) 719-1939. E-mail: HN4923@handsnet. org. Pension Hotline: (800) 355-7714; within New York: (212) 997-7714. This not-for-profit organization provides litigation assistance, legal information, and a resource list of free publications, including Social Security Income (SSI), Medicare, Medigap, and veterans' entitlements.

National Academy of Elder Law Attorneys, Inc., 1604 N. Country Club Road, Tucson, AZ 85716. Voice: (520) 881-4005. Fax: (520) 325-7925. This organization provides referrals and publishes a free brochure, "Questions & Answers When Looking for an Elder Law Attorney." You can purchase a national directory of elder-law attorneys for $25.

National Association for Hispanic Elderly, 3325 Wilshire Blvd., Suite 800, Los Angeles, CA 90010. Voice: (213) 487-1922. Fax: (213) 385-3014. This group provides job-training information for men and women over fifty-five years of age, low-income housing information, and resources. The main office is in Los Angeles, but you can get referrals to offices in thirteen other states.

The National Alliance for Caregiving, 472 Montgomery Lane, Suite 642, Bethesda, MD 20814. Voice: (301) 718-8444. Fax: (301) 718-0034. This organization conducts research and develops national programs that support family caregivers of the elderly. It will direct you to national resources only.

National Association for Home Care, 228 Seventh St. S.E., Washington, DC 20003. Voice: (202) 547-7424. Fax: (202) 547-3540. E-mail: webmaster@nahc.org. This is a member/trade organization with interest in promoting quality care. You can write or call for a free consumer guide detailing how to choose a home care agency and for statistics about home care.

National Association of Geriatric Care Managers, 1604 N. Country Club Road, Tucson, AZ 85716. Voice: (520) 881-8008. Fax: (520) 325-7925. This professional membership organization for geriatric caregivers also provides consumers with a local care-manager referral service. You can receive up to three referrals in your area or send a self-addressed, stamped, business-size envelope to receive more specific information.

National Caucus and Center on Black Aged, 142 K St. N.W., Suite 500, Washington, DC 20005. Voice: (202) 637-8400. Contact this organization to find out what kind of resources it can provide.

National Center for Home Equity Conversion, 7373 147th St. W., Suite 115, Apple Valley, MN 55124. Information on how to get a reverse mortgage. Send $1 and a self-addressed, stamped, business-size envelope for the booklet "Reverse Mortgage Locator" to find a reverse mortgage lender in your area. Also available is a booklet, "Retirement Income on the House."

National Council on Aging/National Institute on Adult Daycare, 409 Third St. S.W., Washington, DC 20024. Voice: (800) 424-9046. Fax: (202) 479-0735. E-mail: info@ncoa.org. The Council has a wealth of information and referrals, and can provide information on adult-care centers in your area.

National Family Caregivers Association, 9621 E. Bexhill Drive, Kensington, MD 20095-3104. Voice: (800) 896-3650 or (301) 942-6430. Fax: (301) 942-2302. Internet: www.nfcacares.org. This membership organization offers peer support to caregivers, including a support network. It also publishes a resource guide for

$12.95 that is available to members at a 30 percent discount. Also available are a caregiver newsletter and referrals and information about local support groups.

National Hispanic Council on Aging, 2713 Ontario Road N.W., Suite 200, Washington, DC 20009. Voice: (202) 265-1288. Fax: (202) 745-2522. Call about resources for your family.

National Hospice Organization, 1901 N. Moore St., Suite 901, Arlington, VA 22209. Voice: (800) 658-8898. Fax: (703) 525 5762. Internet: www.nho.org. This professional membership organization also provides phone referral services, Medicare information, and literature.

National Pacific/Asian Resource Center on Aging, Melbourne Tower, 1511 Third Ave., Suite 914, Seattle WA 98101. Voice: (206) 624-1221. Call for information on services.

The Older Women's League (OWL), 666 Eleventh Street N.W., Suite 700, Washington, DC 20001. Voice: (202) 783-6686 or (800) TAKE-OWL. Fax: (202) 638-2356. OWL is the first national organization to recognize the huge role women play in caregiving. The organization offers a free packet of information that includes practical tips for caregivers.

Well Spouse Foundation, P.O. Box 28876, San Diego, CA 92198-0876. Offers support and information plus a newsletter for partners of chronically ill people. A membership organization.

Hotlines

The Alzheimer's Association: (800) 272-3900. Call for local support groups and referral for assistance in your area.

Alzheimer's Disease Education and Referral Center: (800) 438-4380. Call for free publications on Alzheimer's and related disorders and to get in touch with Alzheimer's research centers nationwide.

The American Association of Homes and Services for the Aging: (800) 508-9442. Call to find out about housing options.

Association of Jewish Family and Children's Agencies: (800) 634-7346. Call to find out about geriatric care managers in your area.

Choice in Dying: (800) 989-9455. Call for information about state-specific living wills and durable power of attorney forms.

Eldercare Locator: Voice: (800) 677-1116. This national service will refer you to local resource services for elders and their caregivers. The local service center may be able to refer you to a geriatric care manager.

Eldercare Help Line: (800) 25-ELDER. Information, advice, and referrals for a number of services.

The Family Caregiver Alliance: (800) 445-8106. Call for information on caregiving.

Medicare Hotline: (800) 772-1213. Call for information about the ins and outs of Medicare.

National Council on Aging/National Institute on Adult Daycare: (800) 424-9046. Will provide information on adult-care centers in your area.

National Hospice Organization: (800) 658-8898. Can help you find information about hospices.

Pension Hotline: (800) 355-7714. Call this legal service with your questions about pensions.

Social Security Administration: (800) 772-1213. Call this number to get information about becoming a representative payee, to find out your future Social Security benefits, or to apply for Medicare.

Periodicals

Answers, The Magazine for Adult Children of Aging Parents. P.O. Box 9889, Birmingham, AL 35220-0889. Voice: (800) 750-2199. This magazine covers all aspects of looking after an elderly parent, including how to deal with your feelings and where to get help if you need it.

The Capsule, newsletter of Children of Aging Parents, 1609 Woodbourne Road, Suite 302-A, Levittown, PA 19057-1511. This bimonthly newsletter for CAP members addresses practical concerns of caregivers and offers many other resources.

The Sandwich Generation, Box 132, Wickatunk, NJ 07765-0132. This quarterly publication is for you if you are taking care of aging parents or relatives and raising children all at the same time. It covers many relevant subjects, including communicating with your parents and your children, dealing with anger, and coping skills.

Books

Cappy Capassela and Sheila Warnoch. *The Share Care: How to Organize a Group to Care for Someone Who Is Seriously Ill.* New York: Simon and Schuster, 1995. This book details a unique approach that the authors themselves used to organize a powerful caregiver team. It's a book that will help you take action.

Rosalynn Carter. *Helping Yourself Help Others: A Book for Caregivers.* New York: Random House, 1996. The former first lady shares her own experiences with caregiving. She offers advice and provides a list of elder-care resources.

Equitable Foundation and Children of Aging Parents. *Aging Parents and Common Sense— A Practical Guide for You and Your Parents.* This is a helpful guide for adult children facing new roles as caregivers for their aging parents. The Equitable Foundation worked with Children of Aging Parents (CAPS), a national caregiving organization, to put this resource guide together. The guide covers many aspects of caregiving for aging parents, including medical care, living arrangements, financial and legal concerns, and basic communication issues. A glossary and directory of resources are included. For a copy of this guide, write to the Equitable Foundation, Box B, 787 Seventh Ave., New York, NY 10019.

Nancy R. Hooyman and Wendy Lustbader. *Taking Care: Supporting Older Women and Their Families.* New York: Free Press, 1986. More ideas for coping, including caregiving in diverse families—from the nuclear family to gay and lesbian families.

Nancy L. Mace, M.A., and Peter V. Rabins, M.D. *The 36-Hour Day: A Family Guide to Caring for Persons with Alzheimer's Disease, Related Dementing Illness, and Memory Loss in Later Life.* New York: Warner Books, 1992. A basic book about dementia and how to deal with problems arising from daily care, how to cope with an impaired person's false ideas, and how to get financial and legal help. This book also includes helpful resources.

Harriet Sarnoff Schiff. *How Did I Become My Parent's Parent?* New York: Penguin, 1996. A comprehensive book of personal stories that explore how we learn to deal with the role reversal between parent and child that occurs as we grow older and our parents grow older still.

J. Shapiro. *The Big Squeeze: Balancing the Needs of Aging Parents, Dependent Children and You.* Bedford, MA: Mills & Sanderson, 1991. If you've got parents growing older and kids growing up, this helpful eight-step survival plan may help you handle the demands of both roles.

William Thomas, M.D. *Life Worth Living: How Someone You Love Can Still Enjoy Life in a Nursing Home.* Acton, MA: Vander-Wyk and Burnham, 1996. This book offers alternatives to standard nursing home care. It is written by a doctor who is an administrator of a nursing home and developed a "lush, lively and human habitat" called Eden Alternative. The nursing home became a place of life that included children, animals, and accessible gardens. Includes how-to's and resources.

Audio/Video

You'll find good tapes on caregiving at some of the agencies listed in Organizations and Services, above. **AARP** and the **Older Women's League (OWL)** both have videos for caregivers.

Innovative Caregiving Resources. Voice: (800) 246-5600. This organization has a catalogue of twenty videos researched by the university of Utah that provide entertainment and hold the attention of Alzheimer's patients so the caregiver can get a respite. The videos are geared to different needs, and some are interactive.

Videos

Survival Tips for New Caregivers. Available from AARP. Caregivers discuss how they cope with the physical and emotional demands of caregiving. The tape also covers good nutrition and exercise for the care receiver, managing another person's finances, and household safety tips.

A Matter of Life and Death. Available from OWL. This video addresses planning in advance for health care decisions at the end of life and using living wills and durable power of attorney. It offers resources, and materials that can be copied for handouts.

Complaints of a Dutiful Daughter, by Deborah Hoffman. Available from Women Make Movies, 462 Broadway, Suite 500, New York, NY 10013. Voice: (212) 925-0606. This documentary film, nominated for an Academy Award, is a thoughtful and inspirational look at the impact of Alzheimer's disease on sufferers and caretakers.

Video Respite. Available from Innovative Caregiving Resources. This interactive video gives caregivers of Alzheimer's patients an opportunity for short breaks.

Online

If you are feeling isolated as a caregiver, you'll feel more like part of a community after you tap into the wealth of resources on the Internet. You'll find online support groups, magazines, and a growing caregiver network of resources and ideas. Help is out there! The following listings barely scratch the surface of what you'll find.

NEWS GROUPS

For general emotional support, try **soc.support.misc** or **soc.support.family.**

WEB SITES

Elderweb, www.ice.net/~kstevens/ELDERWEB.HTM, is a good place to start. It has links and information on health care; living arrangements; aging, death, and dying; social, mental, spiritual, and financial issues; law and legislation; statistics, demographics, and research; regional information; and more.

Caregivers Survival Resources Home Page, www.caregiver911.com/Athens/ 1330, is a warm site and a good place for caregivers' self-care. It has lots of caregiver links—local, regional, and state sources—and a regularly updated clearinghouse of links to caregiver resources available on the Internet. For your needs, you'll find Ask Dr. Caregiver, support services, and books and videos.

The **National Association for Home Care** site, www.nahc.org, has information about home care and hospice care and ways to find local references. **MotherHeart: Unconditional Love Nurtures All,** www.gnv.fdt.net/~mother—the most nurturing site on the Internet—includes many resources for caregiving and caregivers. You will feel better here.

Online newsletters include **Caregiving Newsletter,** www.caregiving.com/newsletter, which calls itself "the support group that arrives at your door every month"; **Today's Caregiver: The Magazine and Web Site for Those Caring for Loved Ones,** www.caregiver.com, has "resources, support, information, empowerment tools, advice and insight, and when the technology allows it—a big warm hug." You'll find **Eldercare Forum Newsletter** at www.mindspring.com/~eldrcare/newsmenu.htm.

16

GETTING HELP

*Support, Counseling, and a
Little Help from Your Friends*

Taking Care of Business

I've spent a lot of time worrying about my daughter's safety, and it's getting out of hand. I know deep down that the fear I feel for her safety is really coming from me, and I don't want it to affect her. I've decided to go into therapy for a short time, to see if I can find out where this fear is coming from. These feelings have come and gone in the past, but this is the first time I've felt strong enough to work on it. I feel this overwhelming need now to clear out some things from the past so I can move on to other levels.   *Lorraine, 49*

Midlife can be a precious time for sorting out, a time to look inward and come to terms with the past. This can be an unsettling task. Our physical changes let us know in no uncertain terms that time is indeed moving on. As we've seen, other changes and losses may accompany our experience of biological loss at menopause—a change in role or self-image, a loss through divorce or death of a spouse, a loss of parents, a change in relationships. In addition we may have children leaving home, and we may have to acknowledge missed opportunities. It's not surprising that women at this time find themselves going though all sorts of confusing feelings.

Sometimes we need help to sort through these issues or to get moving when an emotion lingers a bit too long. This help can come from a number of sources: from friends and family, from support groups, and from professional counselors and therapists. Women thrive in relationships of mutual support, and we do much of our self-discovery in the company of other women. At this crucial time of change, it's especially important to seek out compassionate and mutually supportive relationships. You are not alone on this journey.

> I know menopause is not just a trivial little change whose rough spots can be eased with a little hormone treatment, on the other side of which I will still have a good figure, and a good mind, still be sexy and sexual. . . . I don't want to get around it, I want to live it. I don't want to "treat" it or "cure" it, though I do want to honor it with curiosity, and with "therapy" (*therapaeia*), attention of the kind one devotes to sacred mysteries.
>
> CHRISTINE DOWNING, *Journey Through Menopause*

 ## PACKING FOR THE JOURNEY

Why Would I Need Support Now?

For some reason, we seem to think that if we're not happy all the time, there's something wrong with us. In fact, our natural feelings of anger, sadness, fear, and joy are fluid and changing as we meet the challenges of life. Moods come and go. That's life. The difficulty comes when you get stuck in a particular feeling and can't seem to move beyond it. At times like these the support and understanding of another person can ease the painful feelings that arise.

At midlife some women feel as if they're walking on shifting sands. As in adolescence, changes are happening inside and outside, and everything is changing all at once. A crisis may prompt us to seek out professional counseling so that we can sort out confusing feelings, or we may use counseling to get through a transition or to better understand and be understood. Here are some of the issues that come up for many women at this time.

CHANGE   The physical changes of midlife can be very unsettling. You can't ignore them; you're reminded every time you look in the mirror. It can help to talk to other women of the same age, or to women a little older, about ways of dealing with the emotions that arise at this time. You may also be dealing with other changes that accompany this passage, including shifting social status, an empty nest, your relationship to your partner or your children, and your career path.

OUTGROWN PATTERNS At midlife you may suddenly become aware of behavior patterns that are holding you back: fear of trying new things, problems dealing with authority figures, lack of self-confidence, giving to everyone but yourself, or enabling destructive behavior in loved ones. Support and understanding from someone else may be just what you need to make the leap to a more assured way of relating to the world.

UNFINISHED BUSINESS Many women nearing the end of a pregnancy find themselves suddenly involved in nesting behavior—cleaning, throwing things out, getting the house ready for the new person. In the same way, women at midlife often begin to resolve unfinished business or mourn ungrieved and unacknowledged losses. Over a lifetime, unattended and unexpressed issues can lead to a buildup of stress that may lead to anxiety or depression—in other words, the discomfort just doesn't want to go away! You may want to explore past events that still trouble you and integrate their meaning into your present life.

insight The power or act of seeing into a situation.

RUNAWAY EMOTIONS In this time of heightened emotions, you may be surprised by a seemingly uncontrollable surge of anger or sadness. It's tempting to blame these reactions on "hormones," but it can also be valuable to explore your feelings more deeply in order to understand their meaning. If you find yourself preoccupied with sadness, regret, anger, guilt, or any other emotion, professional help may be able to help you unblock and move on.

GUIDED TOUR: *Getting Help*

Midlife can be a precious time for sorting out, a time to look inward and come to terms with the past, to resolve old issues and grieve for our losses. Sometimes we need help to sort through these issues or to get moving when we're stuck in an emotion that lingers a bit too long. This help can come from a number of sources: friends and family, support groups, professional mental health providers.

WESTERN MEDICINE

For some women, hormone replacement therapy helps with mood swings; for other women, however, progesterone and progestin can contribute to mood swings and depression. If you are suffering from clinical depression or extreme anxiety that makes it impossible for you to function in your daily life, consider consulting a psychiatrist who can prescribe antidepressant or anti-anxiety medication.

COMPLEMENTARY THERAPIES

Acupuncture, acupressure, massage, and similar mind–body approaches may help even out your moods. St. John's wort may help mild to moderate depression; essential oils such as lemon, marjoram, neroli, orange, patchouli, peppermint, rose, rosewood, thyme, and ylang ylang are said to calm mild anxiety.

EXERCISE

Regular exercise can help relieve stress, release tension, and even out mood swings.

MIND–BODY

Meditation may give you a perspective that helps calm mood swings. T'ai chi, qi gong, yoga, and similar practices are aimed at creating balance between body, mind, and spirit.

NUTRITION

Eat a balanced diet. Foods that help calm mild anxiety include pasta and whole grains; foods that provide energy include light protein. Avoid or moderate your use of alcohol, caffeine, and sugar. Eat throughout the day to maintain your blood sugar levels.

Hold That Mood Swing: Transforming Heightened Emotions

In midlife many women find that they react to life in a new way: They may feel more frustrated, more impatient, more deeply sad. Instead of feeling you have to "cure" yourself of the strong emotions of midlife, use them. Here are some ways you can transform powerful emotions into positive ways of dealing with the world.

Frustration: You do not need to seethe silently or wound others with the sword of frustration. What you think and what you have to say are important. Convert your frustration into directness, firmness, and certainty. Use its power to help you speak your mind, to ask for what you want and need with confidence.

Impatience: The farther along the road we get, the less patience we seem to have with incompetence and meaninglessness. Instead of being consumed by impatience, use it as a cue to rid yourself of baggage (physical or emotional) that no longer serves you or you just don't have time for.

Sadness: At this time of life you may find yourself overcome with sadness about the state of the world or the human condition. This sadness is a barometer of deep empathy and compassion. Use it positively close to home, to support friends and family, or channel it into action for change in the world at large. Above all else, feel compassion toward yourself during this time of change.

Fear: If you've ever ridden a roller-coaster, skied down a slope, or made a successful airplane trip, you know that fear can be converted into the thrill of excitement. Try to transform your fear of the unknown—whether it be fear of change, of new beginnings, or of going to a party—into a sense of adventure and hopeful anticipation about what you might find around the next turn.

What Is Grief?

Grief is a reaction to loss. As Chapter 1, "Endings and Beginnings," makes clear, feelings of loss and separation are a natural part of midlife. Clinical social worker Mona Reeva works with women at midlife and beyond, specializing in loss and grief experiences. She classifies losses as personal (such as the realization that you've already lived more years than you have left, loss of some physical abilities, new vulnerabilities involving the physical changes of menopause) and contextual—things outside ourselves, in whose midst we live (such as divorce, death, career plateaus, and financial insecurities).

Reeva points out that you can grieve over many things in addition to the death of a loved one: The loss of a spouse through divorce, the loss of a job, and the loss of your ability to bear children all need to be worked through. Grieving is a natural part of the healing process; grief wants to be expressed. If you deny it or hold it at bay, your body may express it as illness. Allow yourself to feel your emotions, but don't hesitate to get help if your grief makes it hard for you to carry on with daily living. Grief is a process: It doesn't last forever. It's important to remember that you're not alone. Seek help if you can't seem to move beyond the pain.

> I would say to those who mourn . . . look upon each day that comes as a challenge, as a test of courage. The pain will come in waves, some days worse than others, for no apparent reason. Accept the pain. Do not suppress it. Never attempt to hide grief from your self. Little by little . . . the bereaved, the widowed, will find new

strength, new vision born of the very pain and lone-liness which seem, at first, impossible to master.

DAPHNE DU MAURIER

What Are the Stages of Grief?

Grief moves through stages: shock, denial, numbness, pain (anger, guilt, sadness), bargaining, getting on with life (acceptance), reintegration (if it's the loss of a person, you allow that person to live on in your heart and mind), and moving on. It's important to recognize that these stages are not necessarily linear—the feelings may come in waves. You may experience each stage separately, or you may go through several simultaneously. Give yourself time and compassion. Being aware that these stages are part of the process can make grieving bearable.

Honor your loss and treat yourself with kindness and respect. Value your personal and cultural ways of dealing with loss, and remember that we don't all have the same ways of expressing grief.

Does Menopause Have to Mean Mood Swings?

Some women experience mood swings around the time of menopause, and some don't. If your moods are in flux, there may be a good reason. Interrupted sleep patterns can have a huge influence on mood. Hormonal ups and downs accentuate feelings (remember adolescence?), and increased PMS is common at this time. More life stressors, the unsettling unpredictability of physical changes, the realizations that you are not the same person you were ten years ago—with all this going on, who *wouldn't* have mood swings? Cut yourself some slack. This can be a difficult period.

TRAVEL TIP
Revise Your Life Story

"You are the narrator of your own story," says therapist Mandy Aftel in *The Story of Your Life: Becoming the Author of Your Own Experience.* "In fact, whether you are aware of it or not, you probably can't help telling your story. We tell stories to anyone who will listen: about ourself to our listening self, to intimate friends, and to the outside world. Even if we think we're telling the same story to everyone, it will differ according to who's listening."

If the story you've been telling yourself about yourself is no longer constructive, revising your story may give you a new perspective:

"It may be that the way we reacted to an event at the time was the only reaction possible, and then the situation becomes a fixed story in our repertoire. (For example, as a child you thought you were 'too demanding' because you wanted your self-absorbed parents to show you some real concern and attention.) ... Revisiting these experiences again allows us to revise them again, with all our accumulated self-knowledge.

"1. Write a paragraph describing one of these 'fixed stories' in your repertoire.

"2. Now revise the paragraph with an open mind, based on your accumulated self-knowledge. (For example, were you 'too demanding,' or were you demanding what was rightfully yours but impossible for your parents to give?)"

How Can I Even Out My Moods?

The time-tested methods that keep you active and healthy will also help smooth out your mood swings. A quick rundown:

GET SOME EXERCISE Regular aerobic exercise can stimulate release of endorphins, decreasing tension and anxiety and allaying or preventing depression. A recent study at Tufts University found that resistance training can also alleviate depression in older people.

EXERCISE YOUR MIND AND BODY Mind–body practices like yoga, qi gong, and t'ai chi are aimed at balancing mind, body, and spirit.

AVOID OR MODERATE COMSUMPTION OF ALCOHOL, CAFFEINE, SUGAR, SEDATIVES These substances may seem calming or mood-lifting in the short term, but they can actually provoke more anxiety or depression in the long term. When they wear off, you're back where you started or worse.

GRAZE You can avoid sudden highs and lows by "grazing"—eating small meals throughout the day to keep your blood sugar on an even keel.

EAT CALMING FOODS Try to include whole grains and other foods containing B-complex vitamins, and eat smaller servings of protein.

TRY AN ALTERNATIVE TREATMENT Acupuncture, acupressure, massage, and similar mind–body approaches may help even out your moods.

TRY HERBAL TREATMENT St. John's wort (*Hypericum perforatum*) is popular in Germany for mild to moderate depression and is currently being researched here.

TRY HRT Some women find that HRT helps with mood swings. For other women, however, progesterone and especially progestin can contribute to mood swings and depression. Check with your health practitioner to rule out risks, and make an informed decision if you decide to try it.

TAKE A BREAK Doing something completely different may help you break your cycle of ups and downs.

TRY AROMATHERAPY Take a moment out to inhale the scent of oils said to calm anxiety, such as lemon, marjoram, neroli, orange, patchouli, peppermint, rose, rosewood, thyme, lavender, and ylang ylang.

MEDITATE Taking time out to be present and clear in the moment is the perfect antidote to worrying about the past and future.

TALK IT OUT Connect with others who are experiencing what you're going through. They may have some good ideas, and you won't feel so alone.

Why Am I So Anxious?

The instabilities of midlife can make anxiety a concern at this time of life or they can make underlying anxiety of more concern. According to Karen Johnson, M.D., in *Trusting Ourselves*, "Anxiety is second only to depression in prompting women to seek the care of mental-health professionals." For women, anxiety may take a number of forms: worry, panic

Oh Yeah?

When something bothers me at work these days, I can't seem to keep it to myself any more. I have to say something about it, and I know some of my co-workers are starting to think I'm a real bitch. And sometimes, I have to say, the depth of my anger scares me. But it's kind of thrilling, too. This way of acting isn't me, but it *is* me, you know? *Myra, 44*

POINT OF INTEREST
The Signs of Clinical Depression

Clinical depression is different from passing feelings of sadness or having the blues. If five or more of the following symptoms persist for longer than two weeks and make it difficult for you to live your life, you may want to seek professional help. These signs of clinical depression are derived from the *DSM-IV*, a diagnostic tool used by some mental health professionals to identify depression. Remember, these symptoms indicate clinical depression if they are not transitory; they have a persistent quality:

- Persistent sad mood
- Excessive feelings of guilt, worthlessness, and helplessness
- Loss of interest or pleasure in ordinary activities, including sex
- Fatigue or loss of energy almost every day
- Difficulty sleeping
- Weight loss or gain
- Feelings of restlessness or being slowed down
- Difficulty concentrating
- Thoughts of death or suicide or suicide attempts

Women, Menopause, Mood Swings, and Depression

Many women in midlife feel a strong link between hormonal changes and mood, and studies support this. But mood swings are just that: an unpredictable movement between any number of feelings—happiness, sadness, enthusiasm, anger, regret, and on and on. Depression, as we have seen in this chapter, is a lingering state.

A link between menopause and depression has long been accepted as general wisdom, but current research seems to indicate otherwise. In fact, the women most vulnerable to depression are those who experienced depressive episodes before menopause. As reported in *Hot Flash*, in 1989 a long-term study of 2,300 women by the New England Research Institute came up with some interesting results: The majority of women studied, 85 percent, reported no depression accompanying menopause; 10 percent reported occasional depression. The remaining 5 percent had been depressed before menopause, and that depression continued. The most-mentioned cause of depression was family-related problems. Women who were divorced, separated, or widowed, or who had less than twelve years of education, were most depressed around menopause. The least depressed were single women with more education and close friendships or family ties.

Clearly, although we may sometimes feel sad or at the mercy of our capricious hormones, menopausal depression is *not* a given. In fact, many women report what anthropologist Margaret Meade called "postmenopausal zest"—a renewed feeling of energy, enthusiasm, and directedness far greater than in their younger years.

attacks, fears about one's health, preoccupying thoughts. The causes of anxiety are also various—you may have a biological or inherited tendency toward it, or you may have a treatable medical condition that promotes anxiety. Life changes, social issues, and television news can all leave you feeling anxious. Caffeine can intensify anxiety, and so can some medications. If you are taking several different medications, ask your pharmacist about side effects and interactions among them or about interactions with over-the-counter drugs you may be taking.

What Can I Do About Anxiety?

If anxiety is getting in the way of how you live your life, get help. For extreme anxiety, a psychiatrist may prescribe tranquilizers or anti-anxiety medication as a short-term solution to help break the grip of anxiety. Identifying the source of your anxiety (for example, a job that asks more than you can do, a demanding life partner) may help you overcome it or work out new ways of dealing with the problem. Many of the same things that will help you deal with mood swings will help calm anxiety: Eat calming foods, such as whole grains and pasta; avoid or reduce your use of alcohol, drugs, and caffeine; try meditation or relaxation techniques; get plenty of vigorous exercise; take as many breaks as you can; take time out to play; and remember to *breathe*.

What Is Depression?

Feeling sad or "having the blues" is a common response to painful events and may even be part of a larger picture of growth. But when feelings of sadness linger or feelings of hopelessness seem to drain all color from your life, this is a sign that something needs attention! See the Point of Interest "The Signs of Clinical Depression" for symptoms.

What Causes Depression?

Depression is a complex issue. According to the American Psychological Association's Task Force Report on Women and Depression, "Women truly are more depressed then men, primarily due to the experience of being female in our culture. In other words, depression by women is not due primarily to biological causes, as was once believed, but to a variety of biological, social, and psychological issues."

The mix of issues, of course, is different for everyone. All of the following factors may trigger depression. *Biology:* a family history of depression; possible biochemical factors and certain physical illnesses (including thyroid disorder, hypoglycemia, allergies, and diabetes). *How you deal with life:* the meaning you give to events (do you see the glass as half-empty or half-full?); your ability to express your wants and needs (depression is often thought of as anger or sadness that has been held in); a tendency toward selfless giving to others at your expense. *Outside causes:* problematic or traumatic life events such as divorce, death, or past or present sexual or physical abuse; an unhappy primary relationship or lack of intimacy; feelings of powerlessness related to a drop in social status or issues of aging, minority status, poverty, and work.

Lack of support from the people we love and depend on may also lead to depression and immobilization. According to Jean Baker Miller, M.D., and Irene Stiver, Ph.D., of the Stone Center, as noted in *Hot Flash*, "Women are often not permitted by society, friends, or family to feel sad about their real constraints, losses, deprivations, and the discrimination against them."

If you are feeling depressed, it's a good idea to get a medical evaluation and talk to your doctor about any medications you are taking, including

Walk Therapy

Several of my dog-owning friends and I seem to have formed an accidental support group around our dogs' need to walk and our need to talk things out. We walk fairly regularly, rain or shine, watching our dogs play and sharing our experiences. Walking seems to loosen stuff up in a way that sitting and talking doesn't begin to touch. It's amazing how much comes up and gets worked out over the course of walking your dogs together for a year. And we're in much better shape!

Sharon, 43

Is This the Therapist for Me?

An ethical therapist expects an interview and mutual evaluation before beginning a professional relationship. Don't be afraid to ask questions. You may be able to ask some questions on the phone to see if you even want to make an appointment for an initial consultation. Even if the person has impressive credentials, if something makes you uncomfortable, don't be afraid to keep looking. In some urban areas there are many practitioners and you may have abundant choices.

Here are some questions you might want to ask:

1. Are you familiar with the issues of midlife? Have you ever worked with midlife women?
2. What is your theoretical orientation? What is your approach toward problem solving?
3. What is your education? Your credentials?
4. How much experience have you had?
5. Are therapy groups an option?
6. What does it cost? Is there a sliding scale fee? Will my insurance pay for it?
7. How long do you expect therapy to last?

What's your intuitive feeling? You are not wedded to a therapist just because you have had a consultation session. Trust in your intuitive feelings. If you feel a level of distrust or misgiving, move on. Here are some questions to ask yourself, suggested by the authors of *When Talk Is Not Cheap, or How to Find the Right Therapist When You Don't Know How to Begin:*

1. Did the therapist seem to understand what you were trying to say?
2. Was the therapist someone you could learn to trust?

(continued)

herbs, vitamins, and prescription or over-the-counter drugs. Alone or in combination, these may be a factor. And don't forget that alcohol and other substances can also play a role in depression. If you're drinking or using other substances to lift your mood, you may be creating just the effect you're trying to avoid.

What Can I Do About Depression?

Depression is treatable. Even though depression may make you want to pull the covers over your head and just be left alone, the most important way to combat depression is to take positive action. Often, someone else needs to pull us to our feet. If you're mildly depressed, the persistence of a friend or family member may make all the difference. Support groups or talk therapy are a wonderful way to reconnect with your life. If you're clinically depressed, a psychiatrist may recommend drug treatment to lift your mood enough for you to be able to see a light at the end of the tunnel. The drugs can make it possible to do the work of therapy more easily.

What Kind of Support Is Available?

You may be surprised at how much support is available once you begin to look. Here's an overview:

FRIENDS AND FAMILY   According to a report in *Ms.* magazine, "Researchers Phyllis Kernoff Mansfield and Ann Voda surveyed more than 500 women aged thirty-five to fifty-five in the United States and found that they were more likely to seek information about menopause from friends, the media, or even TV sitcoms than from health professionals." Most women get their information about menopause and aging right from the source: other women. When you're looking for support from a confidante, remember to choose your friends wisely. Not every friend can be supportive without being judgmental or giving unwanted advice, and not every friend is ready to deal with your problems. Advice may be offered, but that doesn't mean you have to take it. Make your own choices.

SUPPORT GROUPS Being part of a support group means you can find a great comfort in discussing your issues; the other members of the group let you know you're not alone. Support groups are a way to break isolation, get support, form social networks, and gather information. In a group where you feel you are valued, you may find it easier to have empathy for your own journey. Support groups are formed around many topics: midlife/ menopause loss, depression, spirituality, illness, creating what you want. Look for ongoing support groups in women's centers, counseling centers, and hospitals. If you can't find an already-existing support group, form one of your own. If you have access to the Internet, online support groups can help you feel less isolated even if you're not quite ready to go public with your confusion.

PSYCHOTHERAPY AND COUNSELING Specialists trained in different areas of expertise provide psychotherapy and counseling. You might choose to work with a social worker, a marriage and family counselor, a counselor or clergyperson at

POINT OF INTEREST (continued)

3. Were you able to clarify your position when you felt misunderstood?
4. Were you able to be honest and direct?
5. Did you feel the therapist was interested in you (not preoccupied with other things)?
6. If you were interrupted, did the therapist handle the interruption in a way that did not interfere with your discussion?
7. Did the therapist give you adequate feedback?
8. Could you and the therapist decide on a fee that was comfortable for both of you?
9. Did the therapist seem flexible?
10. Did the therapist make the rules clear at the outset?

Breaking Denial

At thirty-nine I got the strength to admit my husband is an alcoholic. I am beginning to break the denial and am questioning the future. I go to Al-Anon meetings and feel supported for making changes. I used to think people who were alcoholics or had problems were people on the street; now I see everyone has issues to deal with, and I for one am ready.

Suzanne, 41

How to Start a Midlife/ Menopause Support Group

If you want to work on midlife issues in relationship with other women, but you can't find a support group in your area, why not start one of your own? Here are some ideas for getting started.

How do I start? If you know at least one other woman who is interested in the kind of group you have in mind, work together. Ask friends if they are interested in being in the group, and have them ask their friends. You will probably want to limit the size to between seven and ten women. Everyone should agree to this important rule: Maintain confidentiality. What is said in group stays in group.

What will the meetings be like? One advantage to creating your own group is customizing it to your needs. Discuss together where you will meet (At a cafe? At a different house each week? At a local community center?), how often, and for how long. Decide how you will run the meetings. Will there be a leader? Will leader be a rotating position? You might have a topic of the week, or you might give each woman a chance to check in at the beginning of the meeting. Your group may want to have experts speak on certain topics, learn relaxation techniques, or share ritual activities. If the group lasts for a long time, you may move from personal issues into the greater community, lobbying for better health care for midlife women or developing a lending library.

It may take a few weeks of trial and error to find out what format works best for your particular group. Listen to members' wants and needs. Be flexible and willing to change your original ideas if they no longer work for the group.

your place of worship, a hospital social worker, a crisis counselor, or a psychologist or a psychiatrist who is also able to prescribe medication. Whether therapy is short-term or long-term, learning new coping skills should leave you feeling more confident in your ability to deal with life's inevitable ups and downs. Such action can help you achieve a more hopeful present and future.

How Can I Find a Therapist?

The relationship between you and your therapist is at the heart of the work you do together. Healing requires honesty and intimacy, so it's important to trust and feel supported by your therapist. It may take some time and effort to find a person you feel comfortable working with. Finding a therapist is a lot like finding a health practitioner. Ask a friend or another professional for a referral, check out your local women's center, local college or university, and service agencies; or check the Resources at the end of this chapter. It is good to have several referrals to begin this process so that you can feel comfortable that you've made the right choice.

SIDE TRIPS: OTHER PATHWAYS THROUGH THIS BOOK
· · · · · · · · · · · · · · · · · · ·

CHAPTER 1: ENDINGS/BEGINNINGS   Many of the issues brought up in midlife are complex; we may need assistance to resolve them. Look here for ideas that may help you understand the nature of this transition and feel less alone.

CHAPTER 5: BREATHE EASY   If you're troubled by mild to moderate mood swings, stress may be one cause. Look here for some ways to cope with the stresses in your life.

CHAPTER 17: THE INNER JOURNEY   Exploring your spiritual journey can bring the comfort of a broader perspective. Look here for an introduction to the nature of the inner midlife journey.

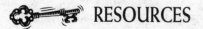 RESOURCES

Organizations and Services

Al-Anon Family Group Headquarters, 1600 Corporate Landing Parkway, Virginia Beach, VA 23454-5617. Voice: (800) 344-2666. Fax: (757) 563-1655. World Directory Meeting Line: (800) 356-9996. Al-Anon is a twelve-step self-help support organization for the friends and families of alcoholics. It will send you free information about the organization geared to either friends, family members, or professionals. You can also get a referral to an Al-Anon support group in your area.

Alcoholics Anonymous, World Services, 475 Riverside Drive, New York, NY 10115. Voice: (212) 870-3400. Fax: (212) 870-3003. Internet: www.alcoholics anonymous.org. AA is a twelve-step self-help support organization for alcoholics. You can call here to get information about AA as well as a referral to a local group.

American Psychological Association, 750 First St. N.E., Washington, DC 20002-4242. Voice: (800) 374-2721. Call this group for a referral to a licensed psychologist in your area. To get the publication "Finding Help: How to Choose a Psychologist," send a stamped, self-addressed business-size envelope to Public Communications at the above address. For a fee, you can order a copy of "Women and Depression: Risk Factors and Treatment Issues."

American Psychological Society, 1010 Vermont Ave. N.W., Suite 1100, Washington, DC 20005-4907. Voice: (202) 783-2077. Internet: psych.hanover.edu/ aps. This nonprofit professional organization can send you research information on mental health disorders.

American Psychiatric Association, 1400 K St. N.W., Washington, DC 20005. Voice: (202) 682-6000 or (800) 368-5777. This group will refer you to your state branch, where you can get a referral to a psychiatrist in your area. Call the 800 number to find out about purchasing information about ethical guidelines.

American Psychiatric Association, Committee on Women, 1400 K St. N.W., Washington, DC 20005. (202) 682-6857. This group's primary goal is to assist women psychiatrists and, by so doing, assist women who need psychiatric help. Call about printed material on women and psychiatric concerns.

American Self-Help Clearinghouse, North West Covenant Medical Center, 25 Pocono Road, Denville, NJ 07834. Voice: (201) 625-7101. Fax: (201) 625-8848. E-mail: ashc@bc.cybernex.net. Internet: www.cmhc.com/selfhelp. This clearinghouse has a national database of support groups. It can put you in touch with national groups or with a clearinghouse in your state, or it can refer you to agencies that will help you find support groups in your area. For a low fee, the clearinghouse will send you a source book listing all the national groups. Also available is information on how to set up your own support group. A real find.

American Association of Marriage and Family Therapy, 1133 15th St. N.W., Suite 300, Washington, DC 20005. Voice: (800) 374-2638. This is a professional organization of marriage and family therapists. Send a stamped, self-addressed business-size envelope to the attention of Mr. Johnson to get a referral to a counselor who specializes in issues of relationship and family.

American Association of Pastoral Counselors, 9504A Lee Highway, Fairfax, VA 22031. Voice: (703) 385-6967. Fax: (703) 352-7725. E-mail: info@aapc.org. This organization certifies pastoral counselors and accredits pastoral counseling centers. It will refer you to a pastoral organization in your area.

American Foundation of Suicide Prevention, 120 Wall St., 22nd Floor, New York, NY 10005. Voice: (888) 333-AFSP. Fax: (212) 363-6237. Internet: www.afsnet.org. This organization will provide referrals to suicide prevention services and support groups in your area. You can also purchase a directory of centers around the country. AFSP also publishes a newsletter, *Lifesavers.* Your local telephone book will also provide a quick reference to the local suicide prevention/crisis hotline.

American Group Psychotherapy Association, 25 E. 21st St., New York, NY 10010. Voice: (212) 477-2677. Fax: (212) 979-6627. Call for educational material on group psychotherapy and a consumer's guide to group psychotherapy. The association will also refer you to an affiliate society that can make a referral to a group psychotherapist in your area.

Anxiety Disorders Association of America, 6000 Executive Blvd., Suite 513, Rockville, MD 20852. Voice: (301) 231-9350. Fax: (301) 231-7392. Internet: www.CyberPsych.org. This association distributes information on anxiety disorder and can provide you with a list of specialists in your area.

Anxiety Disorder Education Program, 5600 Fishers Lane, Room 7-99, Rockville, MD 20857. Voice: (800) 647-2642. This organization offers free educational material on anxiety disorders for the public and the professional.

Association for Death Education Counseling, 638 Prospect Ave., Hartford, CT 06105-7503. Voice: (860) 586-7503. Fax: (860) 586-7550. Fax on demand: (860) 586-7550. E-mail: ADECoffice@aol.com. This professional organization in bereavement can refer you to a certified grief counselor, or you can get a list from the fax-on-demand number.

Catholic Charities USA, 1731 King St., Suite 200, Alexandria, VA 22314. Voice: (703) 549-1390. Fax: (703) 549-1656. Internet: www.catholiccharitiesusa.org. Call here to get a referral to a Catholic counseling service in your area.

Center for Mental Health Services, P.O. Box 6003, Rockville, MD 20849-6003. Voice: (800) 789-2647. Internet: www.mentalhealth.org. This organization distributes a mental health directory and provides free educational material.

Depression/Awareness, Recognition, and Treatment (D/ART), National Institute of Mental Health, 5600 Fishers Lane, Room 10-85, Rockville, MD 20857. Voice: (800) 421-4211 or (301) 443-4140. This national program is designed to educate the public and professionals about the symptoms and treatments of depressive disorders. The organization provides written and audiovisual educational materials for the public as well as training programs for professionals. To get a copy of "Depression: What Every Woman Should Know" and other free brochures, call the 800 number.

Jewish Family Services, 3086 State Highway 27, Suite 11, P.O. Box 248, Kendall Park, NJ 08824. Voice: (800) 634-7346. Fax: (908) 821-0493. E-mail: ajfca@aol.com. Call here for a referral to your local Jewish Family Service Agency for counseling and support.

Mental Health Policy Resource Center, 1730 Rhode Island Ave. N.W., Suite 308, Washington, DC 20036-3101. Voice: (202) 775-8826. Internet: www.pie.org. This nonprofit public policy organization provides customized research services and maintains an extensive library.

National Association of Social Workers, 7981 Eastern Ave., Silver Spring, MD 20910. Voice: (800) 638-8799. This professional organization has a referral service to help you find a social worker in your area.

National Coalition Against Domestic Violence, P.O. Box 18749, Denver, CO 80218-0749. Voice: (303) 839-1852. Fax: (303) 831-9251. This national information and referral service publishes a national directory of domestic violence programs and will put you in touch with a program in your area. The coalition also has a public policy branch.

National Depressive and Manic–Depressive Association, 730 N. Franklin, Suite 501, Chicago, IL 60610. Voice: (800) 826-3632. This nonprofit advocacy association distributes information on depression and bipolar illness and will provide referrals to support groups or a chapter in your area.

National Domestic Violence Hotline, 3616 Far West Blvd., Suites 101–297, Austin, TX 78731. Voice: (512) 453-8117. Fax: (512) 453-8541. Hotline: (800) 799-SAFE. E-mail: ndvh@admin.inetport.com. Internet: www.inetport.com/~ndbh. This organization provides information, referrals, and resources for victims of domestic violence. It also operates a hotline for emergency information and help.

National Institute of Mental Health, 5600 Fishers Lane, Room 7C-02, Rockville, MD 20857-0001. Voice: (301) 443-4513. Fax: (301) 443-4279. Internet: www.nimh. hih.gov. Ask for free educational material about mental health issues. This group has some information specially geared to women, such as brochures on women and depression and eating disorders.

National Mental Health Association, 1021 Prince St., Alexandria, VA 22314-2971. Voice: (800) 969-6642. Internet: www.worldcorp.com/dc-online/nmha. This is a nonprofit advocacy organization that provides some information on mental health issues and referrals to nationwide organizations.

North American Menopause Society (NAMS), c/o Department of OB/GYN, University Hospitals of Cleveland, 11100 Euclid Ave., Cleveland, OH 44106. Voice: (216) 844-8748. Fax: (216) 844-8708. E-mail: nams@atk.et. Internet: www. menopause.org/all.html. NAMS members include therapists and social workers with interest and experience in working with issues of midlife and menopause. Ask for a list of qualified member therapists in your area.

The Samaritan, 500 Commonwealth Ave., Boston, MA 02215. Voice: (617) 536-2460. Fax: (617) 247-0207. This organization offers befriending, nonjudgmental support by phone. The Samaritan will provide referrals to crisis lines on the East Coast and countries abroad.

Shealy Institute, 1328 E. Evergreen St., Springfield, MO 65803. Voice: (417) 865-5940. Fax: (417) 865-6111. This twenty-five-year-old institute offers the ReGenesis Program for recovering from depression and life crisis. It offers amultidisciplinary approach to recovery, including nutrition counseling, relaxationtechniques, stress management, medical and psychological examinations, and more.

The Stone Center for Developmental Services and Studies, Wellesley College, Wellesley, MA 02181-8293. Voice: (617) 283-2510. The Stone Center deals with Relational Therapy, a new theoretical approach to psychology based on the experience of women. "Works in Progress," its series of publications, deals with a variety of issues. "Women's Groups: How Connections Heal," Works in Progress No. 47, 1990, is particularly interesting. Ask for a list of publications and audiocassettes.

Women's Feminist Therapy Center, 562 West End Ave., Suite A, New York, NY 10024. Voice: (212) 721-7005. This center offers training in object relations theory from a feminist perspective. The Center can refer you to mental health professionals in your area who have participated in its training.

ADJUNCTIVE THERAPIES

American Art Therapy Association, 1202 Allanson Road, Mundelein, IL 60060. Voice: (847) 949-6064. Fax: (847) 566-5480. This organization of professionals holds that the creative process involved in making art is healing and life-enhancing. Call to get in touch with a local chapter that will refer you to an art therapist in your area.

American Horticultural Therapy Association, 362A Christopher Ave., Gaithersburg, MD 20879. Voice: (800) 634-1603. Fax: (301) 869-2397. This professional organization of horticultural therapists specializes in using plants, gardening, and horticultural activities as an adjunct to other therapies to heal body, mind, and spirit. This group develops educational programs, publishes reports and periodicals, and operates a national project for people with disabilities. Contact the AHTA for more information (it does not provide referrals).

National Association for Music Therapy, 8455 Colesville Road, Suite 100, Silver Spring, MD, 20910. Voice: (301) 589-3300. Fax: (301) 589-5175. E-mail: namt@namt.com. This professional organization will provide you with information about adjunctive music therapy. You can request a list of professional music therapists in your area.

Hotlines

National Council on Alcoholism and Drug Dependence: (800) 622-2255.

National Domestic Violence Hotline: (800) 799-SAFE. This twenty-four-hour hotline will refer you to counseling services or battered-women shelters in your area and will do some crisis intervention.

National Mental Health Services Knowledge Exchange Network: (800) 789-2647. Call about informational booklets, articles, and videos or to get a referral to a state or private mental health association near you.

Al-Anon World Directory Meeting Line: (800) 356-9996.

Products and Catalogs

Compassion Books, 477 Hannah Branch Road, Burnsville, NC 28714. Voice: (704) 675-9670. Fax: (704) 675-9687. This is a catalog of resources on death, grief, and loss, including books, videos, and audiocassettes.

Courage to Change: Books for Life's Challenges, P.O. Box 2140, Cranberry Township, PA 16066. Voice: (800) 440-4003. Fax: (800) 772-6499. This is a catalog of books on psychosocial topics.

Medic Publishing Co., P.O. Box 89, Redmond, WA 98073. Voice: (206) 881-2883. Fax: (206) 867-8939. This is a source for two publications by Amy Hillyard Jensen. "Healing Grief," 2d ed., is a twenty-four-page booklet that is helpful and concise in its discussion of grief. It includes a reading list. "Is There Anything I Can Do to Help? Suggestions for the Friend and Relative of the Grieving Survivor" offers clear, simple things you can do to help. You can request a product list that allows you to buy the printed material in bulk or by the copy.

Periodicals

Bereavement: A Magazine of Hope and Healing, Bereavement Publishing Inc., 8133 Telegraph Drive, Colorado Springs, CO 80920. Voice: (719) 282-1948. This bimonthly magazine deals with issues of bereavement. This company also has a catalog of bereavement-related items including cards, brochures, books, and tapes.

Psychology Today, Sussex Publishers, 49 E. 21st St., 11th Floor, New York, NY 10010. Voice: (800) 234-8361. You can find this glossy magazine on many newsstands. Each issue covers a wide range of emotional, intellectual, and mental health issues in a style geared to the general public.

Books

Mandy Aftel, M.A., M.F.C.C., and Robin Tolmach Lakoff, Ph.D. *When Talk Is Not Cheap, or How to Find the Right Therapist When You Don't Know Where to Begin.* New York: Warner Books, 1985. This book offers a lot of practical and straightforward information about finding a therapist, what to expect, and how and when to terminate the therapeutic relationship.

Melody Beattie. *Codependent No More: How to Stop Controlling Others and Start Caring for Yourself.* New York: Harper/Hazeldon, 1987. A how-to book about how to stop the pain that is part of the package of codependency. Written by a recovering alcoholic and codependency counselor.

Carmen Raner Berg. *Coming Home to Your Body: 365 Simple Ways to Nourish Yourself Inside and Out.* Berkeley, CA: Page Mill Press, 1996. Day-by-day quotes and self-exploratory questions and exercises to make you feel good.

Paula J. Caplan. *Don't Blame Mother: Mending the Mother–Daughter Relationship.* New York: Harper & Row, 1989. A look at this important and meaningful relationship. Offers understanding of the sometimes conflicted relationship we have with our mothers. It addresses how mothers and daughters have been taught to think about each other and helps break those bad mother myths.

Mary Ellen Copeland, M.S. *The Depression Workbook, A Guide for Living with Depression and Manic Depression.* Oakland, CA: New Harbinger Press, 1992. This book is interactive and useful in understanding depression.

Mani Feniger, *Journey from Anxiety to Freedom: Moving Beyond Panic and Phobias and Learning to Trust Yourself.* Rocklin, CA: Prima Publishing, 1997. Feniger, a certified clinical hypnotherapist and founder of the Anxiety and Phobia Peer Support Group, gives encouragement and hope to anyone who has ever experienced the terror of a panic attack. Personal stories, her own and others, illustrate how it is possible to work with fear as a teacher and recover from panic and anxiety.

Karen Johnson, M.D. *Trusting Ourselves: The Complete Guide to Emotional Well-Being for Women.* New York: Atlantic Monthly Press, 1991. Dr. Johnson, a psychiatrist, has written a "definitive and comprehensive" book examining all aspects of women and psychology. This is a book that gives an understanding of psychology from a woman's perspective as well as ways to make change and find professional help.

Elisabeth Kübler-Ross. *Death, the Final Stage of Growth.* Englewood Cliffs, NJ: Prentice Hall, 1975. An important book for anyone coping with loss.

Stephen Levine. *Healing into Life and Death.* New York: Anchor Press, 1987. This book contains techniques for working with pain and grief. There are influences from Buddhist, Zen, and other traditions. Finishing business with oneself and others is an aspect of healing and of dying.

Stephen Levine. *Who Dies: An Investigation of Conscious Living and Conscious Dying.* New York: Doubleday, 1982. Stephen Levine teaches workshops for the terminally ill. His work uses guided meditations for healing. Reading this book lessens the emotional pain of dying; it is a source of great compassion.

Linda Schierse Leonard. *Wounded Woman: Healing the Father-Daughter Relationship.* Boston: Shambhala, 1982. Exploring the problematic relationship between father and daughter and ways to heal it.

Jennifer Louden. *The Woman's Comfort Book.* San Francisco: HarperSanFrancisco, 1992. Sometimes it's more difficult to care for yourself than it is to care for others. This book offers 200 soothing recipes and rituals for relaxation, practical self-care, and growth.

Ann Mankowitz. *Change of Life: A Psychological Study of Dreams and the Menopause.* Toronto: Inner City Books, 1984. A Jungian therapist tells of women and their dreams at the time of menopause. This book looks at the wisdom of our dreams and is fascinating to read.

Jean Baker Miller, M.D. *Toward A New Psychology of Women.* 2nd ed. Boston: Beacon Press, 1986. This book describes the life, thoughts, and feelings of women and reflects how their psychological and emotional lives reflect the social and political system. Dr. Miller explores the role of relationships in women's lives and how there can be growth of both self and relationship.

Ernest Morgan. *Dealing Creatively with Death: A Manual of Death Education and Simple Burial.* 13th ed. Bayside, NY: Zinn Communications, 1994. This book offers education about death and dying, bereavement, legal issues, and ceremonies. This concise and informative book offers lots of practical and important information.

Judy Tatlebaum. *The Courage to Grieve.* New York: Harper & Row, 1980. A timeless book on grief and grief resolution. It contains important information about finishing business with self and others and learning to let go; it is written with love and compassion.

Audio/Video

You'll find good tapes on support at some of the agencies listed in Organizations and Services, above, and from **AARP** (see Resources in Chapter 15, "Everybody Needs Me

Now"). For tapes on psychology and spirit, see the catalogs listed in Chapter 7, "The Holistic Kit and Caboodle," and Chapter 17, "The Inner Journey."

New Harbinger Publications, Inc., Self-Help Catalog Books and Tapes, 5674 Shattuck Ave., Oakland, CA 94609. Voice: (800) 748-6273. Quality self-help books and audio- and videotapes on such issues as addiction, depression, and death and dying.

VIDEOS

Taking Control of Depression. Available from AARP (see Chapter 15). This video features physicians from the National Institutes of Mental Health in a comprehensive look at clinical depression.

Online

For many people, communicating with others over the Internet is a first step to breaking isolation and getting help. As you'll see from the listings, there's a human face to cyberspace.

MAILING LISTS

If you're suffering from depression, check out **WALKERS-DIGEST (Walkers in Darkness).** For subscription information, contact Majordomo@world.std.com. For support in the worst of times, try **SUICIDE-SUPPORT.** For subscription information, contact listserv@research.canon.oz.au.

NEWS GROUPS

You'll find a number of news groups around emotional issues, all with descriptive names: **alt.support.anxiety-panic, alt.support.social-phobia, alt.support. depression, alt.support.depression.manic, alt.support.depression.seasonal, soc. support.depression, soc.support.misc, soc.support.treatment, soc.support.crisis, soc.support.family, soc.support.manic, soc.support.seasonal.**

WEB SITES

A good starting place to find information, booklets, magazine articles, and links regarding all types of mental disorders is **WWWMental Health Server** at www.mental health.com. **Mental Health Net** at cmhc.com is another good general site. Check out its **Anxiety Guide** at cmhc.com/guide/anxiety.htm for anxiety- and panic-related links on the net, or its **Depression Guide** at cmhc.com/guide/depress.htm for lots of links to sites dealing with depression, including personal stories.

For questions and answers about depression, see the American Psychological Association's **FAQ About Women and Depression** at apa.org/pubinfo/depress.html. The **Depression Resource List,** earth.execpc.com/~corbeau, is a very good guide to online resources.

You'll find the **APA Guide to Choosing a Psychiatrist,** the American Psychological Association's interesting and informative guide, at apa.org/pubinfor/howto.htm.

17

THE INNER JOURNEY
Spirituality

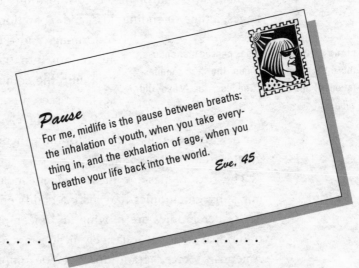

Pause

For me, midlife is the pause between breaths: the inhalation of youth, when you take everything in, and the exhalation of age, when you breathe your life back into the world.

Eve, 45

The midlife journey sweeps you along, whether you're ready to go or not. Along the way, you put a great deal of energy into dealing with the physical changes of midlife and into struggling with questions of illness and wellness and how you are going to live. But it's important to be aware that these changes also reflect changes that are occurring on a deeper level: as an initiation into a new life.

Choosing to live through midlife with this awareness means that you do not suddenly wake up one day and say, "What happened?" You know what happened, because you did the work. As Ursula Le Guin has said, menopause is "a built-in rite of passage" from one stage of life to another. Living this biological process with awareness is a way to consciously participate in the wonder of life and change. This transforming journey is a gift filled with potential. As we leave behind the regenerative power of monthly renewal, we come into the power to be ourselves.

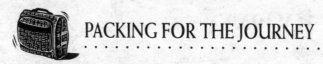

PACKING FOR THE JOURNEY

What Is a "Rite of Passage?"

A rite of passage or initiation honors a person's transition from one phase of life to another, acknowledging its spiritual dimension and connection to all of life. Like transition, a rite of passage has three stages: a time of ending, loss, and separation; a time of unknowing and re-forming; and a time of renewal, when we are reborn into the new life and welcomed back into the community. The rite of passage acts as a sacred container for the fragmented and confusing elements of change, infusing them with meaning and transforming them into a new whole that is greater than the sum of its parts.

crone   A woman who has passed menopause; the third stage of Woman, the third manifestation of the Triple Goddess; the Wise Old Woman.

The rites of passage in our society include confirmations and bat mitzvahs, ceremonies that mark a child's entry into young adulthood. These ceremonies are moving and meaningful; but, in contrast with traditional societies, relatively little is asked of the initiate in modern American society. Traditional societies impose ordeals during rites of passage that may be physically dangerous and painful, reflecting the peril that is at the heart of every transition. Initiates may be taken from the community and turned out into the wilderness. There they wander alone, hungry, thirsty, dependent on their own resources, and at risk of death before they can return. During this time they may enter an altered state in which they feel themselves being taken apart and put back together again in a new way. When finally they return to the community, they are renewed. The community welcomes them back and acknowledges their symbolic rebirth, often giving them a new name to mark the honor.

GUIDED TOUR: *Spirituality*

Menopause incorporates the three stages of transition—ending, unknowing, and renewal. It is an "embodied ritual" because as we progress through its trials with awareness, we also pass through all the stages of initiation into a new life as an older woman. The spiritual work of midlife includes learning to live in the present, feeling one's connection with the infinite, welcoming the self back home, and connecting with the inner wise woman.

MIND–BODY

Meditation, prayer, and mindfulness offer us the opportunity to quiet the mind and go more deeply into ourselves. Our dreams can offer us clues to the nature of our journey. Exploring creative channels is a vital pathway of self-discovery.

Practices such as yoga, t'ai chi, qi gong, and others are designed to work with body and spirit as a whole system. Most of these systems also encourage meditation and mindfulness, and are part of a larger spiritual practice. Many women find that a regular practice involving the mind and body deepens their understanding of the midlife passage.

SUPPORT

Times of change often cause us to reflect on our lives. Find the support you need through friends, others on the spiritual path, a meditation or prayer group, or professional therapy if spiritual awakening becomes spiritual emegency.

COMPLEMENTARY THERAPIES

The physical changes that mark this passage may reflect spiritual changes. Traditional Chinese medicine, Ayurveda, and other old and new treatment systems understand that the separation of mind, body, and spirit can be illusory. You may find relief for discomforts and a new understanding of your body's journey in these traditions.

Design a Croning Ceremony

Reverence for the menopausal process through living it, accepting it, and wanting to honor it may lead you to plan a formalized ritual. In the absence of societal rites of passage, women have begun to make their own rituals to honor each other. One such free-form ritual is the croning ceremony, in which women honor the transition from youth to age. Designing a croning ceremony for yourself or a friend is a vital creative opportunity to recognize this passage. Many women choose to organize a croning ceremony around a birthday and make it the party. You could have a drumming circle, silent meditation, shared feelings about this time of life. Give gifts that symbolize the journey, or honor the new crone with writing, art, and music. And be sure to have a feast! See Resources for more information on midlife rituals.

How Is Menopause an "Embodied Ritual"?

When we choose to honor the biological process of menopause and live it, rather than deny it or manage it out of existence, we become aware that we are on a profound inner journey of transformation. The trials of menopause manifest ritual through our bodies—an embodied ritual—and as we progress through its trials with awareness, we also pass through all the stages of initiation into a new life.

ENDING   In midlife, biology takes us against our will and separates us from the group with which we have identified for most of our lives—sexually potent, attractive young women, potential childbearers. Our menstrual blood, which symbolized potential new life, is lost. Like an initiate, we are thrown into a wilderness of unpredictable change.

UNKNOWING   We spend an unnerving time wandering in this transitional middle ground. We question who we are and wonder what will become of us in this uncharted territory. We undergo disturbing physical ordeals (hot flashes, profuse sweating, flooding or spotting, insomnia) and sometimes painful emotional ordeals that test the new person we are becoming. We live our losses, feel our pain, reclaim long-lost parts of ourselves, and go deep inside for connection and guidance. Anthropologists call this stage *liminal*, a threshold space. We have come to the doorway, but we do not yet know where it leads. This temporary loss of identity is not the cruel trick or senseless punishment it

You're *How* Old?

I feel fortunate to be the age I am at this moment in time. When my mom was my age, not only did she not have a ceremony to honor the wisdom of age, she wouldn't even *tell* her age!

Leslie, 50

may seem: Going through it is vital to the transition. We can't find ourselves unless we are lost. Understanding the process requires, paradoxically, that we first surrender to it.

RENEWAL We enter into stage three having witnessed our rebirth as our true selves: older women, and perhaps wiser women, ready to make a new beginning with the rest of our lives. Instead of bleeding every month, we are said to "retain" our menstrual blood—called by some traditions "wise blood"—for our own use in creating this new life. The post-menopausal body is a new body, a new lived experience that will bring about a different way of being in the world. We have been tested and we have survived; and because of this we are more certain of our strength, our power, and our true nature. We are welcomed into the community of women who have passed into this stage before us, and we see them with new eyes.

> We are all on a pilgrimage of sorts, though it is certainly not necessary to travel physically to sacred places and conduct ceremonies to release our past. It *is* necessary, however, to travel spiritually and to shed the fears that block us from recognizing the beauty in our lives, and to come to a place of healing and self-acceptance. We can take this type of journey daily in the privacy of our own prayers and meditation.
>
> CAROLYN MYSS, *Anatomy of the Spirit*

What Are Some Pathways on the Inner Journey?

You can explore a number of paths on your inner journey. Choose one or all: They are not mutually exclusive.

THE PATH OF DREAMS Dreams can be the doorway into an inner world rich in meaning and a way to connect that rich meaning with our

Welcoming the Fierce Compassionate Feminine

Our Western sacred and mythic traditions are not kind to women in midlife. The mother-in-law, the old hag, the wicked witch, the evil stepmother, the "bag lady"—these are the images that many of us carry with us when we think of aging. On the other end of the spectrum we have only the kindly grandmother, nice but powerless. In Christianity, the dominant religion of the West, we have the Virgin. Mystical Judaism honors the Shekinah, the feminine indwelling spirit of God, but she is mostly lost to modern Jews. Where, then, is our image of wise and powerful old age?

In her earlier traditional incarnations, the Goddess (and the women created in her image) had three faces: the Maiden, the Mother, and the Crone. Some Crone goddesses of the past include Sophia (Wisdom), Minerva (the Roman goddess of wisdom), and Hecate (the Greek goddess of the underworld associated with the dark of the moon). The Crone was a woman past menopause, who no longer shed her "wise blood" but kept it inside as a source of power. According to author Vicki Noble in *The Motherpeace Tarot,* "The Crone represents a stage of life in which wisdom is sought—a time of introspection and spiritual seeking." The Crone also had magical and mystical powers, a woman who walked easily in both this world and the world of the spirit.

Our society venerates the Maiden and honors the Mother, but the Crone seems to have vanished from our consciousness. In the Hindu and Buddhist traditions of the East, the Goddess still retains her fierce aspect and manages to combine it with compassion. Tara, the female Buddha of the Tibetan tradition, also known as the goddess of Compassion, has

(continued)

daily lives. During midlife and menopause, dreams can be particularly helpful guides. Psychologist Carl Jung felt that women were especially adept at using dreams to connect with their inner selves. Dr. Patricia Garfield, an international expert on dreams, says, "Some women can find their internalized menopausal rite of passage in a dream. Awake, they may seek an unexplored direction, a way to revitalize their energy for abundant and luxurious new growth."

While our conscious mind is worrying about whether or not to take HRT or get more exercise, our unconscious is working on the deep issues that underlie this rocky passage. Jungian analyst Ann Mankowitz says, "At crucial times of development, the conscious mind takes a long time to catch up with and integrate both the bodily changes and the unconscious adjustments of the psyche. It often takes a significant dream to do it, and this seems particularly true during the change of life."

Pay attention to your dreams, and consider keeping a dream journal to chart your inner passage. Listen to what you are trying to tell yourself. For example, a fire alarm may symbolize hot flashes; wandering alone in a harsh landscape may symbolize the midlife passage. Every woman has her own personal dream symbolism, and with a little practice you will soon become familiar with yours.

THE PATH OF CREATIVITY

Far too many of us were told early on that we had "no talent," whether it was for singing, dancing, art, writing, poetry, or athletics, and we stopped dead in our tracks. The belief "I am not creative" is not only crippling, it is untrue. Everyone has a well of creativity waiting to be tapped. To discover yours, begin by exploring anything that piques your interest: cooking, gardening, inventing, teaching, being a student, starting your own business. If you think it's too late, think again. Mystery writer P. D. James began at forty; Julia Child learned about French cooking in midlife and published her first book at fifty; Maggie Kuhn organized the Gray Panthers at sixty-five. Opening yourself to your creative potential may open a window that lets new sunlight pour into your life, illuminating parts of yourself you've never seen before. Give yourself time to discover your path.

THE PATH OF MEDITATION AND PRAYER

Meditation and prayer are central to virtually all religious traditions. They allow us to let go of ourselves for a moment—to empty the mind of fear, anxiety, and desire and to allow it to expand and be filled with the clean air of the infinite. Clearing out this mental clutter, even for a few minutes a day, can have far-reaching effects. It's like spiritual housekeeping. Zen Buddhist nun Charlotte Joko Beck says in *Everyday Zen,* "I don't care how many enlightenment experiences you cling to. There's nothing but daily life. *This table is the dharma* [divine truth]. Yesterday, it was dusty; today it's been dusted."

You may have grown up with prayers of supplication—"Please God, if you do this for me, I'll always be good." According to Larry Dossey, M.D., in *Healing Words: The Power of Prayer and the Practice of Medicine,* laboratory experiments indicate that the most powerful form of prayer seems to be nondirected prayer, "an open-ended approach

many different forms. Some of them are beautiful and peaceful, others are fearsome and frightening to behold. In India the goddess Kali, the Destroyer, is also known as Tara, the goddess of Compassion. In India also we find the goddess Durga, the Great Goddess and Warrior Queen, from whose forehead Kali springs. When the world is on the brink of destruction, only Durga is powerful enough to save it. Even the kind and compassionate Virgin Mary is worshiped in many countries of the world as the Black Madonna, a powerful, miracle-working, healing form of Mary. These are images of the sacred fierce feminine, a power we have long forgotten but which is ours to claim in this passage from Mother to Crone.

Sometimes it seems as if our only choice is to be the kindly grandma or the crazy old witch. How can we integrate these seemingly irreconcilable figures? According to China Galland, author of *Longing for Darkness: Tara and the Black Madonna* and the forthcoming *Fierce Compassion,* the key rests in the seemingly paradoxical concept of Buddhism known as *fierce compassion* or *compassionate wrath.* "We must claim the fierce power that so clearly lies within us," she explains, "but we must wield our sword with compassion, for ourselves and for all beings." We can find our examples in goddesses such as Tara/Kali/Durga and her manifestation in ourselves: women such as Mother Teresa; Laura Bonaparte, the courageous founder of the Mothers of the Disappeared in Argentina; and any woman who can draw the line and say "No" to her child or any other human being out of love.

in which no specific outcome is held in the mind. In non-directed prayer the practitioner does not attempt to 'tell the universe what to do.'" A personal prayer of this sort might be, "I welcome whatever is for my highest good." Learning to meditate and find your own inner connection within an established group gives you a context for the feelings and thoughts that inevitably arise. See the discussion of meditation in Chapter 5, "Breathe Easy," for more information.

THE PATH OF MINDFULNESS It's easier to lose ourselves than to find ourselves. No matter how profound a realization you may have about the true meaning of life, sooner or later you may find yourself lost in worries: What's for dinner? How am I going to pay the Visa bill? Mindfulness—remembering to return to ourselves and appreciate the moment—is an easy way to let go of anxiety and allow ourselves to breathe the air of the infinite. It's free, it's easy, and you can do it anywhere. Catching yourself in these moments of worry or concern with the outer world and returning to this larger sense of well-being is a practice that you can easily integrate into daily life. In *Peace Is Every Step*, Vietnamese Buddhist monk Thich Nhat Hanh suggests reciting these lines silently as you breathe in and out: "Breathing in, I calm my body. Breathing out, I smile. Dwelling in the present moment, I know this is a wonderful moment!"

> Deep listening is listening in every possible way to everything possible to hear, no matter what you are doing. Such intense listening includes the sounds of daily life, of nature, of one's own thoughts, as well as musical sounds. Deep listening is my life's practice.
>
> PAULINE OLIVEROS, musician, composer, teacher

What Are the Spiritual Tasks of Midlife?

Because our society does not honor age, it may seem that once we cross the threshold, there will be nothing left for us to do. In traditional societies, however, women past childbearing age are often the social and spiritual leaders of the group. Awareness of the spiritual tasks of midlife can infuse our daily lives with meaning.

LEARNING TO LIVE IN THE PRESENT   All too often in life we are living in either the past or the future—acting from the pain of old wounds, blaming others for our problems, worrying fearfully about what will become of us. But as women in the middle, we have a unique opportunity to look to the past and the future at the same time. In this pause between breaths, we have a real opportunity to learn, finally, to live in the present. In her book *Change of Life*, psychologist Ann Mankowitz tells this story: "One of the most vital people I know is a woman of eighty-four who is still fascinated by her life day by day as it unfolds, and still learns from it and likes to share her insights. She can hardly remember her menopause, but she says she always found changes stimulating, she had raised five children, it was time for something new. . . . 'I stopped looking forward for something wonderful to happen, and learned to live today, this minute.' Since then she has had another full lifetime of thirty years."

FEELING YOUR CONNECTION WITH THE INFINITE   Feeling a connection with the mysteries of life can help break the isolation of this passage. All religious and spiritual beliefs have connection with the unknowable universe at their core. At this time you may choose simply to meditate and find your own inner connection, to return to a religious practice you may have let drop, to go more deeply into the spiritual realms of a religion in which you are actively involved, or to let yourself study and explore a new one altogether.

WELCOMING YOURSELF BACK HOME   Our twenties and thirties—and even, for some, our forties—are years of learning how to make life work for us in a practical sense: years of earning money, living with a partner, living singly, raising a family, making a home—or any combination of these. Meeting these basic needs can sometimes mean that we protect and even sacrifice vital parts of ourselves. In midlife, when we've learned (more or less) to deal with what life gives us, we have the luxury of allowing these more vulnerable and delicate parts of ourselves to reemerge and reintegrate with our more practical parts. This may mean opening to your creativity in any number of ways: hiking, gardening, traveling, cooking, letter writing. . . . Enjoy watching yourself unfold.

CONNECTING WITH YOUR INNER WISE WOMAN   Midlife gives us the opportunity to connect with our inner wise woman, that strong, clear voice within who keeps us on the path. You may be able to hear her voice simply by opening to the possibility, or you may connect with her through dreams and meditation. Listen to what she has to say. She is you.

> There are things the Old Woman can do, say, and think which the Woman cannot do, say, or think. The Woman has to give up more than her menstrual periods before she can do, say, or think them. She has got to change her life.
>
> URSULA LE GUIN, "The Space Crone"

 # SIDE TRIPS: OTHER PATHWAYS THROUGH THIS BOOK

CHAPTER 1: ENDINGS/BEGINNINGS   In many ways the spiritual journey embodies the stages of the midlife transition. Look here to learn more about this powerful period in your life.

CHAPTER 2: WHY IS THIS HAPPENING TO ME?   Menopause is an embodied ritual and a physical fact of life. Look here to learn more about this once-in-a-lifetime experience.

CHAPTER 3: KEEP ON MOVING   Mind–body practices such as yoga and qi gong help us to integrate body and spirit. Look here for an overview.

CHAPTER 5: BREATHE EASY   Meditation is a time-honored doorway to the inner journey. Look here to learn more about how you can begin meditating.

RESOURCES

Organizations and Services

Your community probably has many resources for organized religion, including your local church, temple, synagogue, mosque, or Buddhist meditation center; and community services can be found in places such as the Jewish Community Center. If you're interested in exploring women's spirituality, a women's center and women's bookstore are good starting points.

Center for Women and Religion, Graduate Theological Union, 2400 Ridge Road, Berkeley, CA 94709. Voice: (510) 649-2490. This nondenominational, interfaith group has a number of publications and tapes. Membership will bring you the *Journal of Women and Religion*.

The Community of Mindful Living, P.O. Box 7355, Berkeley, CA 94707. Voice: (510) 527-3751. Fax: (510) 525-7129. CML is a nonprofit religious center that acts as a clearinghouse for the teachings of Thich Nhat Hanh. CML's work includes publishing books and tapes, organizing retreats for the practice of mindfulness, and conducting community programs, including those for veterans of war.

Jewish Women's Resource Center, Project of the National Council of Jewish Women, New York Section, 9 E. 69th St., New York, NY 10021. Voice: (212) 535-5900, ext. 11. Fax: (212) 535-5509. The Jewish Women's Resource Center has been collecting books, periodicals, and other material on Jewish women for twenty-five years; the Center has a reference library of more than 10,000 items. Contact this organization regarding information on any aspect of Jewish women, including books, printed material, and homemade ceremonies dealing with rituals for Jewish women in midlife.

Mind/Body Health, Inc., 393 Dixon Road, Boulder, CO 80302. Voice: (303) 440-8460. This organization was founded by Joan Borysenko, author of *A Woman's Book of Life*. It's a good source for books and tapes, and you can find out where Borysenko is speaking or arrange for her to speak. You can request the free annual newsletter and catalog, *Circle of Healing*, which offers books and tapes by Borysenko.

Spiritual Eldering Institute, 7318 Germantown Ave., Philadelphia, PA 19919. Voice: (888) ELD-RING. E-mail: SprtElder@aol.com. Internet: www.SpiritualEldering. com. The philosophy of the Spiritual Eldering Institute is described in *From Age-ing to Sage-ing*, by Zalman Schachter-Shalomi and Ronald Miller. The Institute works to empower people to age consciously, harvest their life's experience and transmit their wisdom. The Institute offers workshops and leader training seminars around the United States. Some of the basic concepts include life review, forgiveness work, establishing mentoring relationships, and facing our mortality. Ask for a copy of the newsletter.

Wise Woman Center, P.O. Box 64, Woodstock, NY 12498. Voice: (914) 246-8081. This center, run by herbalist Susun Weed, offers one-, two-, and three-day workshops on many topics, including menopause.

Women's Alliance for Theology, Ethics, and Ritual (WATER), 8035 13th St., Suites 1, 3, and 5, Silver Spring, MD 20910. Voice: (301) 589-2509. Fax: (301) 589-3150. E-mail: water@hers.com. Internet: www.hers.com/water. WATER is a feminist educational center, a "think and do tank" co-founded in 1983 by theologian and ethicist Mary Hunt and therapist and liturgist Diann Neu, in response to the need for serious theological, ethical, and liturgical development by and for women. WATER provides programs, projects, publications, workshops, retreats, consulting, counseling, and liturgical creation. The approach to women's spirituality is inclusive, and liturgies may include Native American and Wiccan as well as Christian and other traditional modes of Western religion. Membership in this nonprofit organization brings the journal *WATERwheel*, which includes monthly feminist rituals (the Winter 1996 issue has a ritual called "Change of Life: Journey Through Menopause"), along with many other benefits.

Periodicals

Common Boundary, 5272 River Road, Suite 650, Bethesda, MD 20816. Voice: (301) 652-9495. This bimonthly magazine explores relationships between spirituality, psychology, and creativity.

Creation Spirituality, P.O. Box 8749, Emeryville, CA 94662. Voice: (510) 547-8073. Former Catholic priest Matthew Fox is the editor-in-chief of this quarterly journal, which explores creation spirituality, new science, feminism, and art.

Gnosis, P.O. Box 14217, San Francisco, CA 94114. Voice: (800) 7-GNOSIS. This quarterly journal explores the inner traditions of Judaism, Christianity, and Islam, as well as Paganism and general mystic and occult traditions of the West.

Journal of Women and Religion, Center for Women and Religion, Graduate Theological Union, 2400 Ridge Road, Berkeley, CA 94709. Voice: (510) 649-2490. Free with your membership in the Center for Women and Religion.

SageWoman, P.O. Box 641, Point Arena, CA 95468. Voice: (707) 882-2052. A quarterly Wiccan magazine that celebrates the Goddess.

New Age Journal, 42 Pleasant St., Watertown, MA 02172. Voice: (617) 926-0200. E-mail: editor@newage.com. Internet: www.newage.com. This glossy bimonthly magazine explores New Age spirituality, wellness, and just about every other aspect of life from a holistic perspective. Available on most newsstands. If you have Internet access, the online version has a wealth of information.

The Mindfulness Bell, P.O. Box 7355, Berkeley, CA 94707. This magazine is published three times a year by the Community of Mindful Living. It includes articles by

Thich Nhat Hanh and others about how to practice mindfulness in daily life. You'll also find national and international listings for retreats and mindfulness groups.

Tikkun, P.O. Box 460926, Escondido, CA 92046-9914. Voice: (800) 846-8575. Internet: www.panix.com/~tikkun/index2.html. This bimonthly magazine for Jewish Renewal, founded by Michael Lerner, is a thoughtful and thought-provoking progressive critique of politics and society.

Tricycle: The Buddhist Review, 92 Van Dam St., New York, NY 10013. Voice: (800) 950-7008. Internet: www.tricycle.com/index.html. An award-winning quarterly journal on all aspects of Buddhism and contemporary society, including interviews with American and Asian teachers. Always intriguing.

Books

Joan Borysenko, Ph.D. *A Woman's Book of Life: The Biology, Psychology, and Spirituality of the Feminine Life Cycle*. New York: Riverhead Books, 1996. Borysenko mingles personal stories with a rich mine of information to illuminate the interconnection of women's bodies, emotions, and spiritual nature. This is an intriguing book.

Frederic and Mary Ann Brussat. *Spiritual Literacy: Reading the Sacred in Everyday Life*. New York: Scribner, 1996. A rich sampler of stories, sayings, and observations from an enormous range of sources. A spring of spiritual refreshment.

Susan Cahill, ed. *Wise Women: Over 2,000 Years of Spiritual Writings by Women*. New York: Norton, 1996. Writings by female poets, shamans, visionaries from ancient times to today. This is an inspiring collection for women at any time of life.

Sarah and A. Elizabeth Delany with Amy Hill Hearth. *The Delany Sisters' Book of Everyday Wisdom*. New York: Kodansha, 1994. Sarah and Bessie Delany were among the very first African American professional women. At 100-plus years old, they share their inspiring and intelligent thoughts.

Christine Downing. *Journey Through Menopause: A Personal Rite of Passage*. New York: Crossroad, 1987. "I was at the brink of a centrally important life-change," says Downing, "and had no knowledge of the myths or rituals that had helped women throughout history live this transition with hope, dignity and depth." Her solution was to make a literal journey as a ritual for her passage through menopause. She uses mythology and place to weave a story of this transition that is both personal and universal.

Pamela J. Free. *Come Home to Your Body: A Workbook for Women*. St. Paul, MN: Llewellyn Publications, 1997. This book, based on the Feldenkrais method of bodywork, offers exercises to help connect you more deeply with your mind, body, and spirit. The author also offers inspirational thoughts and encourages using a notebook to record thoughts and feelings.

China Galland, *Longing for Darkness: Tara and the Black Madonna.* New York: Penguin, 1991. The story of Galland's personal journey of spiritual discovery in her search to learn more about Tara, the Buddhist goddess of compassion, and the Black Madonna. Her forthcoming book *Sacred Fierceness* (New York: Riverhead, 1998) is about her search for the sacred fierce feminine as it is embodied in women around the world.

Patricia Lyn Reilly. *A God Who Looks Like Me: Discovering Woman—Affirming Spirituality.* New York: Random House, 1995. A great book if you are looking for a personal and authentic spirituality and are interested in discovering the Wise Old Woman within, no matter what your religion. Full of rituals and packed with ideas.

Rachel Naomi Remen. *Kitchen Table Wisdom.* New York: Riverhead Books, 1996. Remen, a psycho-oncologist, medical director of Commonweal Cancer Help Program, and clinical professor at University of California, San Francisco, Medical School uses storytelling to show how you can enhance your ability to heal yourself and help others do the same.

Rabbi Zalman Schachter-Shalomi and Ronald S. Miller. *From Age-Ing to Sage-Ing: A Profound New Vision of Growing Older.* New York: Warner Books, 1995. Schacter, a rabbi who has also studied the teachings of Sufis, Buddhists, Catholic monks, and Native American elders, is the founder of the Spiritual Eldering Institute. A new vision of what it can mean to be an elder rather than a "senior citizen."

Ann G. Thomas, Ed.D. *The Women We Become: Myths, Folktales, and Stories About Growing Older.* Rocklin, CA: Prima, 1997. Myth is a good mirror in which to see our own faces. Thomas uses familiar and less familiar myths and folktales to explore issues older women must deal with, such as accepting life's limits, relating to the dark feminine, and the reality of death.

RITES OF PASSAGE

Lynn V. Andrews. *Woman at the Edge of Two Worlds Workbook: Menopause and the Feminine Rite of Passage. Exercises, Meditations, and Ceremonies for Transformation and Joy.* New York: Harper Perennial, 1994. Andrews, author of a number of popular books about Native American spirituality and her own quest, offers a number of rituals and meditations for the midlife passage.

S. Levine and Elizabeth Resnick. *A Ceremonies Sampler: New Rites, Celebrations, and Observances of Jewish Women.* San Diego: Women's Institute for Continuing Jewish Education, 1991. Some ideas for Jewish women interested in new ways of honoring their spiritual life.

Denise Shervington, M.D., and Billie J. Pace. *Soul Quest: A Healing Journey for Women of the African Diaspora.* New York: Crown, 1996. A discussion of the process of spiritual healing, with exercises for self-discovery and spiritual healing for African American women.

Edna M. Ward, ed. *Celebrating Ourselves: A Crone Ritual Book.* Portland, ME: Astarte Shell Press, 1992. Croning rituals developed by the Feminist Spiritual Community in Portland, Maine. A good place to get some ideas for creating your own rituals.

RETREAT CENTERS

If you're looking for a peaceful retreat center, these books are a good place to begin.

John Benson. *Transformative Adventures, Vacations, and Retreats: An International Directory of 300+ Host Organizations.* New Millennium Publishing, 1994.

Patricia Christian-Meyers. *Catholic America: Self-Renewal Centers and Retreats.* Junction City, OR: Beacon Point Press, 1989. A guide to Catholic retreat centers.

Roger Housden. *Retreat: Time Apart for Silence and Solitude.* San Francisco: HarperSanFrancisco, 1995. A guide to Christian, Jewish, Buddhist, Sufi, and other peaceful retreats.

Marcia and Jack Kelly. *Sanctuaries: A Guide to Lodgings in Monasteries, Abbeys, and Retreats of the United States.* New York: Bell Tower/Harmony. These are regional guides, including *The Northeast* (1991) and *The West Coast and Southwest* (1993).

Orient Foundation. *A Handbook of Tibetan Culture: A Guide to Tibetan Centres and Resources Throughout the World.* Boulder, CO: Shambhala, 1994.

Stanley Young. *Paradise Found: Beautiful Retreats and Sanctuaries of California and the Southwest.* San Francisco: Chronicle Books, 1995. Features twenty-three gorgeous retreats, from healing centers to Buddhist temples.

Audio/Video

When it comes to spirituality, audiocassettes and videotapes are abundantly available. Rather than recommend an exhaustive list, we suggest you check out these catalogs or visit a women's bookstore or spiritual bookstore to see what's available. You'll find other good catalogs for these tapes, such as **Living Arts, Sound Horizons,** and **Sounds True,** listed in Chapter 5, "Breathe Easy," and Chapter 7, "The Holistic Kit and Caboodle."

New Dimensions Tapes, P.O. Box 569, Ukiah, CA 95482. Voice: (800) 935-8273. Internet: www.newdimensions.org. A catalog of hundreds of audiotapes from the PBS one-hour radio show *New Dimensions,* featuring interviews with such spiritual luminaries as Krishnamurti, Joseph Campbell, Charlotte Spretnak, and Bernie Siegel.

Parallax Press, Books and Tapes for Mindful Living, P.O. Box 7355, Berkeley, CA 94707. E-mail: parapress@aol.com. Voice: (510) 525-0101. Fax: (510) 525-7129. Internet: www.parallax.org. A good source for books and tapes on mindfulness meditation, as well as for Buddhist materials from other publishers.

AUDIO

Wise Woman Archetype: Menopause as Initiation. Jean Shinoda Bolen. Available from Sounds True. Bolen explores the sacred dimension of the wise woman/crone that comes after menopause.

Online

Cyberspace and spirituality are a pretty good match. You can find virtually all the spiritual books ever written somewhere on the Web—and much new thought. Explore and enjoy.

MAILING LISTS

For a woman-to-woman discussion of the personal experience of spirituality, try **COE (Circles of Exchange)**. Subscription address: MAJORDOMO@PUNIX.COM. To learn more about books relating to women and spirituality, try **FEM-BIBLIO**. Subscription address: MAJORDOMO@PUNIX.COM. If you're interested in exploring the relationship between spirituality, health, and wellness, try **IHPNET@INTER ACCESS.COM (the International Network for Interfaith Health Practices)**. Subscription address: MAJORDOMO@INTERACCESS.COM. For wide-ranging information on all aspects of spirituality, try **AAA_ Religion_ Spirituality_ Related_ Web_ Sites**. Subscription address: webscout@webcom.com. For women and men interested in goddess spirituality and the incorporation of feminine/feminist ideas in the study and worship of the divine, try **WMSPRTL@UBUM.CC.BUFFALO.EDU**. Subscription address: LISTSERV@UBUM.CC.BUFFALO.EDU. The MotherHeart web site (see below) has its own mailing list, **MOTHERHEART LIST**. Subscription address: motherheart@fdt.net.

NEWS GROUPS

The major world religions are well-represented. For Buddhism, try **alt.buddha. short.fat.guy** (Zen), **alt.religion.buddhism.tibetan**, **talk.religion.buddhism** (all about Buddhism). For Christianity, try **alt.religion.christian** or **soc.religion.christian, soc.religion.christian.bible-study** (Christianity and the Bible). For Hinduism, try **alt.hindu, soc.religion.hindu** (Hindu dharma, philosophy, and culture). For Islam, try **alt.religion.islam** and **soc.religion.islam**. For Judaism, try **soc.culture.jewish** (Jewish culture and religion).

For other religions, explore **alt.pagan** (Paganism and religion), **soc.religion. paganism** (networking for Pagans), **alt.religion.orisha** (African-based religions), **alt.religion.shamanism** (shamanism), **soc.religion.eastern** (various Eastern religions), **soc.religion.quaker** (the Religious Society of Friends), **soc.religion.unitarian-univ** (Unitarian–Universalism and non-creedal religions), **talk.religion.misc** (religious, ethical, and moral implications), and **talk.religion.newage** (esoteric and minority religions and philosophy).

WEB SITES

Check out **Spirit WWW** at www.spiritweb.org for an overview of the many spiritual paths, including yoga, out-of-body experiences, channeling, healing, meditation, Gnosis, Kaballah, mysticism, Sufism, and *many* more. **MotherHeart,** located at gnv.fdt.net/~mother, is a web site with a compassionate heart of gold. Explore numerous links under these headings: community, real life, spirituality, birth, children and parenting, caregiving, health and wholeness, and caring for Gaia.

DharmaNet, at www.dharmanet.org, calls itself the gateway to Buddhist resources. This is the place to find information on meditation retreats, news groups, lists, chats, online dharma libraries, and other spiritual resources and tools.

Visit **Sacred Transformations** at www.well.com/user/bobby to read personal stories of spiritual transformation—out-of-body, near-death experiences, mystical and religious awakenings—and submit your own.

part 2

YOUR PERSONAL COMPANION

By the time it was all over with, she would certainly not have chosen to have had it differently: yet she could not have chosen it for herself in advance, for she did not have the experience to choose, or the imagination. No, she could not want what was going to happen, although she did stand under her tree, the tray in her hands, thinking: It does go on and on! That's what's wrong: There must be something I could be seeing now, something I could be understanding now, some course of action I could choose. . . .

DORIS LESSING, *The Summer Before the Dark*

18

BRINGING IT TOGETHER
Gathering Information

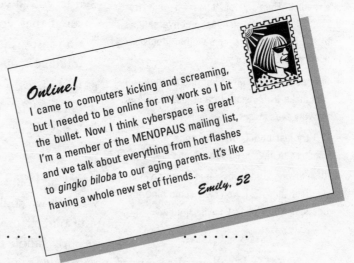

Online!
I came to computers kicking and screaming, but I needed to be online for my work so I bit the bullet. Now I think cyberspace is great! I'm a member of the MENOPAUS mailing list, and we talk about everything from hot flashes to *gingko biloba* to our aging parents. It's like having a whole new set of friends.

Emily, 52

When you're trying to make a decision on a particular issue, gather as much information as you can. Fear and confusion often dissolve in the face of hard data. Your search can be wide-ranging or straight to the point, depending on your time and inclination. For the most part, finding information really isn't difficult. It's just a matter of knowing where and how to look. Here are some of the things we learned in putting together this book:

1. *Define your questions.* Before you begin, make sure you know what you're looking for. If you can state your question clearly, you're that much closer to finding an answer. For example, are you really trying to decide whether or not you should take hormone replacement

Get Your Information in the Form That's Best for You

When the information just doesn't seem to be getting through to you, it might have something to do with the form in which you're getting it. Some people are readers; some are listeners. For example, Melene finds she understands better by listening to what people have to say. She attends lectures, talks with other women in groups, and listens to tapes. Then she mulls things over and lets her decision rise naturally to the top. Naomi, on the other hand, finds that the information goes directly to her brain when she reads it. Then she lets it sit for a while, trying out all sides of a question in conversations with friends. Here are some other decision-making styles:

- "I need to have a lot of information before I can make a decision. I can't just plunge in with my eyes closed."

- "I'll try just about anything once. If I don't like it, I can always do something else."

- "I've always prided myself in being an independent thinker. I won't do something just because some 'expert' says I should."

therapy for the rest of your life, or are you trying to determine how to deal with the hot flashes you're experiencing right now?

2. *Don't be afraid to ask.* You are probably not the first person to ask your particular question, and you won't be the last. Believe it or not, most people are happy to help. You can start close to home—your friends may already have the answers you are looking for. Government and private agencies have a wealth of good information, much of it free, and they are more than happy to send it to you. If you need to go further, rest assured that you can find enough information easily and quickly to enable you to ask intelligent questions of experts.

3. *Keep current.* Make sure your information is up to date. Yesterday's laughable idea is today's accepted wisdom.

How Can I Find Local Resources?

We wish we could have included a local insert of resources for your community. Fortunately, it's fairly simple to compile your own personal list of local resources, whether you live in a small town or an urban area. Begin with the strategies we just discussed, and add the following.

ASK NATIONAL RESOURCES ABOUT LOCAL BRANCHES OR RESOURCES Many organizations are set up to do this. For example, the North American Menopause Society will send you a list of health practitioners in your area who are interested in working with midlife women.

CHECK YOUR LOCAL EXTENSION SCHOOL, LIBRARY, HEALTH CENTERS, AND HOSPITALS Extension schools and community colleges are often great information sources. Libraries are in the information business, and most librarians love sharing the wealth. Many local hospitals offer classes on health issues that affect midlife women, and they often have informative booklets free for the asking.

LET YOUR FINGERS DO THE WALKING Sometimes finding information is as easy as looking it up in the yellow pages. It seems too simple to be true, but it works.

CHECK BULLETIN BOARDS Check the bulletin boards at your gym, library, natural food store, and women's center for notices on classes, groups, seminars, and many other subjects. The natural food store, for example, is a good place to begin looking for complementary health practitioners.

VISIT LIBRARIES AND BOOKSTORES Browse through your library and check your local bookstore: An amazing amount of information is available in printed form. If you can't find the book you're looking for, ask to have it ordered.

VISIT CYBERSPACE The Internet is a big place, but you can meet people from your hometown. If you can't find a news group specific to your area, try a posting that begins, "I'm from Springfield. Does anyone know where I can find . . . ?" It may bring you just what you're looking for. If you don't have a computer with Internet access at home, but you want to check out some of the web sites you see in this book, visit your local library. Many libraries have computers you can use.

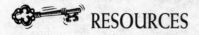 **RESOURCES**

. . . .

Organizations and Services

Federal Information Center, P.O. Box 600, Cumberland, MD 21510-0600. Voice: (800) 688-9889. This is an information clearinghouse for the national government. Looking for the right government agency to help you with your problem? Or the right person in that agency? Start here. Recorded messages include information on federal taxes and jobs, government publications, and other government services.

Feminist Bookstore News, P.O. Box 882554, San Francisco, CA 94188. Voice: (415) 626-1556. Send $1 to receive a list of feminist bookstores throughout the United States. You may even find one in your community that you didn't know about.

National Council for Research on Women, 530 Broadway at Spring St., 10th Floor, New York, NY 10012. Voice: (212) 274-0730. Fax: (212) 274-0821. This network of more than seventy women's research centers and educational institutions may be able to help direct you to just the resource you need. The Council publishes a quarterly journal and newsletter, and it has a directory series, including a directory of women's media, international centers, and opportunities for research and study.

National Women's Mailing List, P.O. Box 68, Jenner, CA 95450. Voice: (707) 632-5763. Fax: (707) 632-5589. E-mail: info@electrapages.com. Internet: www.electra pages.com. If you're interested in women's issues and want to find out what's going on, this is the place. This is something of an introduction service. If you are interested in receiving more mail from a particular source, you let that group know. Register with the National Women's Mailing List, and specify what areas you're most interested in. You can even indicate that you only want to receive mail of interest to midlife women. Rest assured: You will *not* end up on hundreds of mailing lists! You will get mailings from organizations, but they can use your address only once, and they cannot sell it to another organization.

Hotlines

National Health Information Center: (800) 336-4797, or P.O. Box 1133, Washington, DC 20013-1133. Call for a list of 100 hotlines for health referral services.

Books

Robert Berkman. *Find It Fast: How to Research Anything.* New York: HarperCollins, 1994. The name says it all. This book is a great step-by-step guide to information gathering. It demystifies every aspect of the process, from defining your problem, to using the library, to finding the organization you need, to finding experts to talk to and asking the right questions.

Deborah Brecher and Jill Lippitt, eds. *The Women's Information Exchange National Directory.* New York: Avon Books, 1994. If you're looking for a women's service, organization, institution, or program, this list of more than 2,500 addresses and phone numbers is a great reference to have on hand. Look up what you need to know in a wide variety of areas, including arts and the media, professional women's organizations, religious groups, and health.

Shawn Brennan and Julie Winklepleck, eds. *The Resourceful Woman.* Detroit: Visible Ink, 1994. This big book of resources is helpful and interesting. You'll find hundreds of organizations, books, events, videos, and more on everything imaginable pertaining to women of all ages. Each page is adorned with quotes and essays.

Lisa Di Mora and Constance Herndon, eds. *The 1995 Information Please Women's Sourcebook.* New York: Houghton Mifflin, 1994. This book covers just about everything, with phone numbers and addresses, interesting facts, statistics, graphs, and tables. Where to find out what you want to know about just about anything from work and education to family to sexuality.

Thomas Mann. *A Guide to Library Research Methods.* New York: Oxford University Press, 1990. How to search for anything in the library easily and efficiently.

Ilene Rosoff. *The Woman Source Catalog and Review: Tools for Connecting the Community of Women.* Berkeley, CA: Celestial Arts, 1995. A wonderful catalog along the lines of the Whole Earth Catalog, but for women only. Books, organizations, products, and more for just about everything a woman needs. Useful and great fun to read.

Online

To search for a topic or a specific item, use a search engine such as Yahoo (www.yahoo.com), HotBot (www.hotbot.com), Lycos (www.lycos.com), or the system your Internet service provider offers.

News Groups and Mailing Lists

Liszt, www.liszt.com, is a searchable resource that makes it easy to sort through thousands of mailing lists and Usenet news groups to find the one you want.

Web Sites

If you're looking for a magazine to subscribe to, an organization to join, or a business to buy things from and if it's owned by women or aimed at women, you'll probably find it in **ElectraPages, the Women's Resource Locator** at electrapages.com. This database includes more than 7,500 organizations. Search by geographical area, type of service, or name. A project of the Women's Information Exchange.

19

TAKING STOCK

Finding Your Own Path on the Midlife Journey

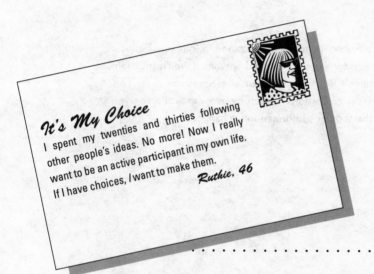

It's My Choice
I spent my twenties and thirties following other people's ideas. No more! Now I really want to be an active participant in my own life. If I have choices, I want to make them.
Ruthie, 46

Our position as women in the middle gives us the perfect opportunity to pause for a moment and survey the territory: where we've been, where we are, and where we want to go. We're fortunate to live in a time that offers us many choices and many paths. Sometimes, however, the sheer abundance of choice can be daunting, and it's a bit of a chore trying to figure out what road to take. This chapter includes an inventory designed to help you see what you've packed for your journey: your physical and emotional needs, your inner and outer support systems, your hopes and dreams, your ideas for action. As you think about the questions, you'll begin to connect with aspects of your life you may not have thought much about, but which will play a part in the decisions you need to make. And as you connect, you'll begin to clear away the debris and the obstacles so that you can find your path and walk on it.

YOUR PERSONAL INVENTORY

Filling out your personal inventory requires a pencil or pen, some time to yourself, and the willingness to answer honestly. Answer in any way you like: This worksheet is for your eyes only. You can fill out all of it or only the parts you feel will be most helpful to you. For example, you may just want to fill out the checklist of medical tests, and your personal and family health history (parts V and VI) so you'll have a good basis for working with your doctor. You may want to write in a journal if these pages don't offer you enough room to explore your thoughts.

A word of permission: You already have enough going on in your life—please don't put more pressure on yourself! This inventory is simply a planning tool, not a prescription for perfection. You'll be answering a lot of questions and raising a lot of issues you may not have thought about. Don't be overwhelmed, and don't feel as if you have to change everything. None of us are ever going to be perfect, nor should we be.

Before you begin you may want to take a few deep breaths, close your eyes, and relax. Take this opportunity to go inside and let your personal wisdom come forth. When you feel centered and ready, begin.

I. Assessing Where You Are Now

1. What aspects of your life do you feel really good about?

_____

_____

_____

_____

_____

_____

2. List the people, groups, or communities you feel are important to and supportive of you.

_____

_____

_____

_____

_____

_____

3. How do you see yourself living in the next five years? In the next ten years? Consider the following issues:

Residence: _____

_____

Work: _____

_____

Finances: _____

_____

Physical and Emotional Health: _____

_____

4. What situations in your life need immediate attention?

_____

_____

_____

_____

_____

5. Is there anything limiting or troubling you? If you can't pin down the cause of your unease, try to list the ways in which your life is being adversely affected.

_____

_____

_____

_____

_____

II. Transitions: Work and Relationships

Work/Retirement/New Horizons

1. How do you feel about your current work situation? (If you are a homemaker, this is work too.)

_____

_____

_____

_____

_____

_____

2. Do you envision your work changing in the near future?

_____

_____

_____

_____

_____

_____

3. What changes would you like to make?

_____

_____

_____

_____

_____

_____

4. What plans, savings, or pensions do you have for your retirement?

_____

_____

_____

_____

_____

_____

5. How many more years do you see yourself working?

_____

_____

6. What changes would you like to make in your work life or plans for retirement?

Work: _____

_____

_____

Retirement: _____

_____

_____

Relationships

1. If you are married or in a serious relationship, what are your feelings about your current situation?

_____

_____

_____

_____

_____

_____

_____

2. What issues in your relationship need to be addressed?

_____

_____

_____

_____

_____

_____

_____

3. If you have recently been widowed or divorced, how are you feeling right now? What practical matters need attention?

_____

_____

_____

_____

_____

_____

4. If you are single or not in a relationship, what are your feelings about your current situation?

_____

_____

_____

_____

_____

_____

5. When you think about your primary relationship, are you satisfied or would you like to make changes? If so, list the changes.

_____

_____

_____

_____

_____

_____

6. How would you describe your support network of friends and relatives?

_____

_____

_____

_____

_____

_____

New Horizons

1. What new areas of interest would you like to explore?

_____

_____

_____

_____

_____

_____

2. What steps can you take to begin your exploration?

_____

_____

_____

_____

_____

_____

III. Menopause

1. Are you currently experiencing perimenopausal or postmenopausal discomforts? If so, can you identify them?

_____

_____

_____

_____

_____

_____

2. What treatment options have you explored?

_____

_____

_____

_____

_____

_____

3. What needs attention now?

_____

_____

_____

_____

_____

_____

IV. Lifestyle: Exercise, Nutrition, Stress

Exercise

1. How much and what kind of exercise do you get? (Include workouts, walks, and daily tasks like gardening.)

_____

_____

_____

_____

_____

_____

_____

2. Does your exercise routine include aerobic exercise, stretching, and strength training? If so, list these activites.

_____

_____

_____

3. What changes would you like to make in your exercise program? Is there anything new you would like to explore?

_____

_____

_____

_____

_____

_____

Nutrition

1. How would you characterize your eating habits?

_____

_____

_____

_____

_____

2. What kinds of food do you include in your diet?

_____

_____

_____

_____

_____

3. What changes would you like to make in the way you eat? Is there anything new you would like to explore?

_____

_____

_____

_____

_____

Stress

1. What, if any, are your environmental stresses (geography, neighborhood, worksite)?

_____

_____

_____

_____

_____

2. What, if any, are your emotional stresses (family responsibility, career crisis, and so on)?

_____
_____
_____
_____
_____
_____

3. What, if any, are your physical stresses (health problems)?

_____
_____
_____
_____
_____
_____

4. Which of these stresses need attention?

_____
_____
_____
_____
_____
_____

5. What steps can you take to alleviate some of this stress?

_____
_____
_____
_____
_____
_____

6. What stress-management techniques would you like to explore?

_____

_____

_____

_____

_____

_____

V. Your Personal Health History

1. When was the last time you visited the doctor, and why?

_____

_____

_____

_____

_____

_____

2. How would you describe your current health?

_____

_____

_____

_____

_____

3. What are the basics of your personal health history?

Serious illnesses: _____

_____

_____

Surgeries: _____

_____

_____

Chronic illness: _____

_____

_____

_____

Allergies: _____

_____

_____

_____

Medications and supplements: _____

_____

_____

_____

Alcohol, smoking, other substance use: _____

_____

_____

_____

4. Do you have any health matters that need attention?

_____

_____

_____

_____

_____

_____

_____

5. Are there any complementary therapies you would like to explore?

_____

_____

_____

_____

_____

_____

_____

6. Your checklist of medical tests

Be sure to keep good records of the health tests every woman should have in midlife. You may want to record monthly and yearly exams in a separate notebook, due to the space limitations here.

Breast Self-Exam (once a month):

Date: _____

Results: _____

Mammogram (once a year, age 40 and over):

Date: _____

Results: _____

Pap Test/Pelvic Exam (once a year):

Date: _____

Results: _____

Blood Pressure (once a year):

Date: _____

Results: _____

Lipid Profile (baseline after 50):

Date: _____

Results: _____

Colorectal Cancer Screening:

Date: _____

Results: _____

Bone Density Test (if at high risk for osteoporosis):

Date: _____

Results: _____

VI. Your Family Health History

What is your family health history? List serious diseases, cause of death, emotional or mental health problems, alcohol or substance abuse problems. Be sure to include all cases of breast cancer (for the women), heart problems and osteoporosis (both men and women), and age of onset.

Mother: _____

_____

_____

_____

Father: _____

_____

_____

_____

Maternal grandparents: _____

_____

_____

_____

Paternal grandparents: _____

_____

_____

_____

_____

Aunts: _____

_____

_____

_____

Uncles: _____

_____

_____

_____

Siblings: _____

_____

_____

_____

VII. Caregiving

1. Are you currently providing care for a relative or friend? If so, what kind of information or services might be of value to you now?

_____
_____
_____
_____
_____
_____

2. Do you have adequate support and assistance? If not, what steps can you take to find that help?

_____
_____
_____
_____
_____
_____

3. If you are not currently caring for someone but think you may be in the future, what steps can you take now to prepare?

_____
_____
_____
_____
_____
_____

VIII. Support

Personal

1. Are there patterns or behaviors in your life that no longer serve you? If so, can you describe them?

_____
_____

_____

_____

_____

_____

2. What steps can you take to change these patterns?

_____

_____

_____

_____

_____

Relationship

1. Do you feel you have adequate support in your life?

_____

_____

_____

_____

_____

2. Do any of your friends or family abuse you or undermine you, emotionally or physically?

_____

_____

_____

_____

_____

3. If you answered yes to question 2 above, what steps can you take to change this situation?

_____

_____

_____

_____

_____

_____

4. What steps can you take to find more support?

_____

_____

_____

_____

_____

_____

Emotional

1. Can you identify any current or past unacknowledged losses that need attention?

_____

_____

_____

_____

_____

_____

2. If so, what support do you need? What action can you take?

_____

_____

_____

_____

_____

_____

3. Are you experiencing mood swings that interfere with your daily life? If so, how?

_____

_____

_____

_____

_____

_____

4. Are you experiencing feelings that linger and interfere with your daily life? If so, what kinds of feelings are they and how do they disrupt your life?

_____

_____

_____

_____

_____

_____

5. If you answered yes to questions 3 or 4 above, what steps can you take to get support in dealing with these disruptive feelings?

_____

_____

_____

_____

_____

IX. Spirituality

1. Were you raised in a traditional religious environment? If so, describe the values it gave you that you find useful in your life today.

_____

_____

_____

_____

_____

_____

_____

2. Does your childhood religion still fulfill your religious and spiritual needs? If not, what are you seeking?

_____

_____

_____

_____

_____

_____

3. What new dimensions would you like to bring into your spiritual life? What steps can you take to do this?

_____

_____

_____

_____

_____

_____

4. What new areas of creativity would you like to explore?

_____

_____

_____

_____

_____

_____

_____

REFLECTIONS

You can use the information you got in touch with in the previous section to begin to plan your journey. Before you begin to think about your destination and the path you will take to get there, however, take some time to reflect on your answers and consider the following areas:

- Your needs: What do you need and want in your life?
- Your lifestyle: What values do you hold dear?
- Reality check: What do you have to work with in terms of your health and practical resources?

BE TRUE TO YOURSELF   It all begins and ends with you, so try to stay true to your values and your lifestyle. For example, when it comes to your health, are you comfortable taking medication, or would you rather avoid taking pills? Are you more comfortable with conventional medicine, with complementary medicine, or with a combination? Can you really afford to care for your aging aunt at home, or would another arrangement work better for both of you?

GET IN TOUCH WITH YOUR INTUITION   If you're still not clear on what path is best, let your intuition guide you. Sometimes all you have to do is listen. Find a quiet space and take some time for yourself. Center yourself in whatever way you choose—meditate, take a relaxing bath, light some candles, go for a walk in nature. Then say good-bye to your chattering mind and your inner critic and let the wise woman inside emerge. Deep inside, you know what's truly right for you.

TAKE ACTION   When you've reached a decision, the next step is to act on it. You've found the resources you need, you've thought about it, you understand your options, so you should feel pretty good about the option you've chosen. Remember: Few decisions are set in stone. A trial period, if that's feasible, is a good compromise for a tough decision.

Personal Inventory Revisited

Filling out the personal inventory may have given you some different ideas about your vision of the future than you had when you began. To find out, you may want to answer the following questions.

1. Has your vision of yourself in the future changed? If, so how?

_____

_____

_____

_____

_____

_____

2. How do you see yourself living in the next five years? In the next ten years? (Consider residence, work, finances, physical and emotional health.)

_____

_____

_____

_____

_____

_____

PERSONAL COMPANION

Itinerary

This is the place to plan your journey. Where will you go? How will you get there? What resources can you use? Use the following chart to help you clarify your ideas. Here's an example to start you out:

MY DESTINATION	OBSTACLES	STEPS ON THE PATH	RESOURCES	ESTIMATED TIME OF ARRIVAL
Adding strength training to my exercise program.	1. I don't think I have enough extra time. 2. I don't want to go to the gym near my house—it's all men.	1. Take a look at my schedule. I only need about 20 minutes a day, 3 days a week. 2. Look into getting a personal trainer to get me started.	1. Look in the yellow pages to see if there are any coed or women's gyms nearby that I don't know about. 2. Call the YMCA— maybe they have trainers. 3. Call the American Council of Exercise to find out about trainers.	I'll give myself 2 weeks to figure this out.

Have a great trip!

MY DESTINATION	OBSTACLES	STEPS ON THE PATH	RESOURCES	ESTIMATED TIME OF ARRIVAL

PERSONAL NOTES: MY OWN RESOURCES

Use this space to note down your own resources.

☞ Name _____

Address _____

_____

Phone/Fax/E-mail/Internet _____

_____

_____

Notes _____

_____

_____

☞ Name _____

Address _____

_____

Phone/Fax/E-mail/Internet _____

_____

_____

Notes _____

_____

_____

☞ Name _____

Address _____

_____

Phone/Fax/E-mail/Internet _____

_____

_____

Notes _____

_____

_____

Name _____

Address _____

_____

Phone/Fax/E-mail/Internet _____

_____

_____

Notes _____

_____

_____

Name _____

Address _____

_____

Phone/Fax/E-mail/Internet _____

_____

_____

Notes _____

_____

_____

Name _____

Address _____

_____

Phone/Fax/E-mail/Internet _____

_____

_____

Notes _____

_____

_____

➤ Name _____

Address _____

_____

Phone/Fax/E-mail/Internet _____

_____

_____

Notes _____

_____

_____

DON'T FORGET TO WRITE!

We'd love to hear about your journey and the resources you have
found. Drop us a postcard at LuckSmith, 1185 Solano Ave., Box 118,
Albany, CA 94706. If you're online, e-mail us at feedback@lucksmith
.com or visit our website at www.lucksmith.com.

INDEX

Hormones, *see also*
    specific hormones
  dietary, 192
  fluctuation, 192–193
  levels
    decline, 35
    effects, 184
    skin and, 124
  natural, 188–190
  replacement, *see* Hormone
    replacement therapy
Ho shour wu, 42
Hospice, 279
Hot flashes, 38, 44–46
Hotlines, about, xxi
Housing
  advocacy groups, 21
  books, 26
  issues, 12–13
HRT, *see* Hormone replacement
  therapy
Hydrogenated fats, 84, 129
Hypertension, *see* High blood
  pressure
Hypnotherapy, 150
Hysterectomy
  alternatives to, 264–265
  audio/video, 272
  books, 271–272
  catalogs, 271
  controversy, 260
  description, 261
  online, 272–273
  organizations, 269–270
  products, 271
  second opinion, 261–262
  side effects, 262–264
  statistics, 264
  types, 262

I

Impatience, 294
Incontinence, *see* Urinary
  incontinence
Information gathering, 331–335

Inositol, 37
Insomnia, 40–42
Intellectual pursuits, 15
Italian Greens, 221

J

James, P. D., 317
Jobs, *see* Career
Journals, 17
Jung, Carl, 316
Junk food, 84

K

Kali, 205, 317
Kapha, 146
Kegel exercise, 204, 265
Khella, 235
Ki, 142
Kreosotum, 42
Kuhn, Maggie, 317

L

Lachesis, 42
Laser resurfacing, 129–130
Laughter, 109
Lavender oil, 45, 105
Lecithin, 37
Lee, Dr. John R., 222
Le Guin, Ursula, xii, 311, 320
Legumes, 86
LH, *see* Luteinizing hormone
Life story, 295
Lipoproteins, 234
Living will, 281
Lubricants, 201
Lumpy breast, 246
Luteinizing hormone, 35

M

Magnesium
  benefits, 89
  menopause, 44
  in water, 218

Makeup, 133–135
Mammogram, 247–248
Martial arts
  books, 74
Marvin's Room, 8
Massage, 107
  chair, 108
  facial, 130
Medicine, *see* Complementary
    medicine *and* Western
    medicine
Meditation
  emotional problems and, 192
  paths, 317–318
  skin problems and, 130–131
  stress, 109–111
Melatonin, 40
Memory
  menopause and, 37
  tricks, 39
Menopause
  acupuncture for, 193
  aging and, 36
  alcohol and, 40
  alternative therapies, 42
  audio/video material, 52–53
  books, 49–52
  candle lighting ritual, 315
  complementary medicine and,
    152–154
  depression during, 38–39
  description, 32
  diet and, 40–41
  emergency kit, 45
  exercise and, 38
  health issues, 37, 166
  herbal remedies, 39, 153–154
  historical views, 36
  hormone decline, 35
  hot flashes, 44–46
  insomnia during, 40–41
  memory and, 37, 39
  midlife and, 4, 6
  mind–body practices, 43
  mood swings, 295, 297–298
  nutrition and, 38
  online, 53–54

Herbal Remedies for Women

Discover Nature's Wonderful Secrets Just for Women

Amanda McQuade Crawford, M.N.I.M.H.

U.S. $17.00
Can. $22.95
ISBN: 0-7615-0980-1
paperback / 304 pages

As the medical establishment confirms what herbalists have said all along, more and more women are turning to herbs for the prevention, treatment, and cure of ailments. Here are safe and effective alternatives to conventional treatments for:

*Menstrual problems *Migraines *Ovarian cysts *Menopause *Fibroids *Candida and other infections *Breast cancer *And more

For each health concern, this easy-to-follow reference provides you with clear explanations of the causes, symptoms, and conventional medical approaches. Then you'll discover practical and effective herbal treatments, including specific recommendations and dosages. You'll also find a comprehensive herbal glossary, lists of herbal suppliers, and techniques for harvesting, storing, and preparing herbs. These expert nutritional and herbal guidelines present a proven method for natural healing that treats the whole woman.

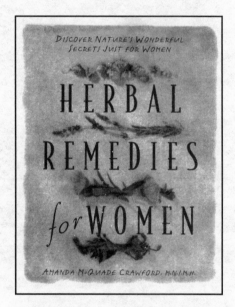

Herbal Prescriptions for Better Health

Your Up-to-Date Guide to the Most Effective Herbal Treatments

Donald J. Brown, N.D.

U.S. $16.00
Can. $21.95
ISBN: 0-7615-1001-X
paperback / 368 pages

Let nature's own remedies work for you! Here's an indispensable guide that introduces you to effective and safe ways to improve your health through the power of herbal medicines. In this insightful book, Dr. Donald Brown recommends specific herbal treatments for dozens of common ailments and provides answers to frequently asked questions. From herbs such as aloe vera, feverfew, ginseng, and goldenseal, you'll find solutions for numerous health conditions, including those related to the heart, digestive system, skin, urinary tract, and more!

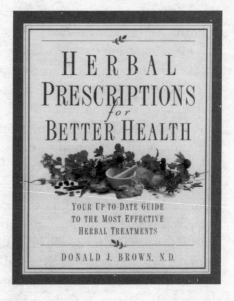

Listening to Your Hormones

From PMS to Menopause, Every Woman's Complete Guide

Gillian Ford

U.S. $18.00
Can. $24.95
ISBN: 0-7615-1002-8
paperback / 496 pages

Nearly all women will suffer from symptoms of hormonal imbalances. Some women become moody and irritable, some have panic attacks, others experience migraines, epilepsy, allergies, skin problems, low thyroid activity, ovarian cysts, or fibroids. For those with a genetic tendency toward hormonal problems, every hormonal event in life—menstruation, pregnancy, menopause—can wreak havoc. In this practical, solution-filled resource, women's health educator Gillian Ford empowers women with the facts. *Listening to Your Hormones* illustrates the pervasive role hormones play in women's lives and reveals how to form a successful partnership with a doctor to find treatments that work.

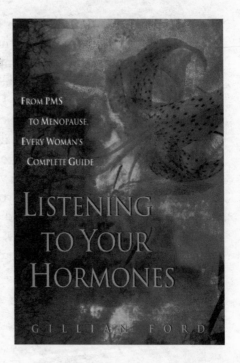

The Women We Become

Myths, Folktales, and Stories About Growing Older

Ann G. Thomas, Ed.D.

U.S. $23.00
Can. $29.95
ISBN 0-7615-0654-3
hardcover / 304 pages

Through discussions with the Old Woman who looks out at her from the mirror, Anne G. Thomas embraces the meaningful journey to old age, confronting the fears that tempt us to deny our aging. She reveals the strength and comfort that are ours if we will only acknowledge and accept ourselves as we are, and as we are becoming. As Thomas interweaves tales from the Brothers Grimm and the Bible with Native American lore and myths from Africa, Europe, and Asia, she embroiders them with insights from modern psychology to illuminate their meaning. In heartwarming style, Thomas renders a true, mythical portrait of the woman looking back at us from the mirror.

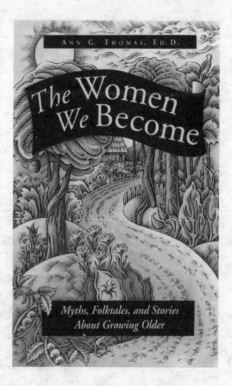

To Order Books

Please send me the following items:

Quantity	Title	Unit Price	Total
_____	_____	$ _____	$ _____
_____	_____	$ _____	$ _____
_____	_____	$ _____	$ _____
_____	_____	$ _____	$ _____
_____	_____	$ _____	$ _____

Subtotal **$** _____

Deduct 10% when ordering 3–5 books **$** _____

7.25% Sales Tax (CA only) **$** _____

8.25% Sales Tax (TN only) **$** _____

5.0% Sales Tax (MD and IN only) **$** _____

Shipping and Handling* **$** _____

Total Order **$** _____

Shipping and Handling depend on Subtotal.

Subtotal	Shipping/Handling
$0.00–$14.99	$3.00
$15.00–$29.99	$4.00
$30.00–$49.99	$6.00
$50.00–$99.99	$10.00
$100.00–$199.99	$13.50
$200.00+	Call for Quote

Foreign and all Priority Request orders:
Call Order Entry department
for price quote at 916/632-4400

This chart represents the total retail price of books only
(before applicable discounts are taken).

By Telephone: With MC or Visa, call 800-632-8676 or 916-632-4400. Mon–Fri, 8:30-4:30.

WWW: http://www.primapublishing.com

By Internet E-mail: sales@primapub.com

By Mail: Just fill out the information below and send with your remittance to:

**Prima Publishing
P.O. Box 1260BK
Rocklin, CA 95677**

My name is _____

I live at _____

City_____ State_____ ZIP _____

MC/Visa#_____ Exp._____

Check/money order enclosed for $ _____ Payable to Prima Publishing

Daytime telephone _____

Signature _____